Preface

Most of the advanced countries are facing serious problems in medical environments due to the aging society, and extension of healthy lifetime is a big challenge for us. In order to tackle these problems, biomedical engineering in addition to life science and medicine is one of the important areas, and innovative technologies concerning minimally invasive treatment, prognosis, and early diagnosis, point-of-care testing, regenerative medicine, and personalized medicine are required to be developed to realize a healthy aging society.

Under these circumstances, the Research Center of Biomedical Engineering (RCBE) was established in April 2016 in collaboration with the Institute of Biomaterials and Bioengineering at Tokyo Medical and Dental University, the Laboratory for Future Interdisciplinary Research of Science and Technology at Tokyo Institute of Technology, the Research Institute for Nanodevice and Biosystems at Hiroshima University, and the Research Institute of Electronics at Shizuoka University, with the support of the Ministry of Education, Culture, Sports, Science and Technology (MEXT). The purpose of the RCBE is to promote interaction and collaboration between engineers and medical researchers to revolutionize future medicine and healthcare through the development of innovative technologies. The four research institutes have their own core competencies in different areas of science and technology, and we aim to integrate and fuse them in the RCBE to strengthen and enhance them. We also seek to foster young researchers in the interdisciplinary field between medicine and engineering through collaboration with advanced research institutes around the world.

This book provides examples of the collaboration research between engineering and life sciences to young researchers and students in the field of biomedical engineering. If the readers can get hints and new ideas from this book for their studies and research in this growing research field, we would be very glad.

Akihiro Miyauchi and Yuji Miyahara
2022

Chapter 1

Biosensors Using Metal Oxides as a Sensing Material

Miyuki Tabata and Yuji Miyahara

Tokyo Medical and Dental University, 2-3-10 Kanda-Surugadai, Chiyodaku, Tokyo 101-0062, Japan

Miyahara.bsr@tmd.ac.jp

Metal oxides, such as SiO_2, Ta_2O_5, and IrO_x, are useful materials for not only electronic devices but also biosensor elements, because they possess a high proton responsiveness. Monitoring of ion dynamics in (/ex) vivo or in (/ex) vitro is important for analyzing various biological reactions, where the proton is the main participant in such reactions. Biosensing based on pH detection provides an understanding of many biological phenomena, and such a detection method might be applied for disease diagnosis in the medical and dental fields. In this chapter, we describe the fundamental pH-sensing mechanisms of metal oxides and their biosensing applications, which include recent examples such as nucleic acid detection and dental caries detection.

Biomedical Engineering
Edited by Akihiro Miyauchi and Yuji Miyahara

ISBN 978-981-4877-63-3 (Hardcover), 978-1-003-14194-5 (eBook)
www.jennystanford.com

1.1 Metal Oxides as a Biosensing Element

1.1.1 Metal Oxides as a pH Sensor

Various biosensors based on an optical [1, 2], thermal [3, 4], or electrical/electrochemical signal change [5, 6] have been reported and developed to detect ions [7], molecules [8], proteins [9], DNA [10–12], and viruses [13]. To detect target biomolecules, the biosensors consist of transducers whose surfaces are factionalized by immobilizing ligand specific substrates. There is a thin membrane on the transducers for specific molecular recognition, and bioassays are performed following labeling processes involving fluorescent dyes, radioactively labeled probes, or redox markers. In the case of electrical/electrochemical biosensors, the physical and chemical stimuli, which result in the molecular recognition reactions on the transducer surface, are converted into electrical signals such as potential, current, and charge change values. The most advanced electrical/electrochemical biosensor is the device based on the working principle of a field-effect transistor (bio-transistor) (Fig. 1.1).

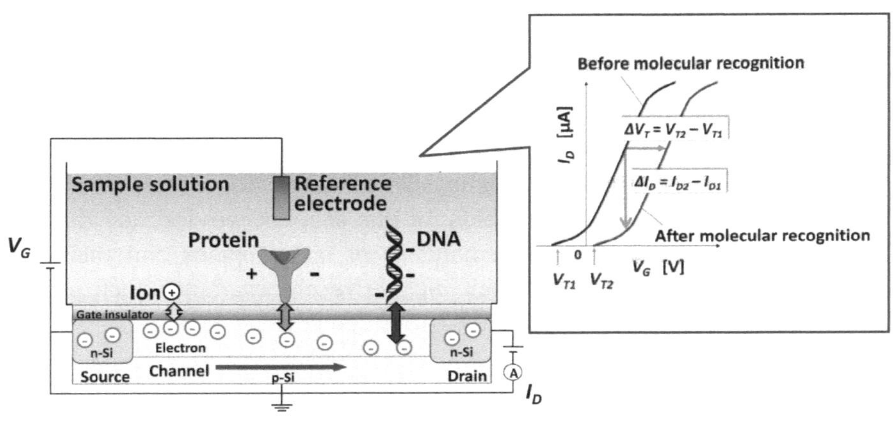

Figure 1.1 Conceptual structures of biosensors based on a field-effect transistor. In the case where the detection target has a negative charge, the electrical output (V_T-I_D characteristics) moves towards the right with respect to V_G after molecular recognition, which results in a decrease in I_D.

While optical detection methods using fluorescence labeling, such as enzyme-linked immunosorbent assay (ELISA) and fluorescence-activated cell sorting (FACS), are mainstream, the label-free biosensing methods that use electrical/electrochemical biosensors are attracting attention because of the simple, cost-effective, portable, and user-friendly systems. Sensitive and specific detection of the ion species involved in a biological reaction is important for practical use, and electrical/electrochemical biosensors achieve a sensitive ion detection in a label-free manner. For example, since the first electrical/electrochemical biosensor (i.e., an ion-sensitive field-effect transistor (ISFET)) was reported by P. Bergveld in 1970 [14], various types of ISFETs and biochemical FETs have been developed, some of which have been commercialized as pH sensors for laboratory, medical, and food uses.

1.1.2 Electrical/Electrochemical pH Detection

Here, the electrical/electrochemical detection principle of the pH is described. Normally, a biosensor, which is able to exhibit a proton response, has a sensitive membrane that responds to protons on the top surface of the transducer, and induces an electrochemical output based on the dissociation state of the hydroxyl groups present on the top surface. As a result of an interaction between the hydroxyl groups and protons, the output signal obeys the Nernst equation, which is expressed by the standard electrode potential, temperature, electron activity, and reaction quotient of the underlying reactions and species (Eq. 1.1).

$$E = E^0 + \left(2.303\, {}^{RT}\!/_{zF}\right) \log a, \tag{1.1}$$

where E^0 is a standard electrode potential, R is an ideal gas constant, T is a temperature in Kelvin, z is a number of moles of electrons, F is the Faraday constant, and a is an ion activity.

$$E = E^0 - 59.16\ \text{pH} \tag{1.2}$$

As shown in Eq. 1.2, when all constants are substituted in Eq. 1.1, the output signal changes by −59.2 mV against one pH unit at room temperature (25 °C).

Typical proton sensing devices used in research experiments and industry include a glass electrode, a light-addressable potentiometric sensor (LAPS), an ISFET, and a metal oxide electrode. To be used as a biosensor, not only are stability and robustness in a liquid required, but also the safety of the sensor material from the viewpoint of application to a living body. Many applications have already been reported for ISFETs and metal oxide electrodes in biosensing. The ISFET, which is the first miniaturized silicon-based chemical sensor, has three terminals: source, drain, and gate. A schematic of the pH detection using an ISFET is shown in Fig. 1.2. The gate used in pH sensing consists of a dielectric material, such as SiO_2, Si_3N_4, Ta_2O_5, and Al_2O_3, and the proton selectivity and pH sensitivity of the ISFET depend on the properties of the solid/liquid interface. The dissociation state of hydroxyl groups on the surface of the dielectric material is dominated by the donation or acceptance of protons, which determines the pH. By following this equilibrium, the drain current value is determined by the proton concentration at the gate. Metal-metal oxide pH electrodes also offer robust and accurate proton measurements, and can be used in a laboratory as an alternative for a glass electrode. In the case of such an electrode, the potentiometric output signal responds to the pH directly, owing to an equilibrium involving the metal and its oxide. The redox reaction involved in the interaction between proton and metal oxide can be described by the following equation (Eq. 1.3):

$$\mathrm{MeO}_x + ze^- + z\mathrm{H}^+ \leftrightarrow \mathrm{MeO}_{x-z}(\mathrm{OH})_z, \tag{1.3}$$

where x is the number of oxygen atoms related to the oxidization state of the metal and z is the activity of the electrons. This reaction follows the Nernst equation, as expressed in Eqs. 1.1 and 1.2. To date, various metal oxides, which include PtO_2, RuO_2, Ta_2O_5, TiO_2, SnO_2, and IrO_x, have been proposed as pH-sensing materials; in particular, it is known that IrO_x shows an excellent pH response. Metal oxides have attracted attention as electrode materials in recent decades, and their preparation methods and properties have been well studied [15]. In general, metal oxides are prepared using a thermal oxidation method or an electrodeposition method by controlling several physical experimental conditions such as treatment time, temperature, and concentration of immersion solution. It is clear that these non-glass membranes of pH-sensing materials show a low interference property of monovalent cation and are not destroyed even at sufficiently high temperature. The interference and selectivity of various metal oxide electrodes (TiO_2, RuO_2, RhO_2, SnO_2, Ta_2O_5, OsO_2, IrO_2, and PtO_2) by adding monovalent cations (Li^+, Na_+, and K^+) in a universal buffer (pH range of 2–12) has been reported in the literature, and the accuracy for the voltage-pH relationships follows the order Ir(IV), Ru(IV), Rh(IV), Pt(IV), and Os(IV). Thus, it has been proven that IrO_x shows a higher proton selectivity compared with the other metal oxides, which can be explained by a simple ion exchange mechanism in the surface layer and a redox equilibrium between two different solids, e.g., an oxide layer and a pure metal layer.

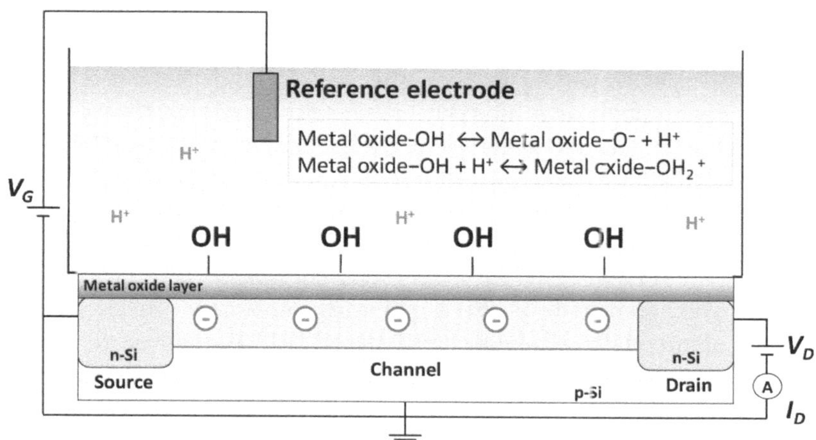

Figure 1.2 Schematic illustration of proton detection in an ISFET. The electrical output (V_T-I_D characteristics) changes according to hydroxyl group dissociation on a metal oxide surface.

A pH sensor using a metal oxide has been well studied and is already widely used. However, the application to biosensing is limited to certain metal oxide materials, such as SiO_2, Ta_2O_5, or IrO_x, from the viewpoints of strength, safety, and robustness. In the following, as examples of biosensors based on pH sensing technology using metal oxide materials, we introduce semiconductor DNA sequencers in commercially available products and micro pH sensors that quantitatively detect caries.

1.2 Nucleic Acids Detection or Sequencing Using Metal Oxide Devices Based on pH Sensing

1.2.1 Semiconductor-Based DNA Sequencer

Nucleic acid detection technology has been applied in various fields, such as medical treatment, administration of justice, and food science. There is no question that the detection technique of nucleic acids provides a very powerful diagnostic tool. Generally, a nucleic acid detection device requires three steps: DNA isolation, amplification, and detection. The real-time polymerase chain reaction (real-time PCR) is a robust nucleic acid detection method because of fluorescently labeled sequence-specific probes, and is already widely used in the clinical field. Recently, there has been increasing interest in electrical and electrochemical detection of nucleic acids for high-throughput and cost-effective DNA detection, as examples, differential pulse voltammetry [16, 17], square wave voltammetry [18], and chronocoulometry [10]. One of the most successful examples of commercialized products is the IonTorrent™, which is an ISFET chip-based DNA sequencer that was launched in 2012 [11, 12]. As shown in Fig. 1.3, the commercially available ISFET-based DNA sequencer achieves massive parallel analysis with highly integrated ISFETs on a Si chip. The ISFET uses Ta_2O_5 for a highly sensitive proton sensing material. In an extension reaction using DNA polymerase, when one of the deoxy nucleotides binds to a synthetic strand, a pyrophosphoric acid and a proton are released as by-products. The high-density ISFET array detects this proton on the transistors during the single-base extension reaction. The sequencer employs microbeads bearing a template DNA, which is amplified by emulsion PCR, to perform accurate sequencing on a transistor.

The extension reaction occurs on the surface of the bead mounted on each ISFET, which detects the protons released during the extension reaction. The ISFETs, which are highly integrated using semiconductor technology, realize massively parallel sequencing, and this technology is being further developed for applications in liquid biopsy or precision medicine.

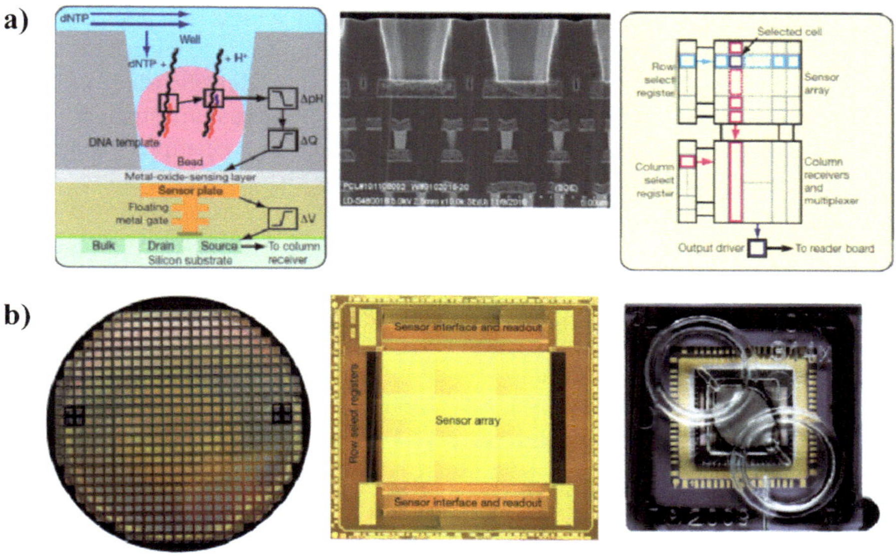

Figure 1.3 Commercialized ISFET-based DNA sequencer. (a) Schematic illustration of sequencing mechanism and electron micrograph showing wells. (b) Ion chip on wafer, dye, and chip packaging. Reprinted with permission from Macmillan Publishers Ltd: ref. 24, copyright 2011.

Liquid biopsy is a diagnosis method using a body fluid sample, such as blood or urine, and is a minimally invasive diagnostic tool. The novel detection candidate in the liquid biopsy is cell-free DNA (cfDNA) or microRNA (miRNA); an understanding of these nucleic acids offers accurate early diagnosis and prognostic monitoring. The Human Genome Project was started in the United States in 1985 and was completed in 2003. It took more than 10 years to analyze the whole human genome sequence using the technology available at that time, which was a DNA sequencer based on electrophoresis. The significant advancement of the DNA sequencing platform has resulted in next-generation sequencers, which are able to perform such an analysis in approximately 1 week. One of the next-generation sequencers is the IonTorrent™, which is a suitable platform for analyzing various regions and various samples at once. To understand an individual's genetic characteristics or predict a risk of disease, liquid biopsy or precision medicine using the semiconductor-based DNA sequencer is underway. The results of semiconductor-based DNA sequencer analysis provide information on single nucleotide mutations, insertions/deletions, and copy number variations in cancer-related genes. It also enables the identification of specific mutations associated with cancer progression, such as tumorigenesis, invasion, and metastasis. For example, the provider of the IonTorrent™ series, Thermo Fisher Scientific Inc., released the "Ion Torrent Oncomine cell-free research Assay" to reproducibly detect gene mutations associated with solid tumors in plasma. This assay evaluates cell-free total DNA (cftDNA) across 52 genes chosen by a clinical trial and literature information using the IonTorrent™ in a massively parallel and high-throughput way. As the semiconductor-based DNA sequencer is already involved in the fields of liquid biopsy or precision medicine, nucleic acid sensing based on pH detection is now playing an innovative role in medical technology.

1.2.2 Simple Detection of Nucleic Acids Using Miniaturized pH Electrodes

Based on the proton detection concept during a DNA extension reaction, ion-selective electrodes have been developed for a liquid biopsy application [19]. Needle-shaped iridium/iridium oxide (Ir/IrO_x), which is a typical proton-sensitive material, was proposed for potentiometric monitoring of primer generation–rolling circle amplification (PG–RCA) [20, 21] in a real-time and label-free manner. The progress in PG–RCA and the detection concept are shown in Fig. 1.4a and b, respectively. Here, PG–RCA is an isothermal amplification method, and is used instead of PCR. PCR requires three steps: denaturation of double strand DNA at 98 °C for 30–60 sec, primer annealing at 50–65 °C for 30 sec, and an extension reaction at 68–72 °C for 60–120 sec, and these steps need to be repeated 25–30 times. This rapid thermal cycling of PCR causes unstable measurements and changes the

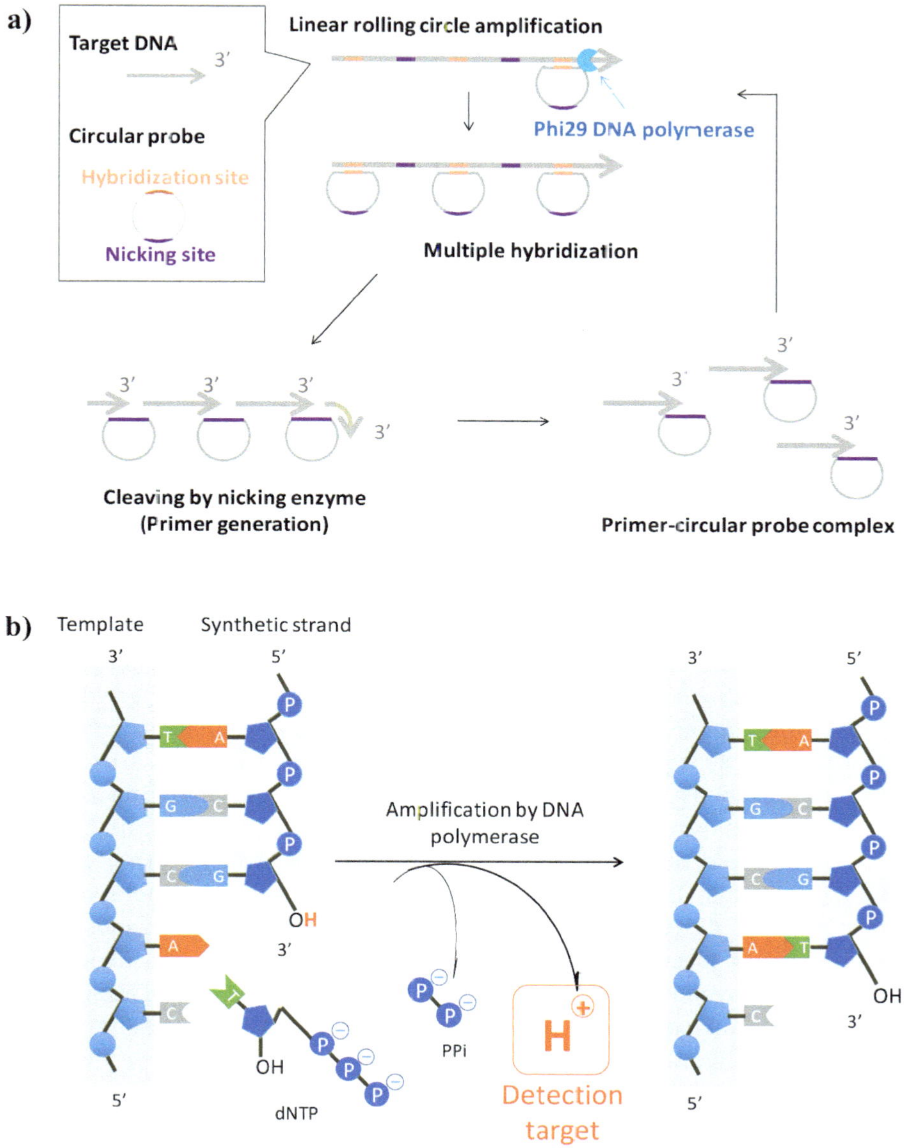

Figure 1.4 Quantitative nucleic acid detection based on pH change during primer generation–rolling circle amplification (PG-RCA). (a) Isothermal amplification of DNA using PG-RCA. (b) A pyrophosphoric acid and a proton are released as by-products.

electrical properties of the electrical/electrochemical sensors. For this reason, isothermal amplification was used instead of conventional PCR, in combination with electrical/electrochemical sensors. The pH sensitivity of the fabricated Ir/IrO_x electrode by thermal oxidation was −57 mV/pH, which is close to the ideal condition. The potentiometric detection of PG–RCA using the Ir/IrO_x pH electrode was also conducted where the proton was the indicator. The target DNA was detected in the range of 10 pM–1 nM.

1.3 Dental Caries Detection Using Ir/IrO_x-Based Micro pH Sensors

1.3.1 General Information on Dental Caries

The Global Burden of Disease Study in 2016 reported that approximately 3.6 billion people suffer from oral diseases [22]. The problem is especially severe in developing countries, where the accumulation of untreated oral diseases in adults often leads to oral disorders arising from the shortage of oral healthcare. The problem is also exacerbated by the aging of society: the world's population of people aged 60 years or older is expected to increase from 900 million in 2015 to 2 billion by 2050. Caries is an infectious disease that people commonly acquire. The degree of caries progression is directly related to our quality of life (QOL), and the maintenance of oral health by using appropriate treatments based on quantitative diagnosis is desirable. At present, diagnostic methods, such as X-ray imaging diagnosis, visual inspection, and palpation, are used as general dental caries diagnosis methods. These diagnostic methods sometimes depend on experience and skill of a dentist, so a diagnosis that is quantitative and non-invasive is required.

Caries bacteria, including *Streptococcus mutans*, *S. sobrinus*, and *Lactobacillus* spp., metabolize sugar and release low molecular organic acids on the teeth. In particular, the accumulated organic acids in the biofilm formed on the teeth lead to mineral dissolution (demineralization), owing to the low pH environment, and finally to tooth decay or tooth loss. The progress of dental caries correlates with the pH of the tooth surface, owing to bacterial activity, and studies on the pH of teeth, saliva, and biofilms have been performed since 1954, but a device for a detailed inspection is still in the developmental stage.

1.3.2 Dental Caries Diagnosis Using pH as a Detection Index

Many visual inspection methods for caries diagnosis, such as dyeing, digital radiography, and fiber-optic transillumination, have been developed. Although there are many qualitative evaluation methods, pH is an index that provides a quantitative evaluation. To confirm the pH decrease in the caries area, a pH microscope [23] and ISFET pH sensor [24] were used. The results showed a correlation between a decrease in the pH and the progression of dental caries; however, it was difficult to apply these systems to the oral cavity from the viewpoint of a device size

For in situ caries diagnosis, Miyahara et al. used Ir/IrO$_x$ wire, which is compact and has excellent workability; for the purpose of being mounted on a dental probe that is generally used by dentists [25, 26]. The typical mapping of caries measured with a micro Ir/IrO$_x$ pH sensor is shown in Fig. 1.5. The Ir wire (with a length of 5 mm and diameter of 0.3 mm) covered with Li_2CO_3 powder was oxidized in an oven at 870 °C for 5 hours. The electrical performance of the Ir/IrO$_x$ pH electrode was evaluated based on the individual pH responsivity and potential drift against an Ag/AgCl reference electrode combined with a salt bridge. The pH responses and calibration curves of the Ir/IrO$_x$ in three pH standard solutions showed nearly an ideal value (−59.2 mV/pH) and the pH drift was less than 1 mV/min at every pH value. Subsequently, the extracted dental caries were categorized into arrested caries, active caries, and the sound root by the dentist based on the activity of the caries. This experiment was approved by the ethics review committee of Tokyo Medical and Dental University (approval number: 725). Among the 18 samples of the extracted human dental caries, there were 7 active caries samples and 11 arrested caries samples. After spot pH measurements on the teeth surface using the Ir/IrO$_x$ pH electrode, the pH values of the arrested caries, active caries, and the sound root were determined to be 6.07, 5.30, and 6.85, respectively. Thus, the caries progression could be quantitatively evaluated based on the pH value in a real-time and label-free manner. This micro-size sensing probe has advantages in clinical use, but the wires still present certain drawbacks. There remain the problems of a feeling of use when the dentist actually holds the wires or discomfort when the device is introduced into the oral cavity of a patient. For these reasons, the possibility of incorporating wireless technology is being investigated for the development of a chair-side device.

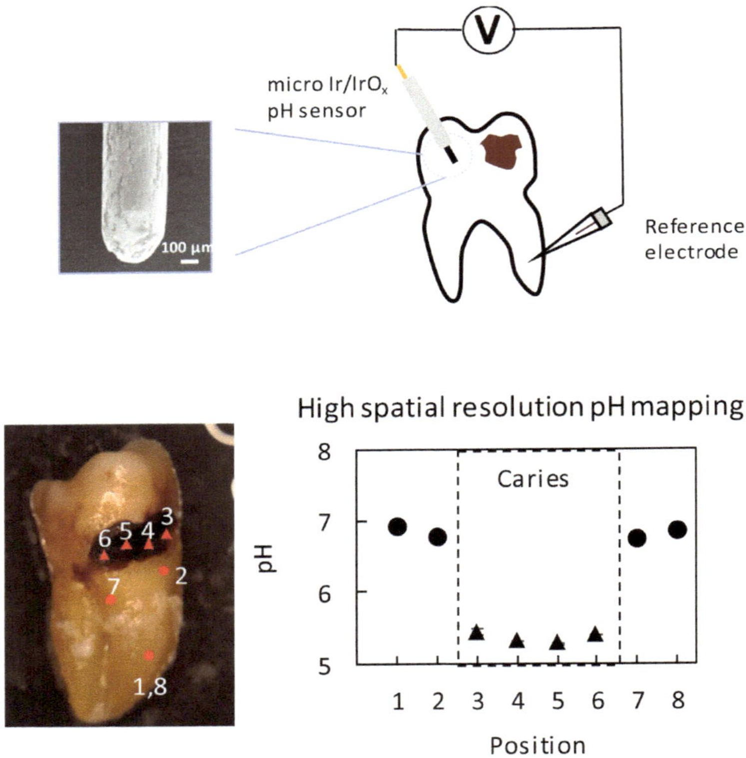

Figure 1.5 Quantitative caries mapping with micro Ir/IrO_x pH sensor.

1.4 Summary

In this chapter, we describe biosensing using metal oxide materials, by taking DNA sequencing and caries detection as examples. Research and development linked to the Internet of Things (IoT) or artificial intelligence (AI) have become popular in the context of modern wireless telecommunications, and the development of sensing devices is required for combining information processing with self-health care, telemedicine, food safety, and environmental monitoring. The current pursuit of the miniaturization and multifunctionality of wearable sensors, which are typified by smart watches, will result in them becoming integral components in our lives. With the evolution of biosensors, a large volume of information will be processed by machine learning, so that the biosensor will be able to provide high-quality information. A biosensor using a metal oxide realizes stable measurements and is advantageous for miniaturization and portability. It is expected that these biosensors combined with IoT or AI will be useful diagnostic platforms for the future of precision medicine.

Acknowledgments

This work was supported in part by the Ministry of Education, Culture, Sports, Science and Technology (MEXT) as part of the Research Center for Biomedical Engineering, the Center of Innovation Program from Japan Science and Technology Agency, JST, JSPS KAKENHI (No. 18K18361), and the research grant of the Nippon Sheet Glass Foundation for Materials Science and Engineering.

References

1. Anker, J. N., Hall, W. P., Lyandres, O., Shah, N. C., Zhao, J., and Van Duyne, R. P. (2008). Biosensing with plasmonic nanosensors. *Nature Materials*, **7(6)**, pp. 442–453.
2. Askim, J. R., Mahmoudi, M., and Suslick, K. S. (2013). Optical sensor arrays for chemical sensing: The optoelectronic nose. *Chemical Society Reviews*, **42(22)**, pp. 8649–8682.
3. Ramanathan, K., and Danielsson, B. (2001). Principles and applications of thermal biosensors. *Biosensors & Bioelectronics*, **16(6)**, pp. 417–423.
4. Calleja, M., Nordstrom, M., Alvarez, M., Tamayo, J., Lechuga, L. M., and Boisen, A. (2005). Highly sensitive polymer-based cantilever-sensors for DNA detection. *Ultramicroscopy*, **105(1–4)**, pp. 215–222.

5. Liu, Y. X., Dong, X. C., and Chen, P. (2012) Biological and chemical sensors based on graphene materials. *Chemical Society Reviews*, **41(6)**, pp. 2283–2307.

6. Gao, A., Zou, N., Dai, P., Lu, N., Li, T., Wang, Y., Zhao, J., and Mao, H. (2013). Signal-to-noise ratio enhancement of silicon nanowires biosensor with rolling circle amplification. *Nano Letters*, **13(9)**, pp. 4123–4130.

7. Schaffhauser, D. F., Andrini, O., Ghezzi, C., Forster, I. C., Franco-Obregon, A., Egli, M., and Dittrich, P. S. (2011). Microfluidic platform for electrophysiological studies on Xenopus laevis oocytes under varying gravity levels. *Lab on a Chip*, **11(20)**, pp. 3471–3478.

8. Matsumoto, A., Sato, N., Kataoka, K., and Miyahara, Y. (2009). Noninvasive sialic acid detection at cell membrane by using phenylboronic acid modified self-assembled monolayer gold electrode. *Journal of the American Chemical Society*, **131(34)**, pp. 12022–12023.

9. Goda, T., Toya, M., Matsumoto, A., and Miyahara, Y. (2015). Poly(3,4-ethylenedioxythiophene) bearing phosphorylcholine groups for metal-free, antibody-free, and low-impedance biosensors specific for C-reactive protein. *ACS Applied Materials & Interfaces*, **7(49)**, pp. 27440–27448.

10. Yao, B., Liu, Y. C., Tabata, M., Zhu, H. T., and Miyahara, Y. (2014). Sensitive detection of microRNA by chronocoulometry and rolling circle amplification on a gold electrode. *Chemical Communications*, **50(68)**, pp. 9704–9706.

11. Toumazou, C., Shepherd, L. M., Reed, S. C., Chen, G. I., Patel, A., Garner, D. M., Wang, C. J. A., Ou, C. P., Amin-Desai, K., Athanasiou, P., Bai, H., Brizido, I. M. Q., Caldwell, B., Coomber-Alford, D., Georgiou, P., Jordan, K. S., Joyce, J. C., La Mura, M., Morley, D., Sathyavruthan, S., Temelso, S., Thomas, R. E., and Zhang, L. L. (2013). Simultaneous DNA amplification and detection using a pH-sensing semiconductor system. *Nature Methods*, **10(7)**, pp. 641–646.

12. Rothberg, J., Hinz, W., Rearick, T., Schultz, J., Mileski, W., Davey, M., Leamon, J., Johnson, K., Milgrew, M., Edwards, M., Hoon, J., Simons, J., Marran, D., Myers, J., Davidson, J., Branting, A., Nobile, J., Puc, B., Light, D., Clark, T., Huber, M., Branciforte, J., Stoner, I., Cawley, S., Lyons, M., Fu, Y., Homer, N., Sedova, M., Miao, X., Reed, B., Sabina, J., Feierstein, E., Schorn, M., Alanjary, M., Dimalanta, E., Dressman, D., Kasinskas, R., Sokolsky, T., Fidanza, J., Namsaraev, E., McKernan, K., Williams, A., Roth, G., and Bustillo, J. (2011). An integrated semiconductor device enabling non-optical genome sequencing. *Nature*, **475(7356)**, pp. 348–352.

13. Velusamy, V., Arshak, K., Korostynska, O., Oliwa, K., and Adley, C. (2010). An overview of foodborne pathogen detection: In the perspective of biosensors. *Biotechnology Advances*, **28(2)**, pp. 232–254.

14. Bergveld, P. (1970). Development of an ion-sensitive solid-state device for neurophysiological measurements. *IEEE Transactions on Biomedical Engineering*, **17(1)**, pp. 70–71.

15. Fog, A., and Buck, R. P. (1984). Electronic semiconducting oxides As PH sensors. *Sensors and Actuators*, **5(2)**, pp 137–146.

16. Zhang, J., Wang, L. L., Hou, M. F., Xia, Y. K., He, W. H., Yan, A., Weng, Y. P., Zeng, L. P., and Chen, J. H. (2018). A ratiometric electrochemical biosensor for the exosomal microRNAs detection based on bipedal DNA walkers propelled by locked nucleic acid modified toehold mediate strand displacement reaction. *Biosensors & Bioelectronics*, **102**, pp. 33–40.

17. Yin, H. S., Zhou, Y. L., Zhang, H. X., Meng, X. M., and Ai, S. Y. (2013). Electrochemical determination of microRNA-21 based on graphene, LNA integrated molecular beacon, AuNPs and biotin multifunctional bio bar codes and enzymatic assay system. *Biosensors & Bioelectronics*, **33(1)**, pp. 247–253.

18. Peng, Y. F., Yi, G. S., and Gao, Z. Q. (2010). A highly sensitive microRNA biosensor based on ruthenium oxide nanoparticle-initiated polymerization of aniline. *Chemical Communications*, **46(48)**, pp. 9131–9133.

19. Tabata, M., Katayama, Y., Mannan, F., Seichi, A., Suzuki, K., Goda, T., Matsumoto, A., and Miyahara, Y. (2016). Label-free and electrochemical detection of nucleic acids based on isothermal amplification in combination with solid-state pH sensor, *Procedia Engineering*, **168**, pp. 419–422.

20. Murakami, T., Sumaoka, J., and Komiyama, M. (2009). Sensitive isothermal detection of nucleic-acid sequence by primer generation-rolling circle amplification. *Nucleic Acids Research*, **37(3)**, e9.

21. Murakami, T., Sumaoka, J., and Komiyama, M. (2012). Sensitive RNA detection by combining three-way junction formation and primer generation-rolling circle amplification. *Nucleic Acids Research*, **40(3)**, e22.

22. Vos, T., Allen, C., Arora, M., Barber, R. M., Bhutta, Z. A., Brown, A., Carter, A., Casey, D. C., Charlson, F. J., Chen, A. Z., Coggeshall, M., Cornaby, L., Dandona, L., Dicker, D. J., Dilegge, T., Erskine, H. E., Ferrari, A. J., Fitzmaurice, C., Fleming, T., Forouzanfar, M. H., Fullman, N., Gething, P. W., Goldberg, E. M., Graetz, N., Haagsma, J. A., Johnson, C. O., Kassebaum,

N. J., et al. (2016). Global, regional, and national incidence, prevalence, and years lived with disability for 310 diseases and injuries, 1990–2015: A systematic analysis for the Global Burden of Disease Study 2015. *Lancet*, **388(10053)**, pp. 1545–1602.

23. Kitasako, Y., Hiraishi, N., Nakajima, M., Nikaido, T., Tagami, J., and Nomura, S. (2002). In vitro surface analysis of active and arrested dentinal caries using a pH-imaging microscope. *Operative Dentistry*, **27(4)**, pp. 354–359.
24. Murakami, K., Kitasako, Y., Burrow, M. F., and Tagami, J. (2006). In vitro pH analysis of active and arrested dentinal caries in extracted human teeth using a micro pH sensor. *Dental Materials Journal*, **25(3)**, pp. 423–429.
25. Ratanaporncharoen, C., Tabata, M., Kitasako, Y., Ikeda, M., Goda, T., Matsumoto, A., Tagami, J., and Miyahara, Y. (2018). pH mapping on tooth surfaces for quantitative caries diagnosis using micro Ir/IrOx pH sensor. *Analytical Chemistry*, **90(7)**, pp. 4925–4931.
26. Ratanaporncharoen, C., Tabata, M., Watanagool, N., Goda, T., Matsumoto, A., Sriyudthsak, M., and Miyahara, Y. (2018). Characterization and optimization of thermally grown iridium oxide and its application to pH sensors. *Sensors and Materials*, **30(5)**, pp. 1175–1185.

Chapter 2

Biosensors Based on FETs Containing Nanostructures

Anri Nakajima

Research Institute for Nanodevice and Bio Systems, Hiroshima University, 1-4-2 Kagamiyama, Higashihiroshima, Hiroshima 739-8527, Japan

anakajima@hiroshima-u.ac.jp

This chapter presents an overview of the biosensors with nanowire field-effect transistors (FETs) and single-electron transistors (SETs) as biosensors with nanostructures for high-sensitivity detection and quantification. Detections and quantifications of biological species are extremely important in medical and life sciences. FETs are sophisticated devices used for the label-free and real-time detection of charged species. Nanowire channels are used for highly sensitive detections of target ion or biomolecule in FET sensors. The high detection sensitivity of nanowire FET sensors is due to the suppression of carrier percolation effect through the channel. SETs are also a promising candidate for achieving high detection sensitivity due to the Coulomb oscillations. However, no reports of an SET-based ion sensor or biosensor

Biomedical Engineering
Edited by Akihiro Miyauchi and Yuji Miyahara

ISBN 978-981-4877-63-3 (Hardcover), 978-1-003-14194-5 (eBook)
www.jennystanford.com

had existed, probably because of the difficulty of the room-temperature operation of SETs and incompatibility of biomolecule solution processes with LSI fabrication processes. Recently, room-temperature SET operations were carried out using a Si multiple-island channel structure and the biosensor based on the SET were realized using the appropriate gate insulator structure for the solution processes. The immunodetection of prostate-specific antigen (PSA) has been achieved using the SET sensor at the required detection level for practical use. Electrically conductive nanoscale organic structures can easily be fabricated with nanoscale lateral size and positional controls by using organic electron beam (EB) resist polymers containing fullerene molecules. The materials have a possibility to be used for the fabrications of sensitive organic biosensors with nanowire FETs or SETs.

2.1 Introduction

Detections and quantifications of biological species are extremely important in medical and life sciences. Various devices have been developed to meet this need. Radioactive or fluorescent markers are used in many of these devices; however, their use involves time-consuming multi-stage processes that are expensive and unsuitable for real-time detection. Problems remain in the use of these makers from the viewpoint of simplicity and speed. Consequently, devices without such markers are desired for detection and quantification.

Field-effect transistors (FETs) are sophisticated devices used for label-free and real-time detections for charged bio-molecules in solutions. Accompanying specific bio-molecular adsorption events, the change of charge on a gate insulator surface modulates the carrier density of the channel, realizing the recognition of the events. The concept was firstly realized by using ion-sensitive FETs (ISFETs) reported by Bergveld [1]. Electrical characteristics of ISFETs change in response to a concentration and valence number of ions present in the aqueous solution on the gate insulator surface. After the publication, biosensors based on Si metal-oxide-semiconductor FETs (MOSFETs) were mainly developed for the detection of various chemical species and biomolecules [2–4]. Later on biosensors having FETs with the channel materials other than Si were also developed [5, 6].

Recently, great interest has been focused on applications of novel inorganic nanomaterials and nanostructures to biotechnology [7]. The size of proteins and lipids constituting cells is on the order of nanometers, which is the same scale as the limits of nanofabrication technology. Therefore, there are possibilities to obtain information effectively on such biological substances by engineering biosensors having nanostructures and/or nanomaterials.

For biosensors based on FETs, several types of semiconductor nanostructures have been applied to detect biological species. Especially, nanowire FETs have emerged as a powerful tool in the field of biosensing [8–18]. Nanowire FETs are recognized as more sensitive than conventional FETs because carriers (electrons or holes) in a very narrow channel are more efficiently affected by charges of nanometer-size biological substances on the gate insulator than those in a wide channel. Another promising FETs having nanostructures used for biosensor are single-electron transistors (SETs) [19–22]. It is noted that SETs are often used as highly sensitive charge sensors in experiments with mesoscopic devices [23].

Therefore, in this chapter, biosensors with nanowire FETs and SETs are introduced as the biosensors based on FETs having nanostructures for highly sensitive detections of biological species. Following this section, first, biosensors with nanowire FETs are described. After the brief introduction, the mechanism of their highly sensitive detection is described from the viewpoint of the effect of percolation for carriers to transfer through the channel. Next, biosensors based on SETs are described. Then, a promising material is introduced for realizing organic nanostructures for biosensors [24, 25] before the summary of this chapter.

2.2 Biosensors with Nanowire FETs

To date, many nanowire FETs have been fabricated for highly sensitive detections of target ions or biomolecules. Biosensors with nanowire FETs fabricated by bottom-up method were realized earlier than those fabricated by the top-down method [22]. Here, bottom-up methods utilize a self-assembled mechanism of atoms and molecules, and top-down methods use electron beam (EB) lithography. Using bottom-up methods, streptavidin [8], a single virus of influenza A [9], interactions between adenosine-5′-triphosphate (ATP) and the protein tyrosine kinase of Abl [10], and prostate-specific antigen (PSA) [11] were detected with various surface modification of Si nanowire in FETs.

Materials other than Si were also used for the bottom-up fabrication of nanowire FET biosensors. Carbon nanotubes are the typical material and were used for label-free detections of several proteins including immunoglobulin E (IgE) [12, 13].

As to the top-down methods, Si nanowires were used in most cases owing to the mature LSI fabrication technique. Mouse-immunoglobulin G and mouse-immunoglobulin A [14], target DNA in solution with the probe DNA (12-mer oligonucleotide) [15], and PSA [16] were detected using highly sensitive biosensors with Si nanowire FETs fabricated by using EB lithography. pH sensors were also fabricated with Si nanowire FETs [17, 18].

2.2.1 Mechanism of High Sensitivity in Biomolecule Detection with Nanowire FETs

The main mechanism of the increase in detection sensitivity in the case of nanowire FETs is considered to be the suppression or enhancement of the effect of percolation for carriers to transfer through the channel. For example, in the case of the same polarity of charges between the target molecule and carrier, much larger channel width than the size of charged target biomolecule can make carriers in the channel possible to avoid the target and to pass through the far regions from the target. Therefore, carriers can transfer through the channel, leading to small change of drain current (I_d) compared to the I_d prior to the attachment. On the other hand, if the channel width is similar or small compared with the size of the target biomolecule, carriers cannot avoid the target and pass through any channel region, leading to the disappearance of the percolation path and large changes of I_d compared to the I_d before the attachment.

The sensitivity enhancement with the decrease in the channel width of ISFET due to the above percolation effect was confirmed by Monte Carlo simulation [26]. Here, the site percolation property of a finite-size two-dimensional square-lattice system was analyzed to investigate the effect of charged substances on the properties of ISFETs. In the simulation, there are L sites along the length direction of the channel and W sites along the width direction. Initially, all sites are conductive. If a charged substance attaches to a site on the channel surface, it is assumed that only the site becomes nonconductive. The size of the charged substance is assumed to be consistent with that of the unit site.

Figure 2.1 shows the dependence of the percolation probability q on the concentration of nonconductive site p at various channel width W with L fixed at 1000. Here, p is proportional to the concentration of charged substances in solutions. It is shown that q starts to decrease at a lower p with decreasing W. When the channel width W is similar to or a little larger than the size of the charged substance (W = 2), the existence of the substance can be detected at the concentration p of the substance lower than 0.01. When W is 100 times larger than the size of the substance, on the other hand, the existence cannot be detected even at a much larger p of 0.3. Consequently, biosensors based on FETs become more sensitive as W is decreased. In other words, to make the sensitivity high at lower concentration of charged target, the channel width must be similar to the size of the target.

The sensitivity enhancement with the decrease in the channel width of ISFET also can be confirmed by three-dimensional (3D) device simulation [27]. In Ref. 27, the dependence of memory characteristics on the number and distribution of the floating dots were systematically analyzed experimentally and numerically for dots-on-nanowire memories with multiple Si nanoscale floating dots. The Coulomb interaction between the charges in the floating dot and the nanowire channel were included in the numerical simulation using MEDICI Taurus Davinci. The operation principle of biosensors with a FET can be considered to be the same to that of floating dot memories as to the threshold voltage shift after the change of the charge on the gate insulator of the channel. This is because the attachment of a charged biomolecule on the gate insulator in the biosensor with a nanowire FET plays the same role as the charge injection of a floating dot in the dots-on-nanowire memories. Detection of a single-electron injection to a floating dot with a single-electron memory reminds us of the analogy between dots-on-nanowire memories and highly sensitive biosensors with a nanowire FET [28–30].

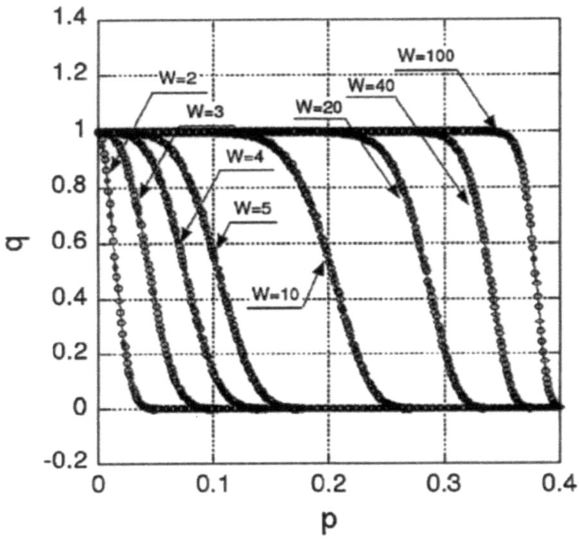

Figure 2.1 Dependences of the percolation probability q on the concentration of nonconductive site p at various channel width W values with the channel length fixed at 1000. Reproduced with permission from [26], Copyright 2009, The Japan Society of Applied Physics.

Following the simulation results [27], the change of threshold voltage from the voltage in the case with no floating dot (Fig. 2.2a) is larger in the case where the width of the channel is the same as the size of floating dot (Figs. 2.2b and 2.3) than in the case where the width is larger than the size of the dot (Figs. 2.2c and 2.4a). This proves the importance of the relative channel width to the size of the target molecule in FET biosensors. The above simulation results can be understood from the numerical potential energy profile (Fig. 2.4b) [27] that the potential energy in the non-existing region of a floating dot was lower than that in the existing region in the case where the width of the channel is wider than the size of the floating dot (Fig. 2.2c), which suggests the existence of a percolation path for electrons to pass through the channel when the width of the channel is wider than the size of the dot.

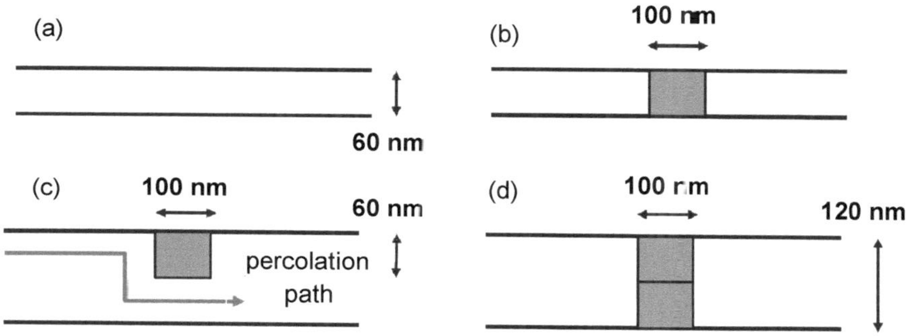

Figure 2.2 Schematics of dot distribution along the nanowire channel. Closed dots represent those filled with electrons. Arrows represent the path of carriers.

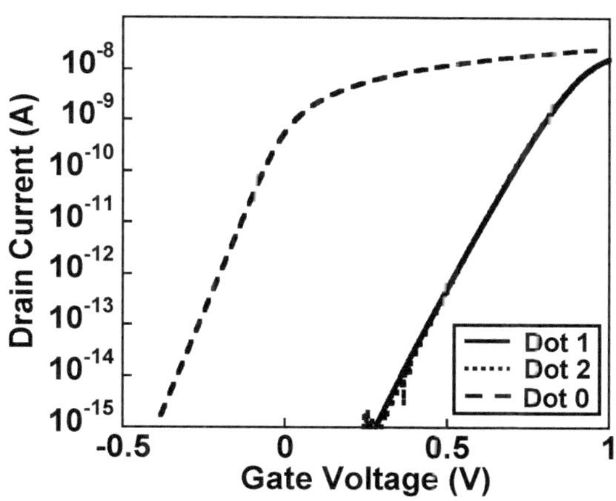

Figure 2.3 Simulation results of drain currents as a function of gate voltage for the devices with no dot (broken), single dot (solid), and double dots distributed in series (dotted). Here, the dot distribution is as shown in Fig. 2.2(a) for the no dot and in Fig. 2.2(b) for the single dot. Reproduced with permission from [27], Copyright 2009, AIP Publishing LLC.

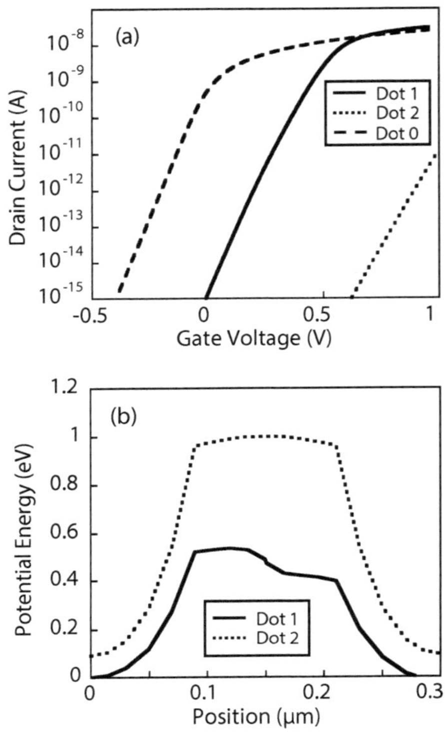

Figure 2.4 Simulation results of (a) drain currents as a function of gate voltage for the devices with no dot (broken), single dot (solid), and double dots (dotted) distributed in parallel and (b) the potential energy profile perpendicular to the channel length direction. Here, the dot distribution is as shown in Fig. 2.2(c) for the single dot and Fig. 2.2(d) for the double dots. Reproduced with permission from [27], Copyright 2009, AIP Publishing LLC.

2.3 Biosensors Based on SETs

Biosensors based on SETs are also a promising candidate for achieving high detection sensitivity due to the Coulomb oscillation. Because of the difficulty of the room-temperature operation of SETs and incompatibility of biomolecule solution processes with LSI fabrication processes, there had been no reports on SET-based ion sensors or biosensors until the series of study published recently. In these studies, a pH sensor [19] and biomolecule sensors for the detection of streptavidin [20, 21] were realized by using Si multiple-island channel structures for the room-temperature operation of SETs and the appropriate gate insulator structure for the solution processes. The immunodetection of PSA has been also demonstrated using an SET [21].

SET sensors should have extremely narrow nanowire barriers for the tunnel current to flow and small islands for sufficiently large single-electron charging energy at room temperature in the channel regions. These make the percolation effect of carriers well suppressed in the SET sensors.

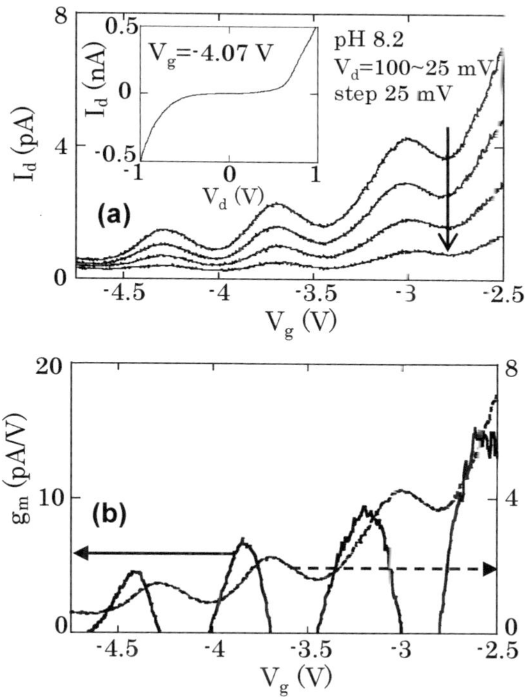

Figure 2.5 Experimental results of SET biosensor in buffer solution. (a) Drain current (I_d)–gate voltage (V_g) characteristics. V_g was applied using a reference electrode. Drain voltage (V_d) was varied from 100 to 25 mV in steps of 25 mV. Back-gate voltage (V_b) was fixed at 0 V. The inset shows I_d–V_d characteristics for valley at V_g of −4.07 V. (b) Transconductance (g_m)–V_g characteristics. I_d–V_g curve for V_d = 100 mV was used, and only positive g_m values are shown. Reproduced with permission from [21], Copyright 2013, AIP Publishing LLC.

Because the Coulomb oscillations is modulated by the change in the tunnel junction resistance of nanowire barrier regions with gate voltage (V_g), the drain current (I_d) and transconductance (g_m) at the corresponding V_g's to their local maximums increase with increasing V_g for the SET sensors. This indicates that the sensitivity of SET based biosensor can be high by increasing V_g.

The above finding was confirmed in detail by theoretical analyses [21, 22]. The fact was also shown by experiments [21]. Figure 2.5a shows the measured I_d–V_g characteristics of a fabricated SET biosensor in buffer solution at room temperature, showing clear Coulomb oscillations in which the peaks of I_d and g_m increase with increasing V_g. Here, V_g was applied by using a reference electrode. The increases of these peaks are due to the increase in the current of the nanowire barrier region at the corresponding V_g's with increasing V_g. The g_m–V_g characteristics (Fig. 2.5b) showed that maximum g_m values appear at the V_g values near the left-side half maximum of each I_d peak in the I_d–V_g characteristics, and that the maximum g_m indeed increases with increasing V_g.

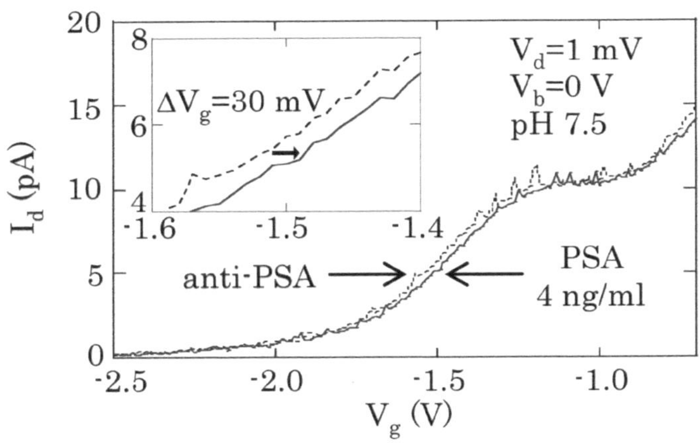

Figure 2.6 Drain current (I_d)–gate voltage (V_g) characteristics of SET biosensor for prostate-specific antigen (PSA) concentration of 4 ng/ml. The inset shows curves in V_g region from −1.6 to −1.4 V. Back-gate voltage (V_b) was fixed at 0 V. Reproduced with permission from [21], Copyright 2013, AIP Publishing LLC.

The immunodetection of PSA has been achieved using an SET sensor [21]. The surface modification of the gate insulator was carried out as described in Refs. 21 and 22. The immunodetection of PSA can be carried out using the specific binding of the antigen and antibody. For the binding event of 4 ng/mL of PSA to anti-PSA, a positive ΔV_g of 30 mV was observed (Fig. 2.6). The positive ΔV_g is consistent with the negative charge of PSA in solution at pH 7.5 due to the isoelectric point (6.9) of PSA. The value of 4 ng/mL is the required detection level for practical use.

2.4 Organic Nanostructures for Biosensors

Channel materials for FET ion sensors and biosensors are not limited to Si. Organic FETs have also been used for label-free detections of many kinds of biomolecules [6]. Organic FETs have unique advantages of low weight, high mechanical flexibility, cost effectiveness, and good chemical structural versatility compared with inorganic devices. However, most of the reported devices are over a micrometer in lateral size. An outstanding issue with organic devices is the difficulty of simultaneously controlling the lateral size and position of structures at nanometer scales. Top-down fabrication using EB lithography is most convenient technique to form various nanoscale structures with enough positional and size control for inorganic nanoscale structures. However, conventional EB lithography techniques have a big problem when they are used for the organic materials. One main reason is that it is difficult to remove only the mask resist which consists of organic material. Organic nanostructures can be fabricated using organic EB resists, however, organic EB resists are not electrically conductive. Therefore, fabrications of nanometer scale organic devices face difficulty in simultaneous control of the lateral size and position of electrically conductive structures in nanometer region.

Recently, organic EB resist polymers containing fullerenes have been developed as materials that allow simultaneous control of the lateral size and position at nanometer scales [24]. In the materials, a positive-type EB resist of ZEP520A was used as the matrix organic polymer and fullerenes are incorporated in it.

The matrix EB resist formed the nanometer scale structure with precise control of its lateral position after the EB exposure and development, and the containing fullerenes made the material electrically conductive. Electrons or holes are transferred through the LUMO or HOMO levels in the fullerenes in ZEP520A, respectively.

Figure 2.7 shows a cross-sectional transmission electron microscopy (TEM) image of ZEP520A containing fullerenes for a nanowire pattern. Here, [6,6]-phenyl-C_{61} butyric acid methyl ester (PCBM) was selected as the fullerene incorporated in the resist. The designed wire width was 200 nm. A very clear pattern was formed and the wire width was observed to be 140 nm.

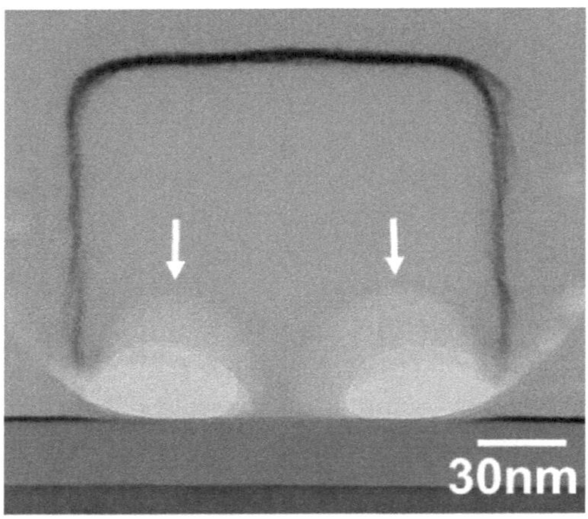

Figure 2.7 Cross sectional TEM micrograph of ZEP520A containing PCBM for a nanowire with the design width of 200 nm. Reproduced from [24].

There are two white regions, indicated by arrows, near the bottom edges of the resist pattern in Fig. 2.7. These regions are considered to be empty, suggesting that the PCBM aggregations existed in these regions before the development and dissolved during the development. Control of the size of the fullerene aggregation is considered to be possible by changing the kind and concentration of incorporated fullerene as well as the baking conditions of ZEP520A containing fullerene.

Although investigations on modifying the surfaces of ZEP520A containing fullerene is necessary, this technique has a possibility to be used for realizing sensitive biosensors having nanowire channels and Coulomb islands in organic integrated chips [25].

2.5 Summary

In this chapter, an overview is given for the biosensors with nanowire FETs and SETs as the biosensors using FETs with nanostructures for highly sensitive detection and quantification. One main reason for the highly sensitive detection of nanowire FET sensors is that nanowire FETs can decrease the percolation effect for carriers to transfer through the channel by decreasing the channel width. This is shown by simulation and experimental results. On the other hand, the mechanism for the high sensitivity in detection of biomolecules based on an SET sensor is explained by the fact that the Coulomb oscillations is modulated by the change in the tunnel junction resistance of nanowire barrier regions with V_g in the SET. This is shown by theoretical and experimental analyses. The immunodetection of PSA has been achieved using an SET sensor at the required detection level for practical use. Finally, organic EB resist polymers containing fullerene molecules are introduced as materials for realizing nanometer lateral-scale electronic devices. The materials have a possibility to be applicable to the fabrications of sensitive organic biosensors with nanowire FETs or SETs.

References

1. Bergveld, P. Development, operation, and application of the ion-sensitive field-effect transistor as a tool for electrophysiology. *IEEE Trans. Biomed. Eng.*, 1972, BME-19, 342–351.
2. Gotoh, M., Tamiya, E., Karube, I., Kagawa, Y. A microsensors for adenosine-5′-triphosphate pH-sensitive field effect transistors. *Anal. Chim. Acta*, 1986, 187, 287–291.
3. Park, K.-Y., Kim, M.-S., Choi, S.-Y. Fabrication and characteristics of MOSFET protein chip for detection of ribosomal protein. *Biosens. Bioelectron.*, 2005, 20, 2111–2115.
4. Kim, D.-S., Jeong, Y.-T., Park, H.-J., Shin, J.-K., Choi, P., Lee, J.-H., Lim, G. An FET-type charge sensor for highly sensitive detection of DNA sequence. *Biosens. Bioelectron.*, 2004, 20, 69–74.

5. Mohanty, N., Berry, V. Graphene-based single-bacterium resolution biodevice and DNA transistor: Interfacing graphene derivatives with nanoscale and microscale biocomponents. *Nano Lett.*, 2008, 8, 4469–4476.
6. Khan, H. U., Roberts, M. E., Johnson, O., Förch, R., Knoll, W., Bao, Z. In situ, label-free DNA detection using organic transistor sensors. *Adv. Mater.*, 2010, 22, 4452–4456.
7. Arima, A., Harlisa, I. H., Yoshida, T., Tsutsui, M., Tanaka, M., Yokota, K., Tonomura, W., Yasuda, J., Taniguchi, M., Washio, T., Okochi, M., Kawai, T. Identifying single viruses using biorecognition solid-state nanopores. *J. Am. Chem. Soc.*, 2018, 140, 16834–16841.
8. Cui, Y., Wei, Q., Park, H., Lieber, C. M. Nanowire nanosensors for highly sensitive and selective detection of biological and chemical species. *Science*, 2001, 293, 1289–1292.
9. Patolsky, F., Zheng, G., Hayden, O., Lakadamyali, M., Zhuang, X., Lieber, C. M. Electrical detection of single viruses. *Proc. Natl. Acad. Sci. U. S. A.*, 2004, 101, 14017–14022.
10. Wang, W. U., Chen, C., Lin, K.-H., Fang, Y., Lieber, C. M. Label-free detection of small-molecule-protein interactions by using nanowire nano-sensors. *Proc. Natl. Acad. Sci. U. S. A.*, 2005, 102, 3208–3212.
11. Zheng, G., Patolsky, F., Cui, Y., Wang, W. U., Lieber, C. M. Multiplexed electrical detection of cancer markers with nanowire sensor arrays. *Nat. Biotechnol.*, 2005, 23, 1294–1301.
12. Chen, R. J., Bangsaruntip, S., Drouvalakis, K. A., Kam, N. W. S., Shim, M., Li, Y., Kim, W., Utz, P. J., Dai, H. Noncovalent functionalization of carbon nanotubes for highly specific electronic biosensors. *Proc. Natl. Acad. Sci. U. S. A.*, 2003, 100, 4984–4989.
13. Maehashi, K., Katsura, T., Kerman, K., Takamura, Y., Matsumoto, K., Tamiya, E. Label-free protein biosensor based on aptamer-modified carbon nanotube field-effect transistors. *Anal. Chem.*, 2007, 79, 782–787.
14. Stern, E., Klemic, J. F., Routenberg, D. A., Wyrembak, P. N., Turner-Evans, D. B., Hamilton, A. D., LaVan, D. A., Fahmy, T. M., Reed, M. A. Label-free immunodetection with CMOS-compatible semiconducting nanowires. *Nature*, 2007, 445, 519–522.
15. Li, Z., Chen, Y., Li, X., Kamins, T. I., Nauka, K., Williams, R. S. Sequence-specific label-free DNA sensors based on silicon nanowires. *Nano Lett.*, 2004, 4, 245–247.

16. Kim, A., Ah, C. S., Yu, H. Y., Yang, J.-H., Baek, I.-B., Ahn, C.-G., Park, C. W., Jun, M. S., Lee, S. Ultrasensitive, label-free, and real-time immunodetection using silicon field-effect transistors. *Appl. Phys. Lett.,* 2007, 91, 103901-1–103901-3.

17. Kudo, T., Kasama, T., Ikeda, T., Hata, Y., Tokonami, S., Yokoyama, S., Kikkawa, T., Sunami, H., Ishikawa, T., Suzuki, M., *et al.* Fabrication of Si nanowire field-effect transistor for highly sensitive, label-free biosensing. *Jpn. J. Appl. Phys.,* 2009, 48, 06FJ04-1–06FJ04-4.

18. Knopfmacher, O., Tarasov, A., Fu, W., Wipf, M., Niesen, B., Calame, M., Schönenberger, C. Nernst limit in dual-gated Si-nanowire FET sensors. *Nano Lett.,* 2010, 10, 2268–2274.

19. Kudo, T., Nakajima, A. Highly sensitive ion detection using Si single-electron transistors. *Appl. Phys. Lett.,* 2011, 98, 123705-1–123705-3.

20. Kudo, T., Nakajima, A. Biomolecule detection based on Si single-electron transistors for highly sensitive integrated sensors on a single chip. *Appl. Phys. Lett.,* 2012, 100, 023704-1–023704-3.

21. Nakajima, A., Kudo, T., Furuse, S. Biomolecule detection based on Si single-electron transistors for practical use. *Appl. Phys. Lett.,* 2013, 103, 043702-1–043702-4.

22. Nakajima, A. Application of single-electron transistor to biomolecule and ion sensors. *Appl. Sci.,* 2016, 6, 94-1–94-14.

23. Veldhorst, M., Yang, C. H., Hwang, J. C. C., Huang, W., Dehollain, J. P., Muhonen, J. T., Simmons, S., Laucht, A., Hudson, F. E., Itoh, K. M., Morello, A., Dzurak, A. S. A two-qubit logic gate in silicon. *Nature,* 2015, 526, 410–414.

24. Nakajima, A., Tabei, T., Yasukawa, T. Fullerene-containing electrically conducting electron beam resist for ultrahigh integration of nanometer lateral-scale organic electronic devices. *Sci. Rep.*, 2017, 7, 4306-1–4306-9.

25. Nakajima, A. Short review on fullerene-containing electrically conducting electron beam resist for organic biosensors with nanostructures. *Adv. Tech. Biol. Med.*, 2018, 6, 1000257-1–1000257-4.

26. Kasama, T., Nakajima, A. Monte Carlo simulation of the two-dimensional site percolation problem for designing sensitive and quantitatively analyzable field-effect transistors. *Jpn. J. Appl. Phys.*, 2009, 48, 100207-1–100207-3.

27. Nakajima, A., Fujiaki, T., Ezaki, T. Impact of floating dot distribution on memory characteristics of self-aligned dots-on-nanowire memory. *J. Appl. Phys.,* 2009, 105, 114505-1–114505-6.

28. Nakajima, A., Futatsugi, T., Kosemura, K., Fukano, T., Yokoyama, N. Room temperature operation of Si single-electron memory with self-aligned floating dot gate. *Appl. Phys. Lett.*, 1997, 70, 1742–1744.
29. Nakajima, A., Futatsugi, T., Kosemura, K., Fukano, T., Yokoyama, N. Si single electron tunneling transistor with nanoscale floating dot stacked on a Coulomb island by self-aligned process. *Appl. Phys. Lett.*, 1997, 71, 353–355.
30. Nakajima, A., Futatsugi, T., Kosemura, K., Fukano, T., Yokoyama, N. Si single-electron tunneling transistor with nanoscale floating dot stacked on a Coulomb island by self-aligned process. *J. Vac. Sci. Technol. B*, 1999, 17, 2163–2171.

Chapter 3

Noble Metallic Pt Coating on Silk Textile by a Supercritical CO_2-Promoted Metallization Technique towards Applications of Biocompatible Medical Wearable Devices

Wan-Ting Chiu,[a] Tso-Fu Mark Chang,[a] Hiromichi Kurosu,[b] and Masato Sone[a]

[a]*Institute of Innovative Research, Tokyo Institute of Technology, 4259 Nagatsuta, Midori-ku, Yokohama 226-8503, Japan*
[b]*Department of Clothing Environmental Science, Nara Women's University, Kitauoya Higashimachi, Nara 630-8506, Japan*
wtchiu@iis.u-tokyo.ac.jp

Highly reliable Pt coating on silk textile was practiced by supercritical carbon dioxide (sc-CO_2)-promoted electroless plating in this study. Electroless plating is a facile method to integrate polymeric and metallic materials, and sc-CO_2 was introduced to the process to enhance the electroless plating characteristics. First, the palladium organometallic complex was inlaid into the silk substrate without damaging the silk structure in the catalyzation step. Second, a smooth and compact Pt layer was realized in the

Biomedical Engineering
Edited by Akihiro Miyauchi and Yuji Miyahara

ISBN 978-981-4877-63-3 (Hardcover), 978-1-003-14194-5 (eBook)
www.jennystanford.com

metallization step. The mechanisms involved in the sc-CO_2-assisted metallization step were focused and discussed in this study. The lowest electrical resistance was found at 50 mΩ in the sample metallized with the optimized conditions. The adhesive test showed robustness of the composite material. Corrosion resistance results revealed the applicability of this silk–Pt composite materials prepared by the sc-CO_2-assisted electroless plating in wearable device technology.

3.1 Introduction

Supercritical carbon dioxide (sc-CO_2) specifies when CO_2 goes beyond its critical point (304 K and 7.4 MPa) possessing the properties midway between a gas and liquid state. Sc-CO_2 shows non-polar property [1], high self-diffusivity [2], and low viscosity [3]. Owing to these advantages, sc-CO_2 is considered as a promising candidate for the development of polymer [2]. Due to the highly demand of next generation technology, wearable devices, which have been developed significantly for decades, suggest the integration of electronic devices with our daily life such as cloth materials and accessories [4]. Electrical conductivity is therefore a fundamental requirement for the applications of wearable electronic devices. Accordingly, cloth materials (i.e., polymers) equipped with electrically conductive characteristics is important topics among the critical wearable devices issues. Sc-CO_2 is non-polar and non-corrosive to most of polymers, which makes sc-CO_2 an ideal solvent in polymer development processes. In this study, we will demonstrate a sc-CO_2-assisted polymer development process for applications in fabrication process of wearable devices.

Electroless plating, which can metallize non-conductive polymer substrates with a thin metal or alloy layer, is utilized for the functionalization of polymers due to the requirement of electrical conductivity in wearable device applications. Electroless plating [5, 6] is also known as auto-catalytic plating or chemical plating. This technique can be accomplished by simple procedures and is operated without external electrical power. In addition, unlike electrodeposition and sputtering, electroless plating is less restricted by the equipment, and the metallization shows conformal properties. Accordingly, electroless plating is considered as a powerful technique to deposit materials on sophisticated structure and non-conductive substrate. There are three major steps in electroless plating, cleaning and roughening the substrate are carried out in the pretreatment step first, activation sites are settled on the substrate to complete the catalyzation step secondly, and the last step is the metallization on the substrate.

Sc-CO_2 is introduced into the catalyzation and metallization steps in the electroless plating system to enhance the properties [7–9]. Since the roughening step can be excluded with the help of sc-CO_2, this technique can simplify the procedures. In the meanwhile, due to the introduction of sc-CO_2, the usage of catalyzation solutions and electrolytes can be reduced [10]. Structure of the polymer substrate is often damaged during the conventional (CONV) catalyzation step, and the catalyst is merely settled on the substrate surface [11]. Due to the low viscosity and non-corrosive property, sc-CO_2 can bring non-polar organometallic complexes to go into the substrate while remains the substrate structure intact after the catalyzation step. This enhancement solves the most challenging issue in the CONV catalyzation step, which settles the catalyst on the substrate surface only by using a corrosive solution [12]. On the other hand, in CONV metallization, reactions are usually accompanied with hydrogen evolutions, which could lead to defects in the metallization layer [13]. In this study, Sc-CO_2 is introduced into the metallization step to enhance the metallization properties. A surfactant is introduced into the aqueous metallization bath to emulsify the aqueous bath and form sc-CO_2 micelles [14]. With the help of sc-CO_2 micelles, it can carry the hydrogen bubbles away from the substrate due to its non-polarity and high self-diffusivity. The metallization layer turns out to be compact and smooth by elimination of the hydrogen bubbles. Therefore, a sc-CO_2-assisted method was further introduced into the metallization process in this study to enhance the properties of the metal film and solve the difficulties from the CONV metallization.

For applications in wearable devices, making the devices user-friendly and biocompatible are the critical issues since there are frequent interaction between the device and human body. From the metallization point of view, common wearable devices are made of Ni metal or its alloys because of their high corrosion resistance [15, 16] and low price. However, there is a high risk that Ni results in allergy due to the non-biocompatible property [17, 18]. Platinum was chosen in this study for having biological inertia [19, 20] and high corrosion resistance [21] to avoid the allergy reactions. Furthermore, platinum also performs high electrical conductivity [22] and high thermal stability. Based on the aforementioned interests, electroless Pt metallization assisted by sc-CO_2 on silk textile was conducted and evaluated in this study.

3.2 Experimentals

3.2.1 Sc-CO_2-Assisted Catalyzation

Palladium(II) acetylacetonate (Pd(acac)$_2$; 99%, Tokyo Chemical Industry Co., Ltd., Japan) organometallic complex and a stir bar were enclosed into a 50 ml stainless reaction cell. Silk substrates with dimensions in 2 cm × 4 cm were hooked from top of the reaction cell. Pd(acac)$_2$ in 25 mg was included into the reaction cell to maintain the Pd(acac)$_2$ concentration at the saturation concentration point throughout the entire catalyzation step. The solubility of Pd(acac)$_2$ in sc-CO_2 is 2×10^{-5} mol/mol [23]. After sealing the reaction cell, CO_2 (99.99%, Nippon Tansan Co., Ltd., Japan) was injected into the reaction cell using a high pressure CO_2 apparatus [24] (Japan Spectra Company, Japan). The catalyzation was carried out under T = 80 ± 1 °C and P = 15 ± 0.1 MPa with agitation for 2 h. No pretreatment or post treatments were carried out after the catalyzation.

3.2.2 Sc-CO_2-Assisted Metallization

50 mL of an acidic platinum-metallization electrolyte consisted of 0.06 M chloroplatinic acid hexahydrate (≥37.50% Pt basis, Sigma-Aldrich, U.S.A), 0.15 M N_2H_4 reducing agent (24–26%, Sigma-Aldrich, U.S.A.), and 0.2 vol.% non-ionic surfactant (polyoxyethylene lauryl ether, $C_{12}H_{25}(OCH_2CH_2)_{15}OH$, 25%, Toshin Yuka Kogyo, Japan) was added into the 50 ml reaction cell. CO_2 was injected into the reaction cell after the cell was tightly

sealed. Metallization was carried out in an isothermal furnace controlled at T = 70 ± 1 °C and P = 15 ± 0.1 MPa with agitation. Various metallization time periods were performed to examine the relationship between lengths of the metallization time and silk–Pt characteristics. No post treatment was conducted after the metallization. An illustration of the sc-CO_2 metallization method is shown in Fig. 3.1.

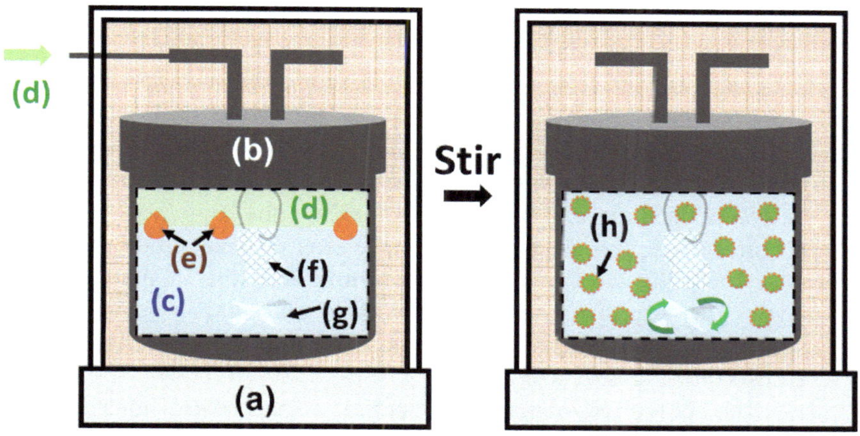

Figure 3.1 Experimental settings of the sc-CO_2 assisted metallization step: (a) A thermal bath that is controlled by an isothermal furnace, (b) the reaction-cell (PEEK-lined SUS316L), (c) Pt metallization electrolyte (80 vol.%), (d) sc-CO_2 (19.8 vol.%), (e) non-ionic surfactant (0.2 vol.%), (f) silk textile, and (g) cross stirrer, and (h) sc-CO_2/surfactant micelles formed when the solution is stirred in the reaction cell.

3.2.3 Analyses of Surface, Physical and Chemical Properties

An optical microscope (OM, VHV-5000, KEYENCE, Japan) and a scanning electron microscope (SEM, JSM-7500, JEOL, Japan) were used to observe morphologies of the silk–Pt. Thicknesses of the Pt layer were estimated by observing cross sections of the metallized silks via SEM and were analyzed by ImageJ (National Institutes of Health, U.S.A.). Metallized silks were cut into two pieces to unclose the cross section of silk–Pt. One piece of the composite material was fixed perpendicularly to the SEM holder surface by carbon tape showing the cross section to the electron beam. The composition and coverage of the Pt layer were measured by energy-dispersive X-ray spectroscopy (EDX, EMAX Evolution, HORIBA, Japan). The phases and crystal structures were identified by an X-ray diffractometer (XRD, Ultima IV, Rigaku, Japan).

Electrical resistances of the samples with dimensions at 1 cm × 0.5 cm (length × width) were measured by an in-line four-point probe (Mitsubishi Chemical Analytech Co., Ltd, MCP-T370, Japan) at room temperature. In the adhesive tests, Pt metallized silks with the same dimension (1 cm × 0.5 cm) was evaluated by 3M tape (3M adhesive tape #810, 3M, USA), which a piece of the tape having dimensions large enough to cover entire surface of the silk–Pt composite was used and firmly stuck to the composite. A 1 kg loading was used to ensure complete adhesion between the tape and the composite, then the tape was peeled off afterward. The electrical resistance was measured before and after the adhesive test to evaluate firmness of the Pt metallized layer. The adhesive test with one cycle and two cycles of the sticking–peeling procedure are named as first adhesive test and second adhesive test.

The potentiodynamic polarization curves were measured by a potentiostat/galvanostat (1287A, Solartron Analytical, UK). The silk–Pt composite prepared by 140 min of the metallization time, a Pt plate, and a Ag/AgCl reference electrode were used as the working electrode, the counter electrode, and the reference electrode, respectively. The testing solutions were 3.5 wt.% NaCl and simulated body fluid (SBF) (r-type) [25]. The 3.5 wt.% NaCl was used to simulate artificial sweat. The SBF was used to simulate the human body fluid. Total surface area of the working electrode, which is a piece of the 1 × 1 cm^2 silk–Pt composite, was calculated by considering surface area of every bundle of the Pt metallized silk fiber in a piece of the textile, and the value was 9.5 cm^2. The Pt counter electrode was cleaned ultrasonically in ethanol and pure water for 1 min, respectively, before the polarization measurement. The scan range was −0.4 to +0.6 V vs. Ag/AgCl at a scan rate of 1 mV/s. Prior to the polarization measurement, the three electrodes were immersed into the solution for 25 min to certify the stability. Similar adhesive tests were also conducted before the polarization measurements to confirm firmness of the Pt layer.

In the immersion test, one piece of the Pt metallized silk composite (1 cm × 1 cm) was immersed into the solution at 37 °C for 3 months. Then the SBF was drawn out and centrifugated for 2 h to remove the redundant particles. Pd and Pt ion concentrations in the solution were analyzed by inductively coupled plasma atomic emission spectroscopy (ICP-AES, ICPS-8100, Shimadzu Co., Ltd., Japan). Both the electrical resistance and the ICP measurements were carried out at least 10 times to provide a reliable average value and calculation of the standard deviation.

3.3 Results and Discussion

3.3.1 Structures and Phases Investigation

Figure 3.2 shows the (a) as-received silk and (b) sc-CO_2 catalyzation-treated silk. Transparent thread bundles and flakes with polygon structures seen in the OM images indicate the silk substrate and Pd(acac)$_2$, respectively. With the help of sc-CO_2 in the catalyzation step, the Pd(acac)$_2$ was successfully inlaid into the silk substrate without damaging the silk structure (Fig. 3.2b). X-ray diffraction patterns of the (a) as-received silk, (b) sc-CO_2 catalyzation-treated silk, and (c) Pt metallized silk are shown in Fig. 3.3. Silk textiles in Fig. 3.3a shows one broad peak at around 2θ = 20° indicating the amorphous structure of the substrate. After the catalyzation, all the diffraction peaks in Fig. 3.3b can be indexed to Pd(acac)$_2$ (diamond) well suggesting the Pd(acac)$_2$ was successfully deposited. X-ray diffraction pattern of the Pt metallized silk is demonstrated in Fig. 3.3c, five diffraction peaks locating at 2θ = 40.2°, 46.8°, 68.4°, 82.4°, and 84.5° can be indexed to (111), (200), (220), (311), and (222) planes of the FCC structure for platinum (circle) (JCPDS #87-0647), respectively. This result indicates that metallic platinum phase was deposited with only trace amount of impurity, and no other phases were observed as well within the X-ray detection limitation. Due to the small amount of reduced Pd metal catalyst, no metallic Pd characteristic peaks were observed after the metallization step.

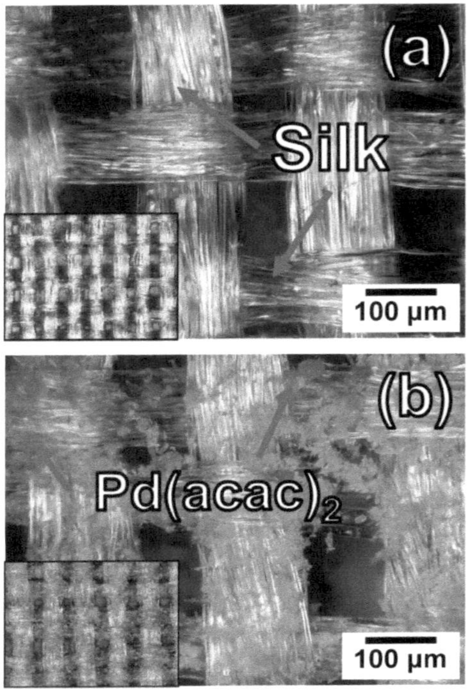

Figure 3.2 OM images of the (a) as-received and (b) sc-CO_2 catalyzation-treated silks.

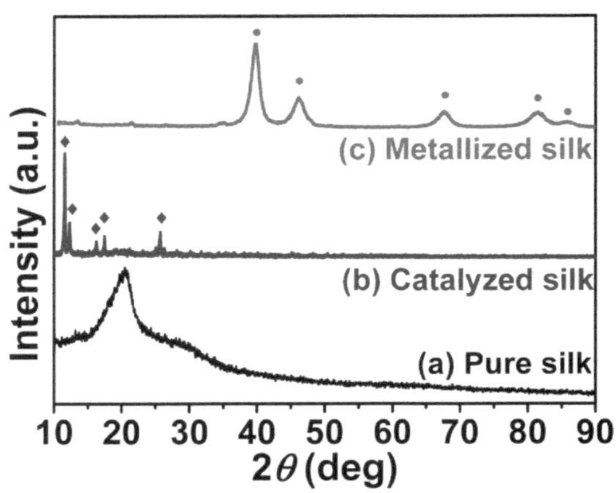

Figure 3.3 X-ray diffraction patterns of the (a) as-received, (b) sc-CO_2 catalyzation-treated, and (c) Pt metallized silks. Diamond: Pd(acac)$_2$; circle: Pt.

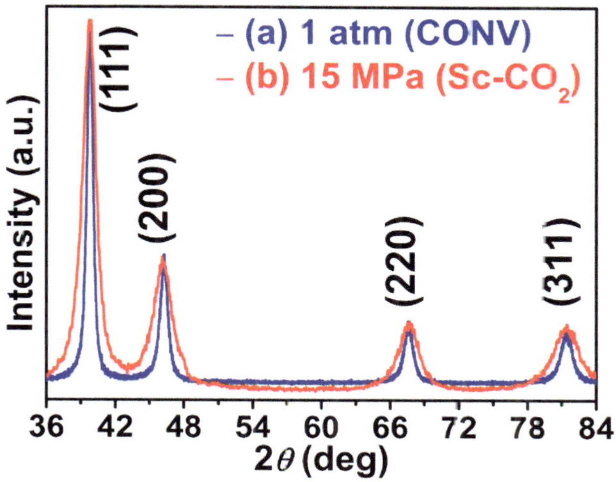

Figure 3.4 X-ray diffraction patterns of Pt metallized silks by the (a) CONV at 1 atm, and (b) sc-CO_2-assisted metallization methods.

Figure 3.4 shows diffraction patterns of the Pt metallized silk by the (a) CONV method and (b) the sc-CO_2-assisted metallization technique. In Fig. 3.4, full width at half maximums of the diffraction peaks of the Pt layer fabricated by the sc-CO_2-assisted technique were clearly wider than those prepared by the CONV method indicating that the sc-CO_2-assisted metallization brings a finer grain size. Influence of the sc-CO_2 on the grain size is shown in Fig. 3.5. In the CONV metallization, concentration of Pt complex around the electrode surface is similar to the concentration in the bulk solution and Pt nucleated on the substrate surface in early stage of the metallization as shown in Fig. 3.5a. As the metallization proceeds (Fig. 3.5b), concentration of the Pt complex around the substrate surface gradually decreases, which favors grain growth instead of nucleation. On the other hand, micelles composed of surfactant and sc-CO_2 would repeatedly bounce on the substrate surface to promote the mixing of reactive species in the solution (Fig. 3.5d). In this case, transfer or diffusion of Pt complex from the bulk solution to the surface of the substrate is enhanced and leads to a higher Pt complex concentration near the substrate than that in the CONV metallization as shown in Fig. 3.5e. When concentration of the reactive species, the Pt complex in this case, is high, nucleation

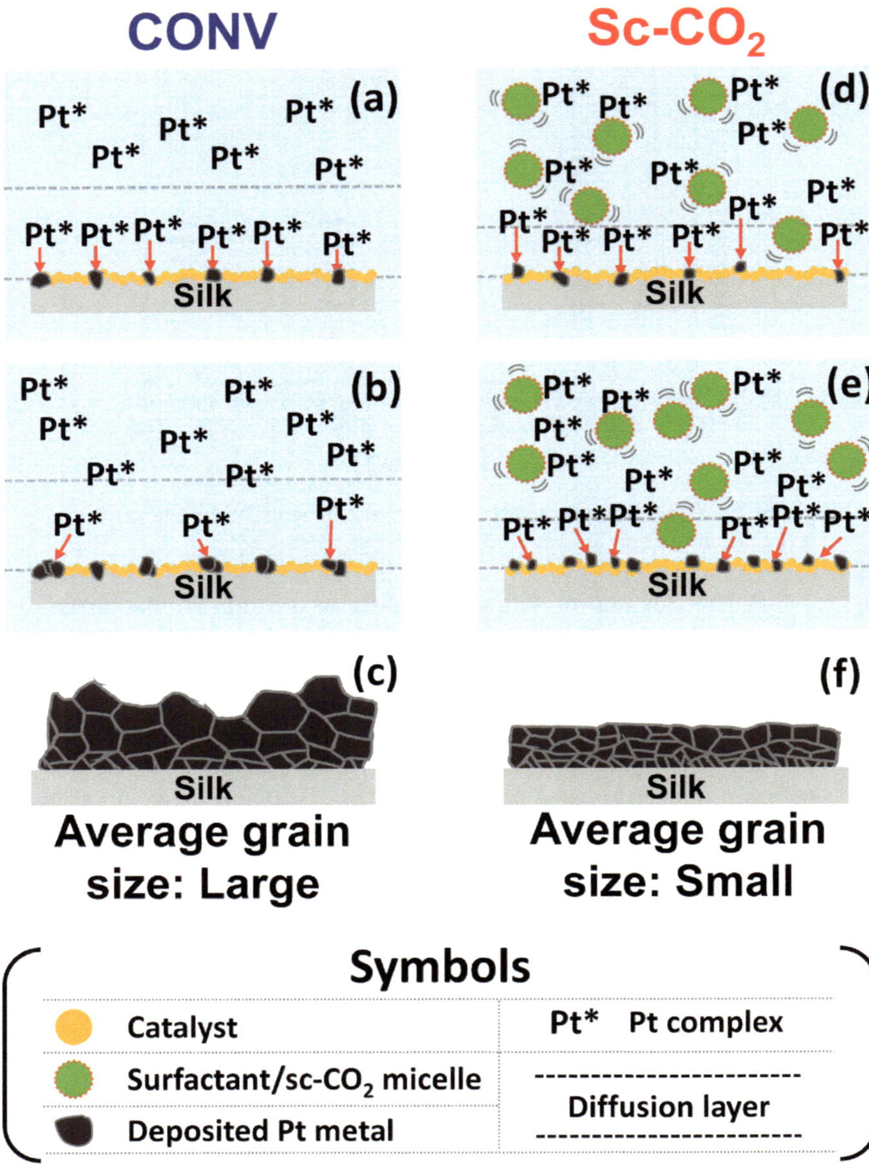

Figure 3.5 Illustration of influences of sc-CO_2 in the metallization step: (a–c) CONV and (d–f) sc-CO_2-assisted metallization methods.

is favored instead of grain growth, thus, high nuclei density and fine grain size are obtained (Figs. 3.5c,f). In addition, high nuclei density also brings about the smooth surface due to even growth rate of the Pt metallization layer on entire surface of the substrate. Since no obvious difference in ratio of the XRD peak intensities was found between the CONV and the sc-CO_2-assisted metallization method, the sc-CO_2 is suggested to have no influence on preferred crystal orientation of the Pt. Influence of the grain size on properties of the silk–Pt composites will be discussed in Section 3.3.

3.3.2 Morphologies of Silk–Pt Composites at Various Metallization Times

Six SEM images of silk–Pt composites metallized at 10, 20, 60, 100, and 140 min are shown in Figs. 3.6a–e to demonstrate the Pt coverage trend. Figure 3.6a reveals surface condition of the silk substrate metallized for only 10 min, and the dark phase is the Pt metallized region. Composition of the dark phase is pure Pt phase with only limited impurities. The bright phase corresponds to the silk, since silk is a non-conductive material which shows charging effect under SEM observation. Some parts of the silk are still non-metallized (pointing by arrows) indicating the Pt layer is not continuous on the silk. Depending on the Pt coverage condition, the metallization results are classified into two stages. This partially metallized silk substrate is classified into the first stage. Figure 3.6b shows a SEM image of the sample metallized for 20 min. A continuous Pt layer was achieved showing gray color on the entire surface, which are characterized into the second stage. As the metallization time extended to 60, 100, and 140 min (Figs. 3.6c–e), the silk substrates were completely covered. It is worth to note that the surface roughness increases as a function of the metallization time in the CONV metallization [24]. On the other hand, since sc-CO_2 gives brightener-like effect during the metallization [15], the surface became smoother than that metallized by the CONV metallization method when sc-CO_2 is applied. Moreover, hydrogen bubbles, which are generated as a side reaction during the metallization reaction, can be removed away from the substrate surface by the sc-CO_2 micelles due to the non-polar and high self-diffusivity characteristics [26], and this eventually leads to smooth Pt layer as shown in Fig. 3.7.

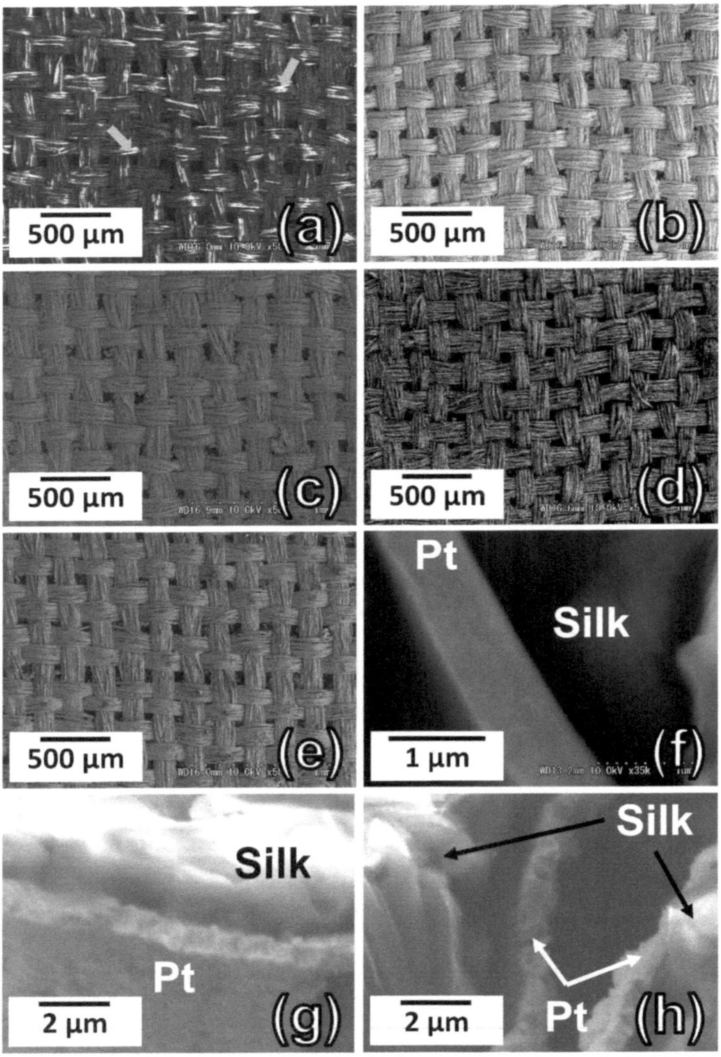

Figure 3.6 SEM images of the Pt metallized silk with (a) 10 min, (b) 20 min, (c) 60 min, (d) 100 min, and (e) 140 min of the metallization time, and (f) cross-section of the silk–Pt by 140 min of the sc-CO_2 metallization, and (g) and (f) cross-section of the silk–Pt by CONV sc-CO_2 metallization.

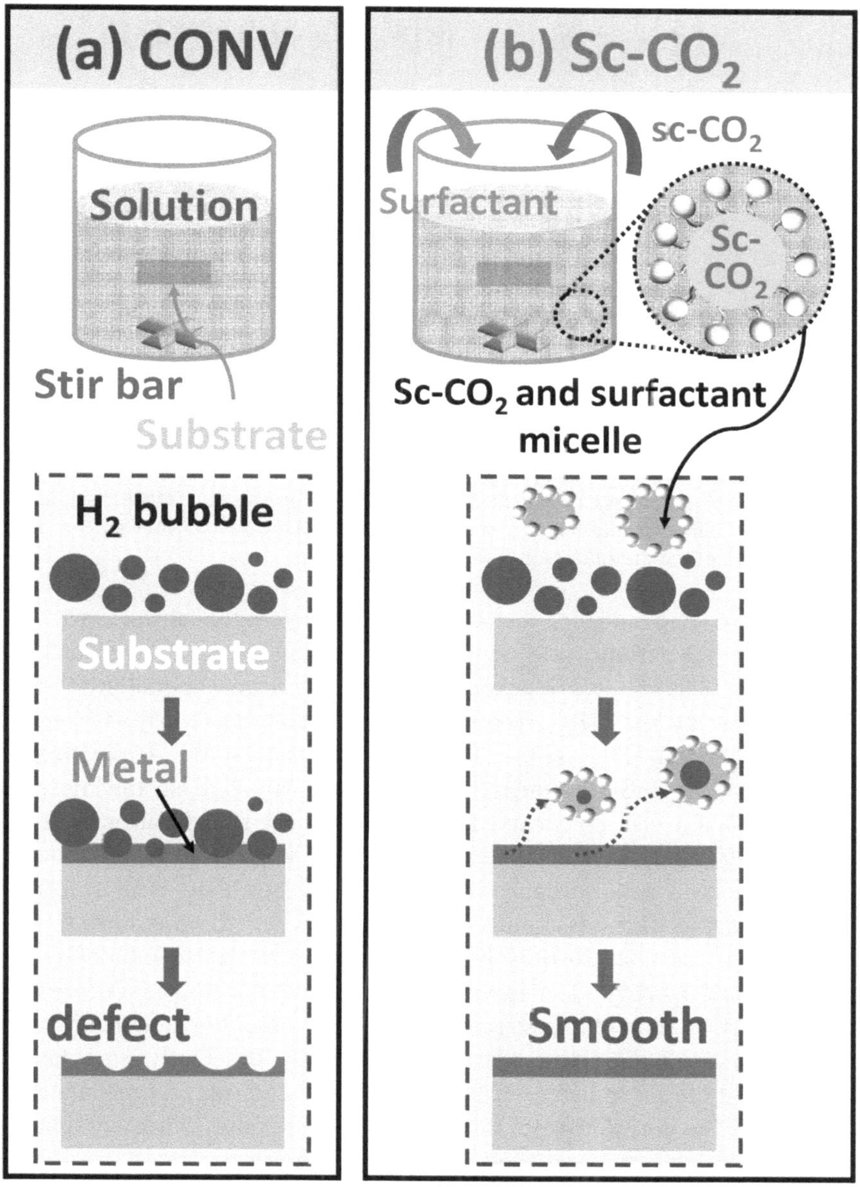

Figure 3.7 Illustration of effects of sc-CO_2 on morphologies of the Pt layer by the (a) CONV and (b) sc-CO_2-assisted metallization.

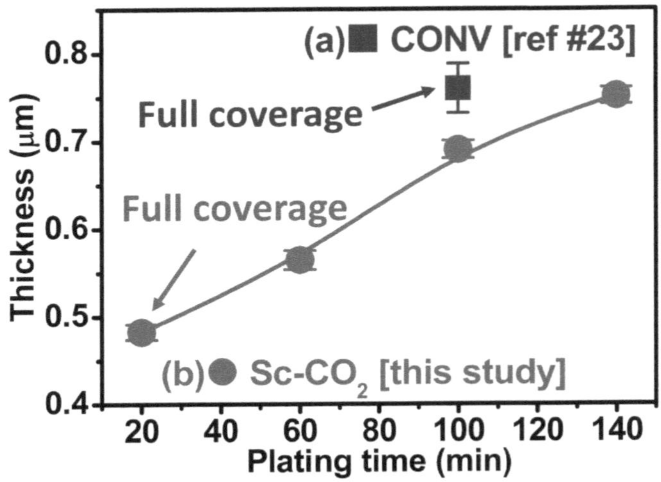

Figure 3.8 Thickness of the Pt layer metallized by the (a) CONV method at 100 min of metallization time and (b) sc-CO_2-assisted method as a function of the metallization time.

The dependences between the Pt layer thicknesses with the metallization time length are demonstrated in Fig. 3.8. Figure 3.8a shows thickness of the Pt layer metallized at 100 min by the CONV metallization [24]. For the sc-CO_2-assisted metallization, Fig. 3.8b, the Pt thicknesses show a positive correlation with the metallization time. The highest thickness at 0.75 μm was constructed with the longest metallization time of 140 min. The average growth rate was at 2.3 nm/min. This result is in accordance with the morphology shown in Fig. 3.6. No reliable thickness could be measured when the metallization time is less than 10 min due to the poor electrical conductivity. The sc-CO_2-assisted metallization prepared specimens entered the second stage (full coverage stage) at 20 min of the metallization time having a thickness at 0.48 μm while the CONV samples entered the second stage at 100 min of the metallization time along with 0.76 μm of the Pt thickness. These results indicated that more Pt sources were used in growth of the Pt thickness instead of covering the silk textile in the CONV case. The full coverage with a thinner thickness can also be attributed to the high nuclei density in the sc-CO_2-assisted metallization (Fig. 3.5) [27]. Based on the aforementioned reasons, through introduction of sc-CO_2, full Pt coverage was achieved with less metallization time and less Pt ion source, which indicates a more efficient metallization.

3.3.3 Electrical Properties

Electrical resistances of the as-metallized and the adhesive test-treated silk–Pt composites as a function of the metallization time are revealed in Fig. 3.9. Samples in the first stage exhibited high electrical resistances, which are mostly due to the incomplete Pt coverage (refer to Fig. 3.6a). On the other hand, at 60 min of the metallization time, the electrical resistance reached 50 mΩ. The electrical resistance remained almost unaffected as the metallization time extended beyond 60 min due to the same degree of Pt coverage and smooth surfaced. This result is in accordance with the coverage shown in Fig. 3.6 indicating that the Pt coverage is one of the critical factors affecting the electrical resistance. After a significant drop of the electrical resistance in the first stage, the electrical resistance for the samples metalized at 20 to 140 min deliberately decreased in the second stage (also refer to Figs. 3.6b–f).

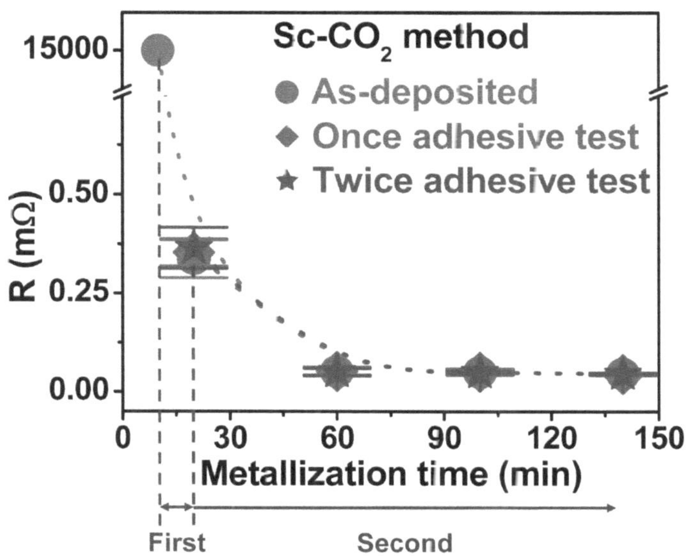

Figure 3.9 Electrical resistance-metallization time curves before and after the adhesive tests.

In the CONV metallization, similar two stages were found; however, the electrical resistance was offset by the increasing roughness as the metallization time went beyond 140 min [24, 28]. On the other hand, the sc-CO_2-assisted metallization gives compact and smooth Pt coatings on the silk (Fig. 3.6f). The electrical resistance thus persisted after 60 min of the metallization time. The second stage was prolonged by the sc-CO_2-assisted metallization, and the region showing the deteriorated electrical conductivity was not found in this study. No experiments were conducted at the metallization time longer than 140 min since the electrical resistances are expected to remain at the same level.

The grain size can affect the electrical resistance, and a finer grain size is expected to result a higher electrical resistance [29]. In Fig. 3.4, finer grain size of the Pt layer via the sc-CO_2-assisted metallization was obtained while comparing to the CONV metallization. However, electrical resistance of the silk–Pt synthesized by the sc-CO_2-assisted metallization method shows a 16% reduction while comparing to those without sc-CO_2 [24]. Roughness of the Pt layer metallized on the silk is suggested to be the cause of the difference in electrical resistance [29]. Cross sections of the samples prepared by the CONV (Figs. 3.6g and h) and the sc-CO_2-assisted metallization methods (Fig. 3.6f) with the optimized metallization conditions clearly demonstrated the difference in roughness of Pt layer metallized on the silk.

3.3.4 Adhesive Tests

Electrical resistances of the adhesive test-treated silk–Pt composites are also shown in Fig. 3.9. No adhesive tests were performed for the samples in the first stage due to the unfeasible high electrical resistance for applications. Impact of the adhesive test on electrical resistance of the sc-CO_2-assisted metallized samples was not obvious. 18% reduction in the electrical resistance after second adhesive was observed in the sample prepared by the CONV method [24]. On the other hand, only 0.5% reduction in the electrical resistance was observed after second adhesive test in this study. The closely packed and smooth Pt coating prepared by the sc-CO_2-assisted metallization method allows the Pt layer to stay intact after the second adhesive test and shows better resistance against the adhesive tests than those prepared without utilizing sc-CO_2.

3.3.5 Corrosion Resistance Measurements in 3.5 wt% NaCl and in SBF

3.3.5.1 Corrosion behavior in 3.5 wt% NaCl solution

Figure 3.10a shows polarization curves of the as-metallized and the adhesion test-treated silk–Pt composites in 3.5 wt.% NaCl solution. Samples prepared with 140 min of the metallization time were chosen for the corrosion resistance evaluations. No significant difference was found between the three polarization curves in Fig. 3.10a revealing excellent corrosion resistance of this Pt layer. The corrosion potential (E_{corr}) and the corrosion current density (I_{corr}) are summarized in Table 3.1 Specimens prepared by the sc-CO_2-assisted metallization show higher corrosion resistance than those by the CONV method [24]. In 3.5 wt.% NaCl solution, the corrosion current density after second adhesive test decreased from 5.93×10^{-7} to 2.17×10^{-7} A/cm^2 when sc-CO_2 was introduced into the metallization step. Decrease in the corrosion current density is suggested to be a result of the smooth surface condition and compact Pt metallization layer when the sc-CO_2-assisted metallization step is applied.

Table 3.1 Corrosion potentials and corrosion current densities of the silk–Pt composites in (a) 3.5 wt.% NaCl and (b) SBF solutions

(a) Samples (in 3.5 wt.% NaCl)	**E_{corr} (V)**	**I_{corr} (μA/cm^2) ± SD**
As-deposited	0.16	0.217 ± 0.005
First adhesive test	0.16	0.220 ± 0.004
Second adhesive test	0.16	0.217 ± 0.004
(b) Samples (in SBF)	**E_{corr} (V)**	**I_{corr} (μA/cm^2) ± SD**
As-deposited	0.25	0.175 ± 0.007
First adhesive test	0.26	0.167 ± 0.006
Second adhesive test	0.25	0.171 ± 0.005

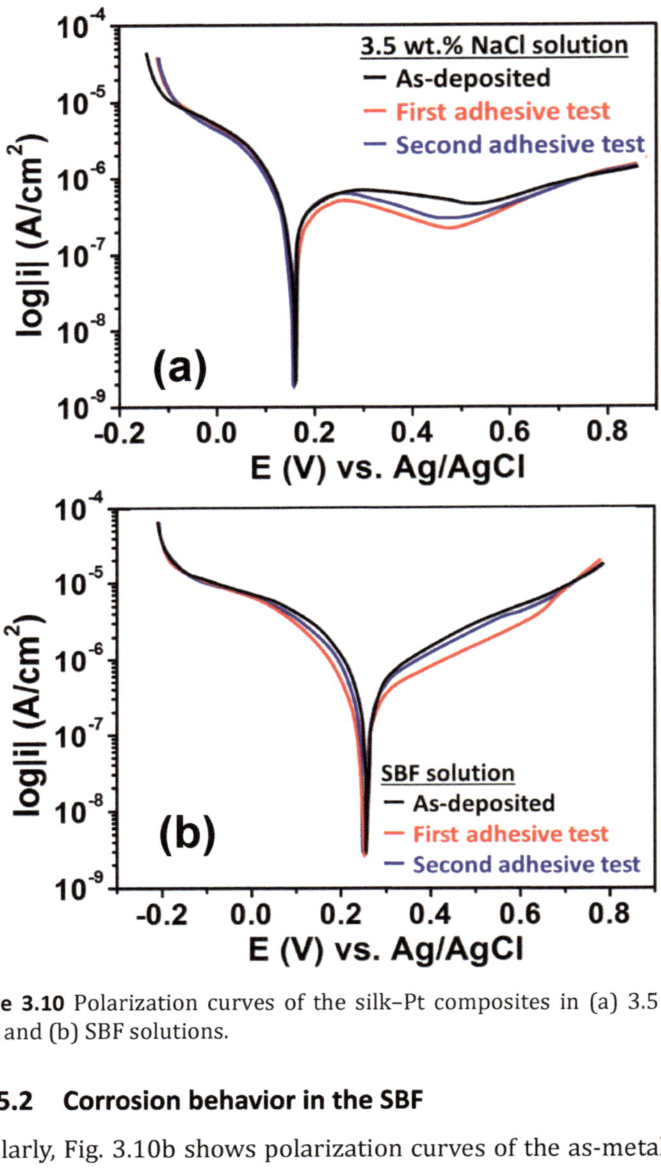

Figure 3.10 Polarization curves of the silk–Pt composites in (a) 3.5 wt.% NaCl and (b) SBF solutions.

3.3.5.2 Corrosion behavior in the SBF

Similarly, Fig. 3.10b shows polarization curves of the as-metallized and adhesion-treated samples in the SBF. In the same way, composites metallized at 140 min were chosen as the working electrode. The E_{corr} and I_{corr} are also listed in Table 3.1, which shows limited standard deviation around ± 0.005 (μA/cm^2). The corrosion resistances are similar to those of bulk Pt metal indicating high corrosion resistance of the Pt metallization layer despite being deposited on a non-conductive substrate. In addition, the corrosion current density after second test decreased from 2.02 × 10^{-7} to 1.71 × 10^{-7} A/cm^2 in the SBF while sc-CO_2 was introduced [24]. Silk–Pt composite shows high corrosion resistance in the corrosion test in both 3.5 wt.% NaCl and SBF.

3.3.6 Immersion Test for Biocompatibility Assessment

Allergy reaction is provoked when there is metal ion released from the environment and transferred into human body as reported by Wataha [29]; therefore, examining metal ion releasing rates in the SBF is a straightforward approach to assess the biocompatibility of the silk–Pt composite. Metal ion concentrations in human body vary with races, environments, and diets. According to several literatures based on different living situations, the average Pt input from diet is 1.44 μg/day, and the Pt output through the feces can be up to 1.79 μg/day [30–32]. The average Pd intake is 2 μg/day, and the average Pd output through the feces can be up to around 2.5 μg/day [33, 34]. In this study, after 3 months of the immersion test in the SBF at human body temperature (37 °C), the Pd and Pt releasing rates were only 0.037 μg/day and 0.057 μg/day, respectively. The releasing rates are too small and can be neglected when comparing to the daily intake and output rates. Despite of the small grain size, which can promote release of metal ions, the corrosion resistance was balanced by the high compactness of the Pt layer.

The silk–Pt composites prepared by the sc-CO_2-assisted catalyzation and the metallization methods showed smooth and compact surface conditions for the Pt layer, decent electrical conductivity, high reliability from the adhesive tests, and high biocompatibility in both of the immersion and polarization measurements. The results further demonstrated practicability of the Pt metallized silks in wearable and medical devices.

3.4 Conclusions

Robust and electrical conductive Pt metallized silks were successfully fabricated via the sc-CO_2-assisted electroless plating technique in this study. In the catalyzation step, the Pd(acac)$_2$ was successfully inlaid into the silk textile without damaging the structure with the help of sc-CO_2. In the metallization step, a compact and smooth Pt layer was metallized. The coverage and thickness of the Pt metallized layer increased as a function of the metallization time. Full Pt coverage on the silk substrate was achieved in merely 20 min of the metallization time, which was shortened significantly while comparing to the metallization method without sc-CO_2. The electrical resistance reached 50 mΩ at 60 min of the metallization time and remained almost unchanged as the metallization time extended to 140 min since the surface was smoothened by the introduction of sc-CO_2. The electrical resistance persisted after the adhesive tests, which also confirmed the great enhancement in the reliability while comparing to those synthesized by the metallization method without sc-CO_2. The silk–Pt composite shows high corrosion resistance before and after the adhesive test in both 3.5 wt.% NaCl and the SBF solutions. The Pd and Pt ion releasing rates were both negligible comparing to the daily input and output of Pd and Pt in human body.

Acknowledgments

This work is supported by Japan Society for the Promotion of Science (17J07395), Japan Society for the Promotion of Science (19F19048), the Grant-in-Aid for Scientific Research (B) (JSPS KAKENHI Grant Number 26282013), the Grant-in-Aid for Scientific Research (B) (JSPS KAKENHI Grant Number 17H01956), the CREST Project (#14531864) operated by the Japan Science and Technology Agency (JST).

References

1. Mukhopadhyay, M. (2000). *Natural Extracts Using Supercritical Carbon Dioxide* (CRC press, USA).

2. Kemmere, M. F., and Meyer, T. (2006). *Supercritical Carbon Dioxide: In Polymer Reaction Engineering* (John Wiley & Sons, USA).

3. Rozzi, N., and Singh, R. (2002). Supercritical fluids and the food industry, *Compr. Rev. Food Sci. Food Saf.*, **1**, pp. 33–44.

4. Patel, M. S., Asch, D. A., and Volpp, K. G. (2015). Wearable devices as facilitators, not drivers, of health behavior change, *Jama*, **313**, pp. 459–460.

5. Mallory, G. O., and Hajdu, J. B. (1990). *Electroless Plating: Fundamentals and Applications* (William Andrew, USA).

6. Shacham-Diamand, Y., Inberg, A., Sverdlov, Y., Bogush, V., Croitoru, N., Moscovich, H., and Freeman, A. (2003). Electroless processes for micro-and nanoelectronics, *Electrochim. Acta*, **48**, pp. 2987–2996.

7. Watkins, J. J., and McCarthy, T. J. (1995). Polymer/metal nanocomposite synthesis in supercritical CO_2, *Chem. Mater.*, **7**, pp. 1991–1994.

8. Adachi, H., Taki, K., Nagamine, S., Yusa, A., and Ohshima, M. (2009). Supercritical carbon dioxide assisted electroless plating on thermoplastic polymers, *J. Supercrit. Fluids*, **49**, pp. 265–270.

9. Chiu, W.-T., Tahara, Y., Chen, C.-Y., Chang, T.-F. M., Hashimoto, T., Kurosu, H., and Sone, M. (2017). Silk–Pt composite integration by supercritical carbon dioxide assisted electroless plating for medical devices application, *Microelectron. Eng.*, **175**, pp. 34–37.

10. Tengsuwan, S., and Ohshima, M. (2012). Electroless nickel plating on polypropylene via hydrophilic modification and supercritical carbon dioxide Pd-complex infusion, *J. Supercrit. Fluids*, **69**, pp. 117–123.

11. Chiu, W.-T., Tahara, Y., Chen, C.-Y., Chang, T.-F. M., Hashimoto, T., Kurosu, H., and Sone, M. (2017). A Supercritical CO_2 Promoted Electroless Ni-P Plating on Silk and Their Fundamental Characteristics Investigations, *J. Electrochem. Soc.*, **164**, pp. D406–D411.

12. Sano, M., Tahara, Y., Chang, T.-F. M., Chen, C.-Y., Hashimoto, T., Kurosu, H., and Sone M. (2016). Metallization of textile by Pt catalyzation in supercritical carbon dioxide and Pt electroless plating for applications in wearable devise, *Microelectron. Eng.*, **153**, pp. 92–95.

13 Chang, T.-F. M., Tasaki, T., Ishiyama, C., and Sone, M. (2011). Defect-free nickel micropillars fabricated at a high current density by application of a supercritical carbon dioxide emulsion, *Ind. Eng. Chem. Res.*, **50**, pp. 8080–8085.

14. Tanabe, M., Chang, T.-F. M., Nagoshi, T., Chung, S.-T., Tsai, W.-T., Hosoda, H., Sato, T., and Sone, M. (2015). Mechanical properties of Sn electrodeposited in supercritical CO_2 emulsions using micro-compression test, *Microelectron. Eng.*, **141**, pp. 219–222.
15. Chang, T.-F. M., Sone, M., Shibata, A., Ishiyama, C., and Higo, Y. (2010). Bright nickel film deposited by supercritical carbon dioxide emulsion using additive-free Watts bath, *Electrochim. Acta,* **55**, pp. 6469–6475.
16. Kucernak, A. R., and Sundaram, V. N. N. (2014). Nickel phosphide: The effect of phosphorus content on hydrogen evolution activity and corrosion resistance in acidic medium, *J. Mater. Chem. A,* **2**, pp. 17435–17445.
17. Sugiyama, T., Uo, M., Wada, T., Hongo, T., Omagari, D., Komiyama, K., Sasaki, H., Takahashi, H., Kusama, M., and Mori, Y. (2014). Novel metal allergy patch test using metal nanoballs, *J. Nanobiotechnol.*, **12**, p. 51.
18. Ashrin, M. N., Arakaki, R., Yamada, A., Kondo, T., Kurosawa, M., Kudo, Y., Watanabe, M., Ichikawa, T., Hayashi, Y., and Ishimaru, N. (2014). A critical role for thymic stromal lymphopoietin in nickel-induced allergy in mice, *J. Immunol.*, **192**, pp. 4025–4031.
19. Lago, N., Yoshida, K., Koch, K. P., and Navarro, X. (2007). Assessment of biocompatibility of chronically implanted polyimide and platinum intrafascicular electrodes, *IEEE Trans. Biomed. Eng.*, **54**, pp. 281–290.
20. Kansu, G., and Aydin, A. (1996). Evaluation of the biocompatibility of various dental alloys: Part 2-Allergenical potentials, *Eur. J. Prosthodont. Restora. Dent.*, **4**, pp. 155–161.
21. John, K., Jänsch-Kaiser, G., and Sharp, D. H. (2008). *Platinum, Platinum Metals, and Their Alloys, Corrosion Handbook* (Wiley-VCH Verlag GmbH & Co. KGaA, Germany).
22. Powell, R., Tye, R., Woodman, and Margaret, J. (1962). Thermal conductivities and electrical resistivities of the platinum metals, *Platin. Met. Rev.*, **6**, pp. 138–143.
23. Yoda, S., Hasegawa, A., Suda, H., Uchimaru, Y., Haraya, K., Tsuji, T., and Otake, K. (2004). Preparation of a platinum and palladium/polyimide nanocomposite film as a precursor of metal-doped carbon molecular sieve membrane via supercritical impregnation, *Chem. Mater.*, **16**, pp. 2363–2368.
24. Chiu, W.-T., Tahara, Y., Chen, C.-Y., Chang, T.-F. M., Hashimoto, T., Kurosu, H., and Sone, M. (2017). Fundamental property assessments of biocompatible silk–Pt composite prepared by supercritical

carbon dioxide promoted electroless plating, *Ind. Eng. Chem. Res.*, **56**, pp. 8864–8871.

25. Oyane, A., Kim, H. M., Furuya, T., Kokubo, T., Miyazaki, T., and Nakamura, T. (2003). Preparation and assessment of revised simulated body fluids, *J. Biomed. Mater. Res. A*, **65**, pp. 188–195.

26. Chang, T.-F. M., Shimizu, T., Ishiyama, C., and Sone, M. (2013). Effects of pressure on electroplating of copper using supercritical carbon dioxide emulsified electrolyte, *Thin Solid Films*, **529**, pp. 25–28.

27. Chang, T.-F. M., and Sone M. (2011). Function and mechanism of supercritical carbon dioxide emulsified electrolyte in nickel electroplating reaction, *Surf. Coat. Technol.*, **205**, pp. 3890–3899.

28. Tang, W., Xu, K., Wang, P., and Li, X. (2003). Surface roughness and resistivity of Au film on Si-(111) substrate, *Microelectron. Eng.*, **66**, pp. 445–450.

29. Chaverri, D., Saenz, A., and Castano, V. (1991). Grain size and electrical resistivity measurements on aluminum polycrystalline thin films, *Mater. Lett.*, **12**, pp. 344–348.

30. Wataha, J. C. (2001). Principles of biocompatibility for dental practitioners, *J. Prosthet. Dent.*, **86**, pp. 203–209.

31. Vaughan, G., and Florence T. (1992). Platinum in the human diet, blood, hair and excreta, *Sci. Total Environ.*, **111**, pp. 47–58.

32. van den Berg, C. M., and Jacinto, G. S. (1988). The determination of platinum in sea water by adsorptive cathodic stripping voltammetry, *Anal. Chim. Acta*, **211**, pp. 129–139.

33. Goldberg, E. D., Hodge, V., Kay, P., Stallard, M., and Koide, M. (1986). Some comparative marine chemistries of platinum and iridium, *Appl. Geochem.*, **1**, pp. 227–232.

34. Goldberg, E. D., and Koide, M. (1990). Understanding the marine chemistries of the platinum group metals, *Mar. Chem.*, **30**, pp. 249–257.

Chapter 4

Biosensors Based on Silicon Photonics

Shin Yokoyama,[a] Yoshiteru Amemiya,[a] Takeshi Ikeda,[a] Akio Kuroda,[a] and Mitsuhiko Ogihara[b]

[a]*Hiroshima University, 1-4-2 Kagamiyama, Higashihiroshima, Hiroshima 739-8527, Japan*
[b]*Filnex Corporation, 1-42-1-1-310 Bessho, Hachioji, Tokyo 192-0363, Japan*

yokoyama-shin@hiroshima-u.ac.jp

4.1 Introduction

In the medical field, detection of various antigen-antibody reactions is used. For example, by measuring the amount of antigen (Table 4.1) [1], which is a tumor marker in blood, the kinetics of cancer can be known. The tumor marker is not useful for early detection of cancer because the dead body of advanced cancer cells has flowed out into the blood, but serves as an index for cancer treatment. In this chapter, biosensors which detect antigen-antibody reactions using silicon photonics [2] are described. It is said that early detection of cancer requires detection of exosomes in blood and miRNAs encapsulated therein [3]. There

Biomedical Engineering
Edited by Akihiro Miyauchi and Yuji Miyahara

ISBN 978-981-4877-63-3 (Hardcover), 978-1-003-14194-5 (eBook)
www.jennystanford.com

are special proteins on the surface of exosomes [4]. Therefore, the biosensor proposed in this study could be applied to a device for early detection of cancer by using a protein that specifically binds to a protein on the surface of exosomes or a complementary miRNA.

Table 4.1 Example of cancer markers with normal concentration in blood, and detectable sickness [1].

Marker	Normal value	Detectable sickness
AFP	< 20 ng/ml	Liver cancer
CEA	< 5 ng/ml	Digestive cancer
PSA	< 4 ng/ml	Prostate cancer
BFP	< 75 ng/ml	Genital cancer
SCC	< 1.5 ng/ml	Lung cancer

Various biosensors are compared in Table 4.2 in the different categories of detection principle [5–15]. Biosensors using light have low noise and high sensitivity. The enzyme-linked immunosorbent assay (ELISA) method [7], which is generally used, is ultra-sensitive, but need labeling, too large in its equipment size, expensive, and not suitable for home use. The label free detection is preferred because the labeling sometimes alters the molecular structure and causes incorrect results. Although the surface plasmon resonance (SPR) [8] is label free and already in practical use, the equipment is still too large for home use.

Table 4.2 Variable biosensors and their characteristics [5–15].

Detection Method	Device	Advantage	Disadvantage	Refs.
Electric	Nanowire Transistor	Compact, Super High Sensitivity	Detection Area is limited by Debye Length, Large Noise	5
	FET[*1]	Compact, High Sensitivity		6
Optic Luminescence	ELISA[*2]	Super High Sensitivity pg/ml	Labeling Necessary, Long Measurement Time, Expensive	7

Detection Method		Device	Advantage	Disadvantage	Refs.
Resonance		SPR[*3]	High Sensitivity, Resistant to Electric Noise	Large Size, Expensive	8
		Silicon Resonator (Ring, PhC[*4])	High Sensitivity, High Integration, Resistant to Electric Noise	Temperature Sensitive	9-12
Magnetic		Magnetic Bead Sensor (Hall Effect Sensor)	Low Noise, Magnetic Washing Possible without Water	Labeling Necessary, Low Sensitivity	13
Mechanic	Mass	QCM[*5]	Low Cost, Real Time	Temperature Sensitive	14
	Stress	MSS[*6]	High Integration, Real Time, Low Cost	Basic research for commercialization is required.	15

[*1]FET: Field Effect Transistor, [*2]ELISA: Enzyme-Linked Immunosorbent Assay, [*3]SPR: Surface Plasmon Resonance, [*4]PhC: Photonic Crystal, [*5]QCM: Quartz Crystal Microbalance, [*6]MSS: Membrane-type Surface stress Sensor

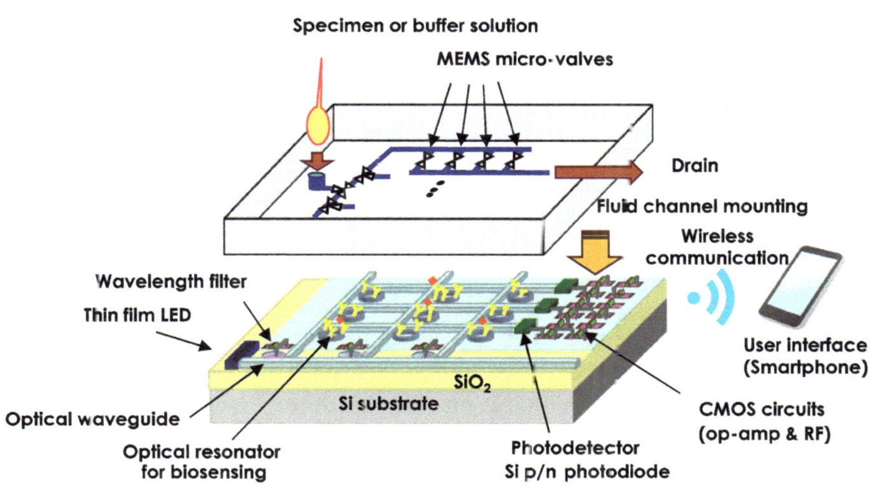

Figure 4.1 Example of the target biosensor chip which we propose.

Figure 4.1 shows an example of our target biosensor chip [16]. By using "Silicon Photonics," which uses mature silicon LSI fabrication technology to optical devices, it is thought that high-performance, label-free compact biosensors that can be used at home could be mass-produced at low cost. This biosensor should be sufficiently sensitive for a screening test, which is a preliminary step, rather than a detailed test. From Table 4.1, the sensitivity of several ng/ml is set to the target sensitivity of the detection.

4.2 Optical Ring Resonator Biosensor

Mach–Zehnder interferometer shown in Fig. 4.2a is a typical method to detect biological materials adsorbed on the optical waveguide. The output light intensity is changed because the phase of the output light is changed by the adsorbed biological materials on the arm. In order to obtain sufficiently large sensitivity, the detection length L must be sufficiently long. As a method to overcome this disadvantage, there is a method to employ a ring resonator shown in Fig. 4.2b.

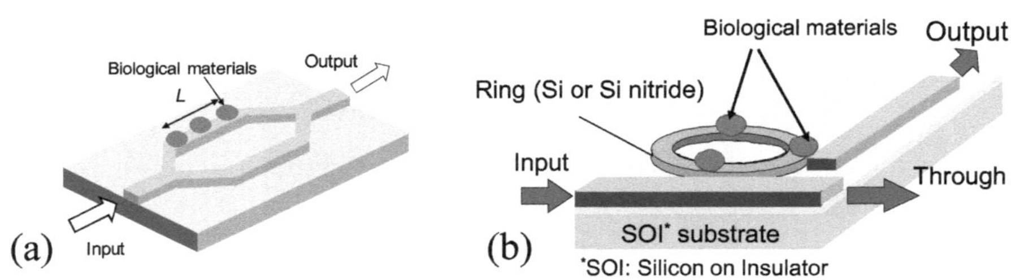

Figure 4.2 (a) Mach–Zehnder interferometer biosensor and (b) ring resonator biosensor.

In this case, since light travels along the resonator for many times, a large sensitivity can be obtained with a small area, which is suitable for dense integration. On the other hand, considering the temperature dependence, in the case of the Mach–Zehnder interferometer, the temperature dependence is canceled by the two arms, but in the case of the single resonator, the output light intensity is directly affected by temperature changes. How to overcome this problem is described in Section 4.4 "Differential Ring Resonator Biosensor."

4.2.1 Operation Principle

The resonance wavelength λ_{res} of the ring resonator is given by

$$\lambda_{\text{res}} = n_{\text{eff}} \frac{L}{m}, \tag{4.1}$$

where n_{eff} is the effective refractive index of the optical waveguide consisting the ring resonator, L is the peripheral length of the ring resonator, and m is the integer. When the wavelength of the input light is close to the resonance wavelength, the output light intensity takes a certain value. When the resonance wavelength is changed due to the attachment of the biological substance, the resonance spectrum shifts so that the output light intensity is changed. The effective refractive index is determined by the refractive index and the amount of the adsorbed substance existing within the range of the evanescent light which is roughly in the order of the wavelength. From Eq. (4.1) the shift of the resonance wavelength, $\Delta\lambda$, when the n_{eff} is changed by Δn_{eff}, is given by

$$\Delta\lambda = \frac{\lambda_{\text{res}} \Delta n_{\text{eff}}}{n_{\text{eff}}} \tag{4.2}$$

There are two types of detection methods. One is observing the shift of the resonance spectrum before and after the adsorption of the biological substance. The other is observing the output change before and after the adsorption of the biological substance, where the input light wavelength is fixed near the resonance wavelength. The latter is used in practical sensors but the former is used in the research phase.

4.2.2 Fabrication Process

Fabrication process of the silicon ring resonator is shown in Figs. 4.3a,b and the scanning electron microscope (SEM) images of the fabricated ring resonator are shown in Fig. 4.3c.

The electron beam (EB) lithography and dry etching are used to obtain accuracy in the order of nanometer. The SiO_2 film is used for the silicon etching in order to obtain nearly vertical side walls of the waveguide, because the side wall steepness is much degraded when the resist is used as a mask.

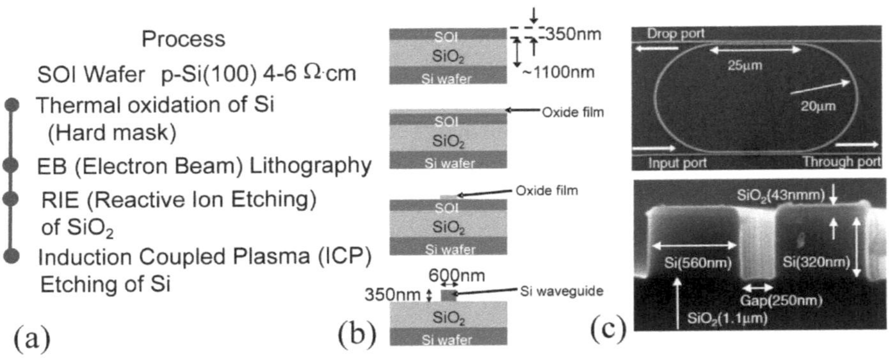

Figure 4.3 (a) Fabrication process of Si ring resonator sensor. (b) shows the scanning electron microscope (SEM) images (plan and cross section).

4.2.3 Measurement

Measurement system is shown in Fig. 4.4. The tunable semiconductor laser is used as the light source. The light is input to the cleaved edge of the input waveguide of the sensor by using a lensed fiber. The output light is captured by the lensed fiber and guided to the InGaAs photodetector. The temperature of the sample stage is stabilized within ±10^{-3} °C using Peltier device because the temperature coefficient of the refractive index of silicon (1.8×10^{-4}/ °C) is very large [17].

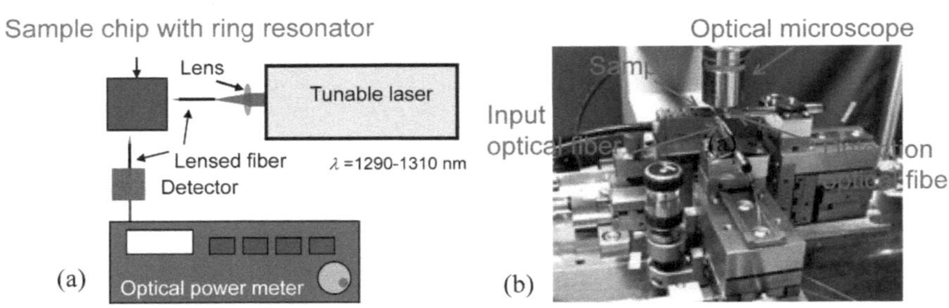

Figure 4.4 (a) Schematic measurement system and (b) its photograph.

The fluid channel required to flow the sample liquid has been made by poly(dimethylsiloxane) (PDMS) and it is shown in Fig. 4.5.

The details are described in Ref. [9].

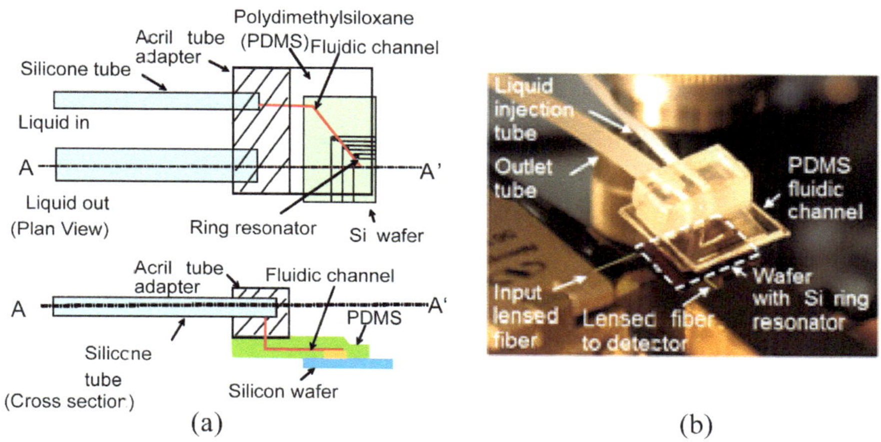

Figure 4.5 (a) Schematic of the fluid channel and (b) its photograph.

4.2.4 Si-Tag and Detection Process

In order to efficiently detect an antigen-antibody reaction, it is necessary to fix the antibodies on the sensor surface in the same direction as shown in Fig. 4.6a, whereas the receptor-directions are random without suitable immobilizer as shown in Fig. 4.6b. For this reason, the conventionally used covalent bonding method requires a complicated chemical modification treatment of the substrate surface. In this study, the target protein is fused with a silicon-binding protein (called Si-tag) by genetic engineering in advance [18]. Then the protein can be quickly adsorbed on the substrate surface only by bringing the solution containing the protein fused with Si-tag into contact with the substrate. By using the Si-tag the detection sensitivity is roughly five times enhanced as shown in Fig. 4.6c [18, 19].

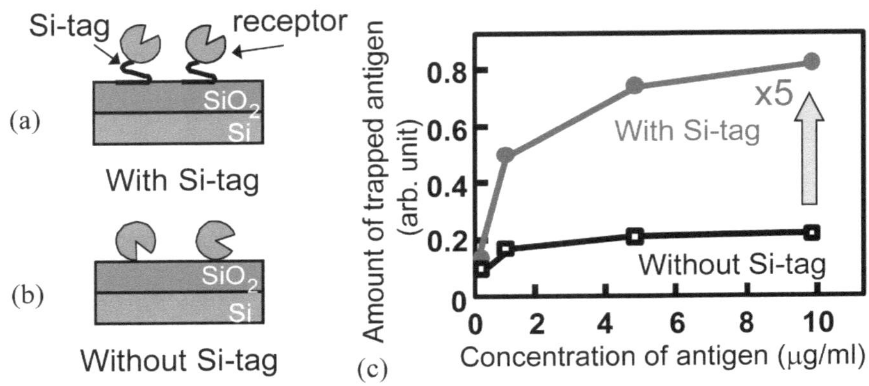

Figure 4.6 Effect of Si-tag. (a) With Si-tag the receptors align in the same direction, but (b) they are random without Si-tag. (c) With Si-tag the detection sensitivity is enhanced about five times [18, 19].

4.2.5 Measurement and Results

We have first evaluated the sensitivity of the fabricated device using sucrose solution and get a resonance wavelength shift rate of 36.5 nm/RIU and next biotin-streptavidin reaction has been detected [9]. And then we challenged the detection of antigen-antibody reaction.

(i) Confirmation of selective reaction of antibody with antigen

We have checked the selective reaction of antibody with antigen by using rabbit antiserum and normal serum [20]. The experimental sequence is shown in Fig. 4.7.

In the antiserum, there exists antibody called "Anti Der f 2 IgG," which is the antibody selectively reacts with the antigen called Der f 2 which is major house-dust mite allergen. On the other hand, there exists no Anti Der f 2 IgG in the normal serum. The fusion protein of Der f 2 with Si-tag was produced by the gene fusion technology [20] and initially adsorbed on the sensor surface. It should be noted that anti-IgG secondary antibody used in step (4) selectively reacts with anti-Der f 2 IgG. The measured resonant spectra after each treatment step for the antiserum and normal serum are shown in Figs. 4.8a,b, respectively.

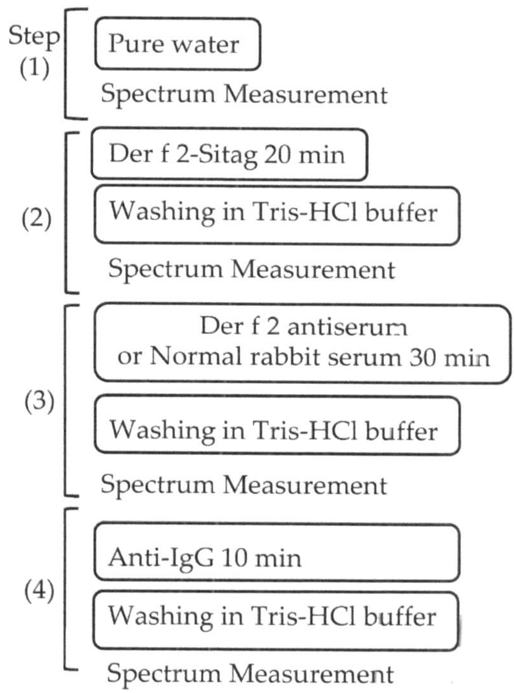

Figure 4.7 Experimental sequence for detection of antigen and antibody reaction. Tris-HCl is $C_4H_{11}NO_3ClH$ for pH adjustment [20].

The final spectrum after Anti IgG exposure is noticeably shifted in case of antiserum whereas the final shift is not observed in case of normal serum. This is reasonably explained by the fact that there exists no Anti Der f 2 IgG in the normal serum. For the normal serum in Fig. 4.8b, the resonance wavelength shift should not occur in the step (3) because there exists no Anti Der f 2 IgG. But a small shift of 0.07 nm is observed. This may be due to the physical adsorption of immunoglobulin (Ig) except by IgG, which is confirmed by no more shift after exposure to Anti IgG.

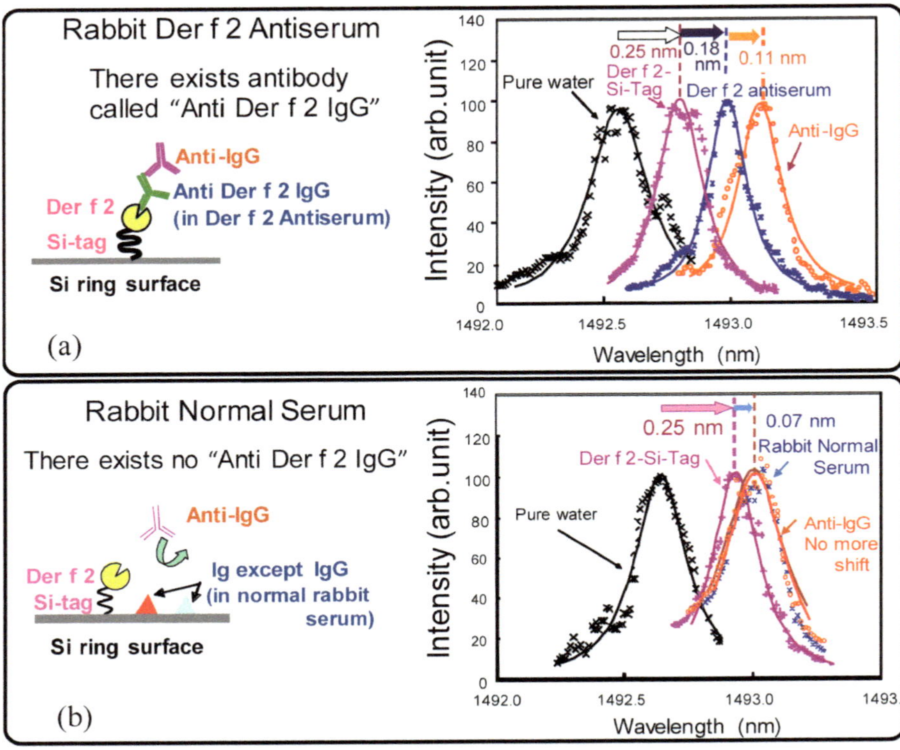

Figure 4.8 Selective detection of reaction of antigen-antibody. (a) The sample is rabbit antiserum. The antiserum is the serum containing antibody called "Anti Der f 2 IgG (Immunoglobulin G)" which selectively reacts with antigen called "Der f 2." (b) The sample is the rabbit normal serum which does not contain "Anti Der f 2 IgG."

(ii) Detection of PSA

Next we have tried to detect prostate specific antigen (PSA) which is a cancer marker of the prostate cancer quantitatively [21]. The detection process is shown in Fig. 4.9.

In this case, the fusion protein of Si-tag and protein A was used for the immobilization of the antibody. The protein A binds to many kinds of mammalian antibodies only by mixing the antibody solution [22].

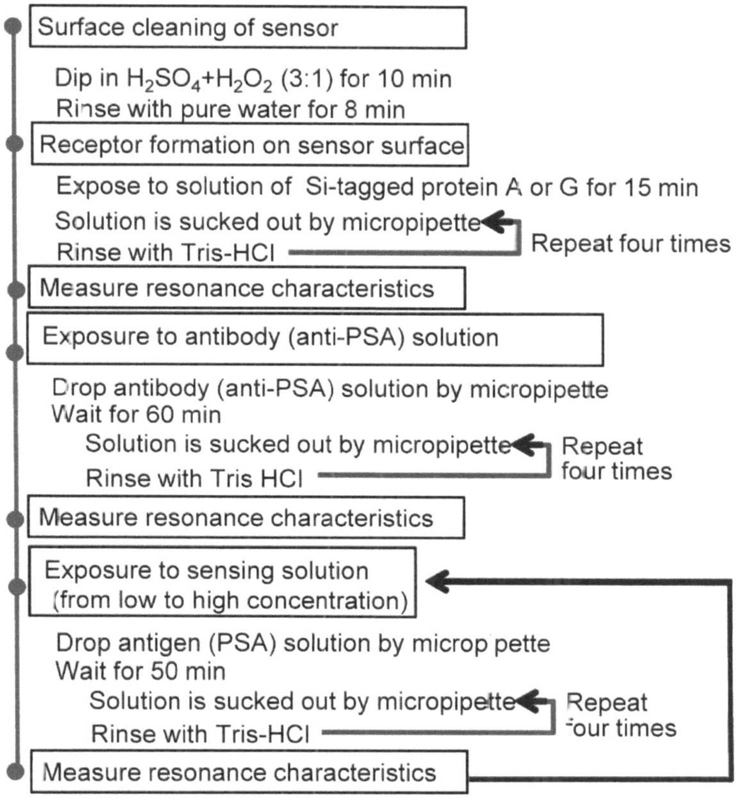

Figure 4.9 Detection process of antibody-antigen reaction.

Figure 4.10 shows the concentration of PSA versus measured resonance wavelength shift. The measured wavelength shift, $\Delta\lambda$, fits well to the Langmuir's equation,

$$\Delta\lambda = \Delta\lambda_{\max}\frac{CK}{1+CK}, \tag{4.3}$$

where $\Delta\lambda_{\max}$ is the maximum wavelength shift, C is the concentration of PSA and K is the constant. The minimum detectable concentration is roughly 10^{-6} g/ml, which is about three orders of magnitude larger than that for the practical use (cf. 4 ng/ml for PSA shown in Table 4.1).

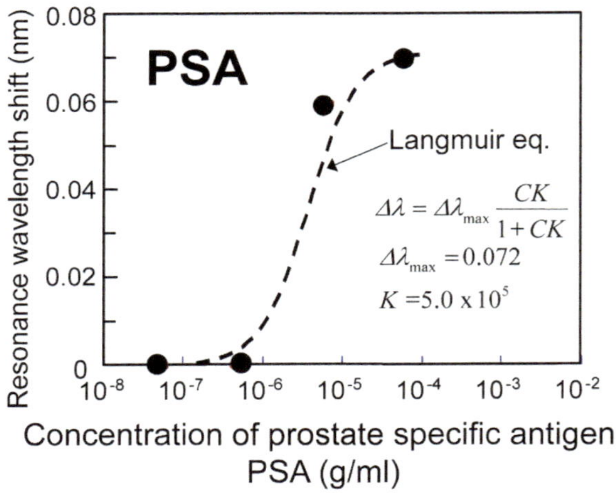

Figure 4.10 Concentration of PSA versus measured resonance wavelength shift.

4.3 Slot Ring Resonator Biosensor

4.3.1 Principle of Enhanced Sensitivity by Slot Ring

As pointed out in the former section, the sensitivity of our simple ring resonator is not good enough to the practical usage (ng/ml). In order to increase the sensitivity, we proposed the slot waveguide ring resonator [23].

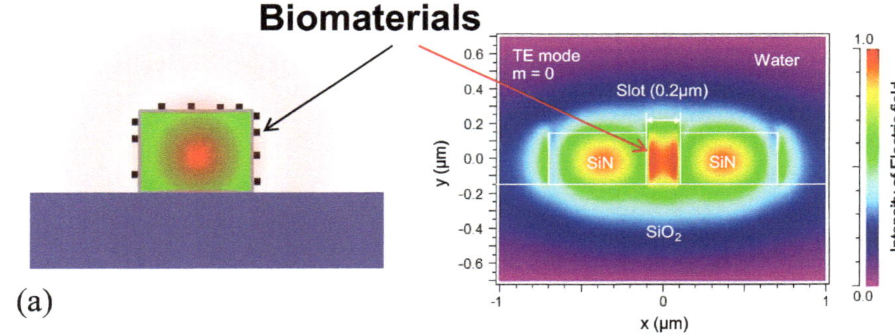

Figure 4.11 Light intensity (electric field component) distribution of (a) normal and (b) slot waveguide ring resonators. For the normal ring only a conceptual light intensity is shown whereas for the slot waveguide the numerically simulated one is shown [23].

Figure 4.11 shows the light intensity (electric field component) distribution of (a) normal and (b) slot waveguide ring resonators. For the normal ring resonator, the light intensity is very weak at the surface of the waveguide where the biomaterial is adsorbed. Therefore, the change in the refractive index is very small. On the other hand, the evanescent light is overlapped and enhanced in the slot where the biomaterial is adsorbed, resulting higher sensitivity in case of the slot waveguide.

4.3.2 Fabrication of Silicon Nitride Slot Ring

Figure 4.12 shows the fabrication process of the silicon nitride (SiN) slot ring resonator biosensor, which is similar to that shown in Fig. 4.3. Here, we employed "two step growth technique," where SiN deposition is divided to two steps after each lithography and etching process so that the mechanical stress in the SiN film is reduced and the crack generation is avoided. The reason for employing SiN is that the thermo-optic coefficient of SiN (2.45×10^{-5}/°C) [24] is much smaller than that of Si (1.8×10^{-4}/°C) [17]. And the thermal independent slot waveguide biosensor using SiN was reported [25].

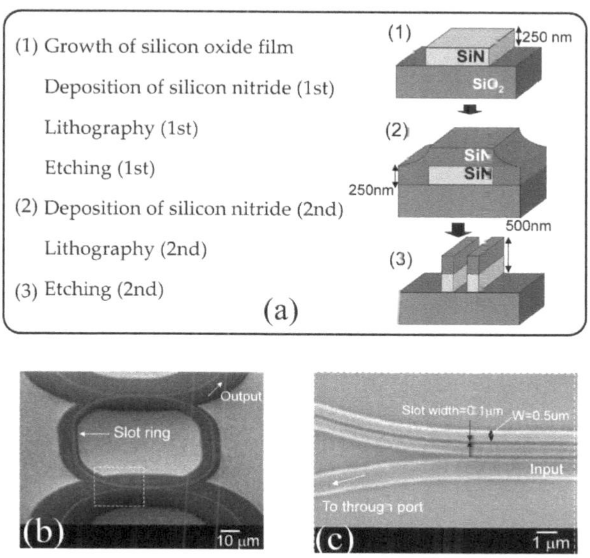

Figure 4.12 (a) Fabrication process of slot ring resonator using silicon nitride by two step growth, (b) bird's eye SEM view, and (c) expanded SEM image of the slot and coupling region [23].

4.3.3 Detection of PSA by Slot Ring Biosensor

The experimental procedure is same as that shown in Fig. 4.9 except by employing protein G instead of protein A. Protein G has stronger binding energy with many kinds of antibody than protein A [22, 26]. It was found that the binding energy between protein A and antibodies is relatively weak and antibodies are dissociated from protein A [21].

Figure 4.13 shows the resonance wavelength shift as a function of the concentration of PSA solution. The result fits to the summation of two Langmuir-equation components with different parameters, presumably due to two different adsorption mechanisms at the slot portion and at the other places in the waveguide. The sensitivity is drastically improved in the small concentration region less than 10^{-6} g/ml by using the slot-ring sensor. It seems that the minimum detection concentration is near 10^{-8} g/ml which is close to the practically required sensitivity of 10^{-9} g/ml. The sensitivity of previous biosensor was only 5 μg/ml [21]. By employing slot-ring, protein G, measurement wavelength of 1300 nm and temperature stabilizer, the sensitivity has been much improved.

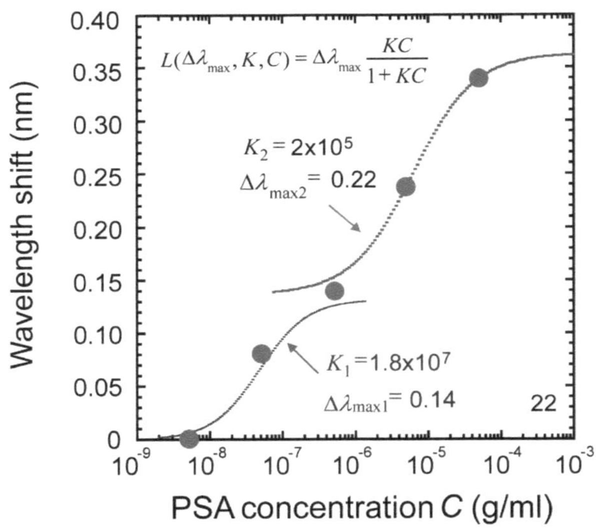

Figure 4.13 Resonance wavelength shift versus PSA concentration for SiN slot-ring biosensor [23].

4.3.4 Temperature Dependence of Resonance Wavelength

The temperature dependences of the resonance characteristics of the SiN slot ring and Si ring without slot are shown in Fig. 4.14.

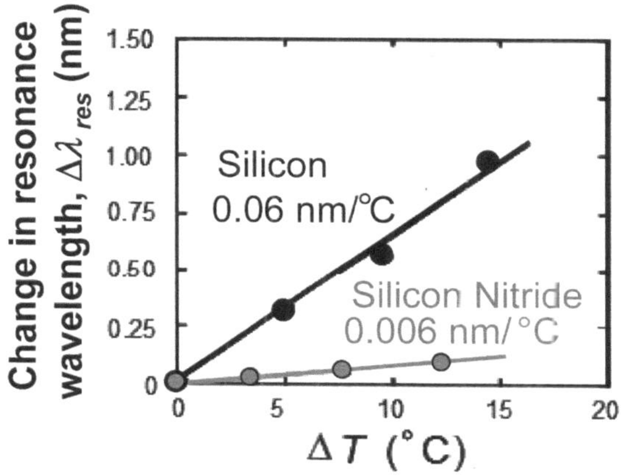

Figure 4.14 Temperature dependences of the silicon-nitride slot-ring resonator and Si ring resonator without slot [23].

The thermo-optic coefficient of the SiN slot ring resonator is 0.006 nm/°C, while that of the Si ring resonator is 0.06 nm/°C, which is one order of magnitude higher than that of SiN. The temperature stability required for Si ring resonator without slot for the detection of 1 ng/ml PSA is ± 0.005°C [27]. On the other hand, the temperature stability required for the SiN ring for the detection of the same concentration of PSA is ± 0.06°C, which may be realized without Peltier device during a period of a few minutes required for the measurement.

4.4 Differential Ring Resonator Biosensor

4.4.1 Operation Principle of Differential Resonator Biosensor

In order to further improve the performance, we have proposed differential ring resonator biosensor [28]. The problems are

(1) temperature sensitive and (2) low sensitivity characteristics of the simple ring resonator sensor.

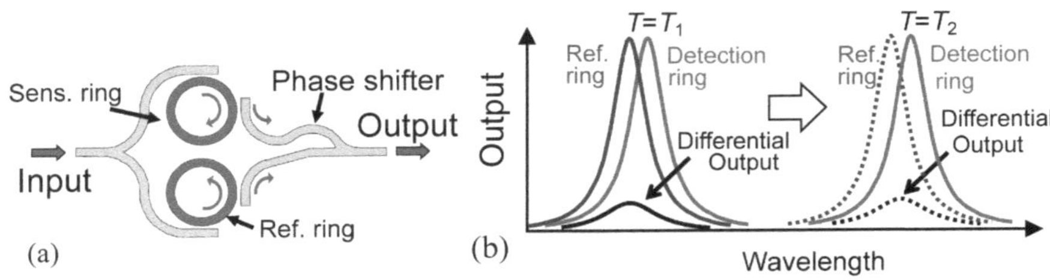

Figure 4.15 (a) Structure of differential ring resonator sensor. (b) Differential output is almost constant even when temperature is changed because both the reference and detection ring characteristics move in parallel.

The structure of the differential sensor is shown in Fig. 4.15a where the input light is incident into two resonators (rings), and one of the outputs is connected to the π phase shifter and then the two outputs are merged again. By using this structure, the differential output becomes insensitive to temperature change because both characteristics of the two resonators move in parallel (see Fig. 4.15b). The only concern is the temperature stability of the π shifter. The temperature change required for the differential output for PSA of 1 ng/ml due to the temperature change of the Si π shifter was calculated to be 6×10^5 °C, which means that the temperature dependence of the π shifter is negligible. The detection sensitivity will be also improved by the differential sensing because the common mode noise, which is induced in the both two resonators in the same phase, will be cancelled.

4.4.2 Fabrication of Differential Ring Resonator

Differential Si ring optical resonator sensors have been fabricated following the process shown in Fig. 4.3.

The SEM image of the fabricated sensor is shown in Fig. 4.16. The π phase shifter is realized by the displacement of the center axis of the output by δ from that of the input waveguide (see Fig. 4.16a). The fluid channel required for the separate flow of the sample and reference liquids to each ring was fabricated using PDMS and thick resist, SU-8, and is shown in Fig. 4.17.

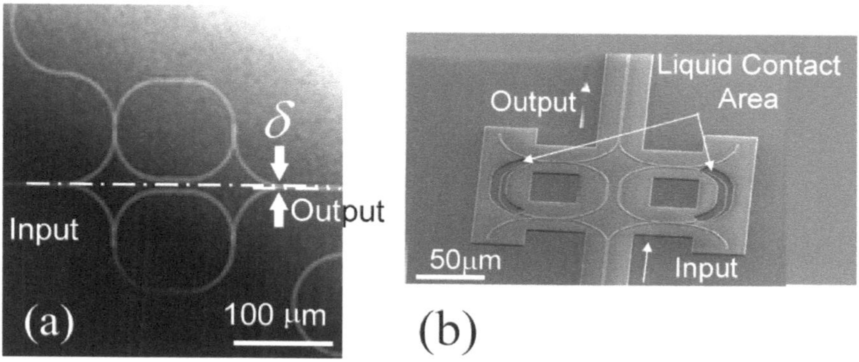

Figure 4.16 (a) SEM image of fabricated differential ring resonator and (b) SEM image after making of the windows for liquid contact in the cover SiN/SiO_2 layer.

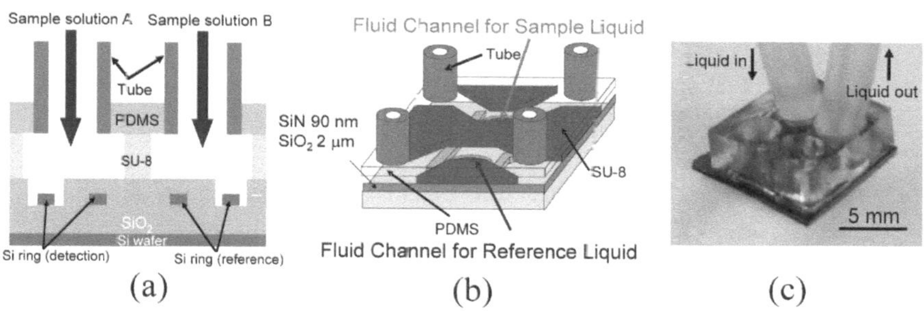

Figure 4.17 (a) Schematic cross section and (b) schematic bird's eye view and (c) photograph of the fabricated fluid channel.

4.4.3 Temperature Dependence of the Differential Output

Figure 4.18 shows the change in differential output when temperature is changed from 25 to 29 °C for the various kind of upper cladding layers [29]. The error bar indicated by "Reproducibility" shows the data scattering when the measurement was repeated four times at 25 °C in the case of air cladding. Even though the differential output intensity is scattered around the average due to the noise, there is no systematic correlation between the differential output and temperature. In addition, the range of the data scattering due to the temperature change is not so different from that of "Reproducibility." This result is consistent with the predicted insensitiveness to the temperature described in Section 4.4.2.

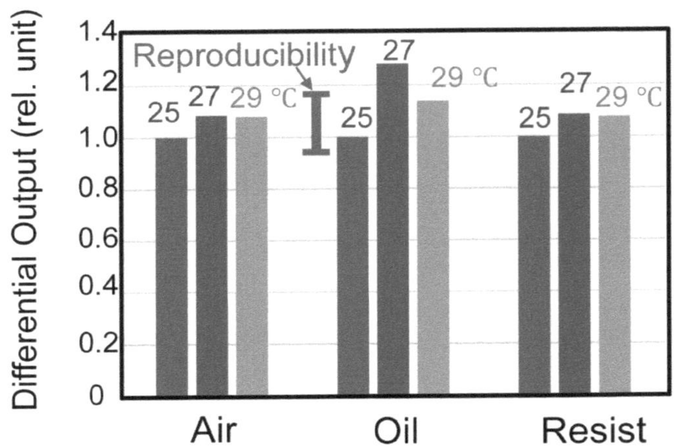

Figure 4.18 Change in differential output when temperature is changed from 25 to 29 °C for the various kind of upper cladding layers.

4.4.4 Detection of Sucrose and PSA by Differential Sensor

Figure 4.19a shows measured differential output spectra when the sensing ring is exposed to sucrose solution with various concentration, where the reference ring is exposed to pure water [28]. The integrated differential output is plotted as a function of the sucrose concentration in Fig. 4.19b, where 10^{-3}~10^{-2} % of sucrose can be detected and it well fits to the simulation. This detection sensitivity corresponds to a sensitivity of a few ng/ml for PSA, which is in the level of practical use. The differential output decreases with increasing the sucrose concentration, which is explained as follows. The resonance wavelength of the sensing ring is initially different from that of the reference ring and they approach by increasing the sucrose concentration.

Figure 4.20 shows the measured results for PSA [30]. The measurement procedure is similar to that in Section 4.3.2, but only the sensing ring is exposed to the sample liquid containing PSA and the reference ring is exposed to the liquid without PSA. The integrated output is changed at the PSA concentration of

~5 × 10^{-10} g/ml, which is in the level of practical use. Also, the simulation result well fits to the experiment. At this stage the error bar is relatively large because the light coupling efficiency at the input/output port (cleaved waveguide edge/lensed fiber is used) is small. This will be much improved by using the spot size converter [31].

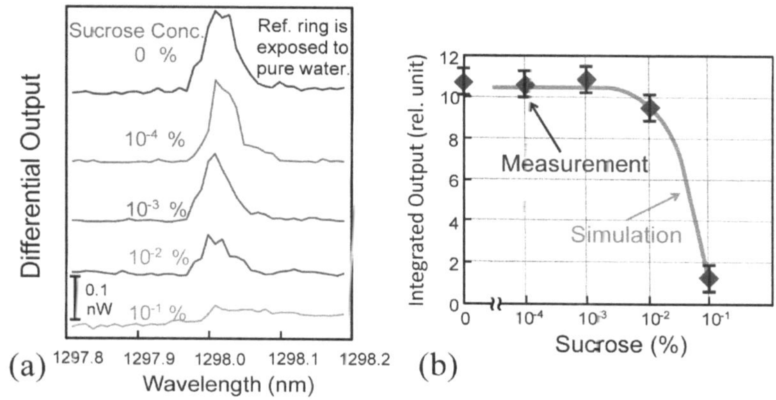

Figure 4.19 (a) Measured differential output when sucrose solution concentration is changed, where the reference ring is exposed to pure water. (b) Integrated differential output versus sucrose concentration with simulation curve.

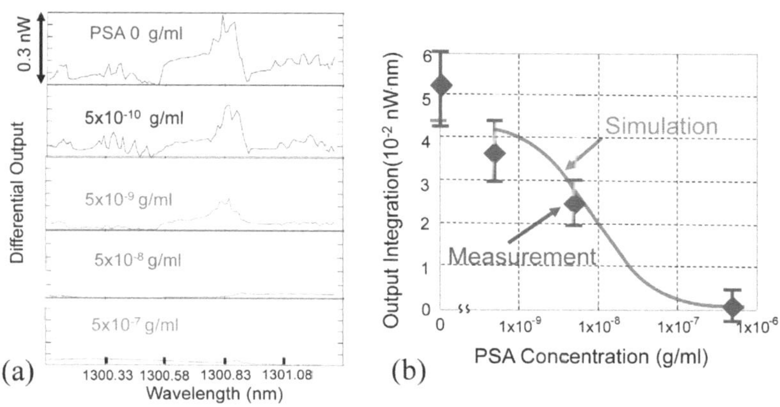

Figure 4.20 (a) Measured differential output when sucrose solution concentration is changed, where the reference ring is exposed to pure water. (b) Integrated differential output versus sucrose concentration with simulation curve.

We have proposed a method to obtain a constant sensitivity irrespective of the scattering of the resonance wavelength of the constituent pair of rings [28]. But we do not discuss about this issue due to the space limitation.

4.5 Photonic Crystal Resonator Biosensor

In order to increase the sensitivity of the biosensor using resonator, it is necessary to increase the quality factor, Q, of the resonator [28]. When we started the research of photonic crystal (PhC) resonator (2014), the highest Q value of ring resonators was 3.9×10^5 [32], while that of the PhC resonator was 9×10^6 [33]. By the way the highest Q value for the ring resonator reported to date (2019) have been realized in silicon nitride ($Q \approx 35 \times 10^6$) [34]. In contrast to ring resonator, the size of the PhC resonator is small, and the light intensity in the cavity hole is relatively higher than that of the slot waveguide described in Section 4.3. Therefore, we have studied PhC resonator as for biosensors.

There are two kinds of PhC resonators. One is cavity type [35], in which the cavity-hole diameter is larger than that of the peripheral holes, and another is defect type [36], in which the holes are missing in the resonance area. The cavity type seems to be suitable because more amount of biomaterial can be adsorbed in the resonance area than slot type resonator. Then we have mainly studied about cavity-type resonators. We have studied single cavity-hole [37] and double-cavity hole resonators [38]. It is expected that the greater the number of cavity holes, the greater the sensitivity, because the sensing area is increased. Here, the results on the double-cavity resonators are explained.

4.5.1 Fabrication and Performance of PhC Resonator

The structure of the fabricated double-cavity PhC resonator is shown in Fig. 4.21 with the simulated light intensity distribution [38]. The radius of the holes near the center cavity holes was varied because it strongly affects the quality factor of the resonator [39]. The fabrication process and measurement method are same as in the case of the differential ring resonator. The both of the center cavity holes (designed each diameter is 420 nm, and actually fabricated one is about 457 nm) are connected to the surrounding neighbor holes (design diameter is 65 nm, actual one is 68.5 nm). The simulated and experimental Q-factors as a function of neighbor hole radius are shown in Fig. 4.22.

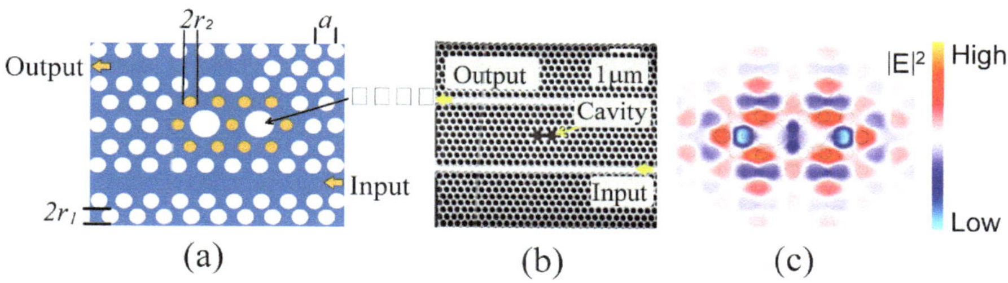

Figure 4.21 (a) Schematic structure of the photonic crystal double-cavity resonator, (c) SEM image of the fabricated one, and (c) simulated light intensity distribution [38]. In the simulation the diameter of the neighbor hole, $2r_2$, is 65 nm.

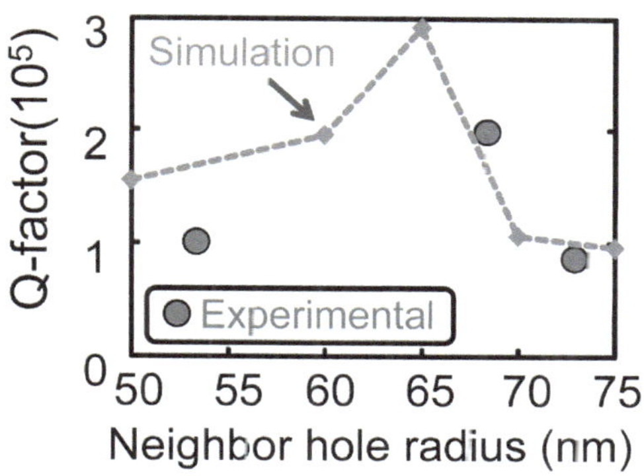

Figure 4.22 Simulated and experimental quality factor versus neighbor hole radius.

At neighbor hole radius of 65 nm, the simulated Q-factor goes highest. From Fig. 4.21c, it is recognized that the light intensity is localized around the neighbor holes. Therefore, it is expected that the neighbor-hole size strongly affects the performance of the resonator. The trend of experimental Q-factor is consistent with the simulated ones as shown in Fig. 4.22. The performance of the fabricated sensor was measured by using sucrose solution and the top-class sensitivity was obtained among of many studies concerning PhC resonator sensors [38].

4.5.2 Detection of PSA by PhC Resonator Sensor [40]

The experimental process is same as in Section 4.4.4. Figure 4.23a shows the resonance spectra for various concentration of PSA. Figure 4.23b shows the resonance-wavelength shift as a function of the PSA concentration and its Langmuir's fitting curve. We succeeded in detection of the PSA concentration as low as 0.01 ng/mL (312.5 pM). This detection sensitivity is as high as that (233 pM of anti-biotin) of the top class of PhC resonator biosensors [41].

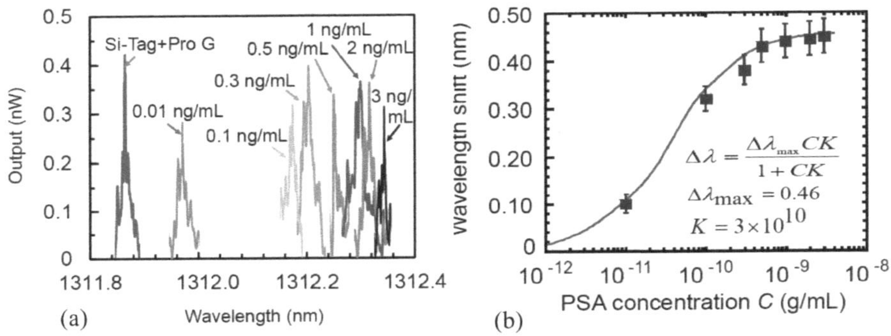

Figure 4.23 (a) Resonance spectra for various concentration of PSA and (b) resonance wavelength shift versus PSA concentration with Langmuir fitting curve [40].

4.6 Total Sensing System

In order to realize the total sensing chip as shown in Fig. 4.1, the following technology must be developed in addition to the resonator: (1) technology for integration of CMOS amplifiers, photodetectors, and waveguides (resonators) on the same chip, (2) sample-liquid supply system including micro valves, and (3) light-emitting diode (LED) mounting technology. These issues are discussed in this section.

4.6.1 Implementation of CMOS Operational Amplifiers, Photodetectors, and Waveguides on a Single Chip

We have developed a simple integration technology for optical waveguides and photodiodes using evanescent light [42]. The previous integration technology uses micromirror [43] or grating coupler [44].

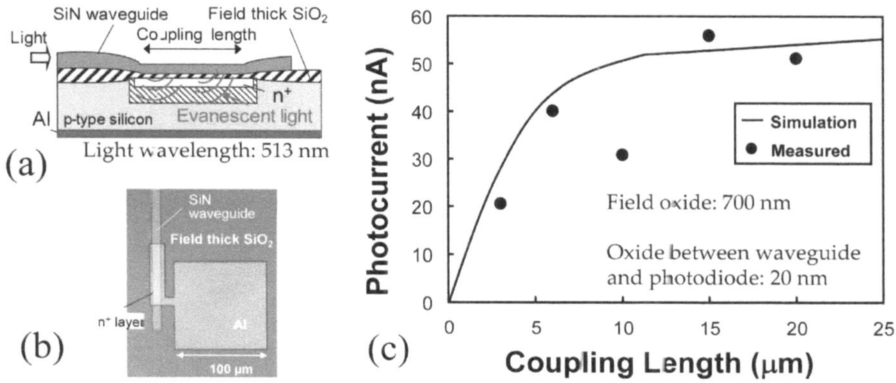

Figure 4.24 (a) Cross section of the waveguide with n^+/p photodiode using evanescent light coupling. (b) Optical micrograph of the fabricated waveguide/photodiode. (c) Photocurrent versus coupling length.

Figure 4.24 shows (a) cross section of the waveguide with n^+/p photodiode using evanescent light coupling, (b) optical micrograph (plan view) of the fabricated waveguide/photodiode, and (c) photocurrent versus coupling length behavior with fitted simulation curve [42]. The fabrication process is CMOS compatible and details are described in Ref. [42]. As the light propagates along the SiN waveguide, a part of the light is transferred to the photodiode through thin SiO_2 (20 nm) as the evanescent light and at certain distance from the edge of the photodiode, the light energy is almost completely transferred to the photodiode. This behavior is shown by the simulated solid curve in Fig. 4.24c. The experimental data almost fit to the simulation result except by the data at the coupling length L = 10 μm, which may be due to some defects (particle, damaged cleaved edge of the waveguide, etc.). Here, the width of the waveguide is 10 μm and the width of the photodiode is 17 μm. The photocurrent is measured under the reverse bias at 2 V.

Next, CMOS operational amplifiers (Op Amp) and photodiodes were fabricated on the same chip, and the photocurrent was amplified. The circuit diagram of the CMOS Op Amp is shown in Fig. 4.25 which is imported from Ref. [45].

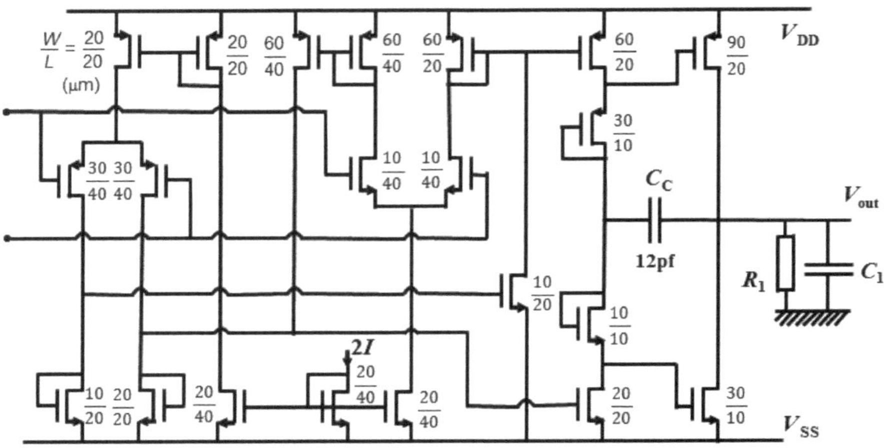

Figure 4.25 Circuit diagram of the fabricated CMOS operational amplifier, which is completely same as in Ref. [45].

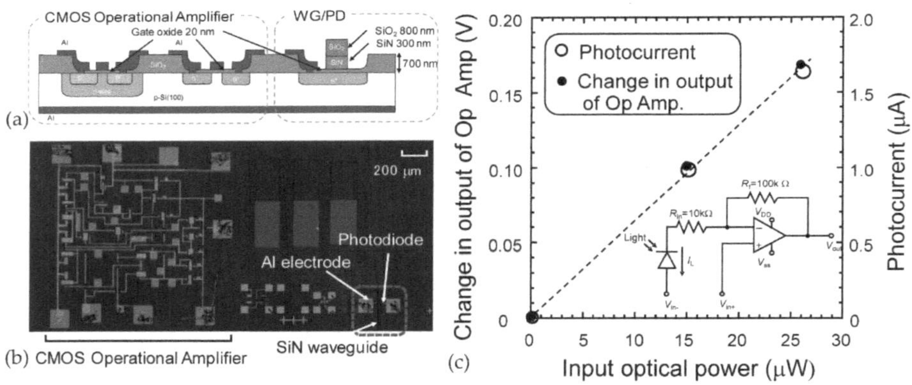

Figure 4.26 (a) Cross section of CMOS Op Amp, photodetector, and SiN waveguide on the same chip. (b) Optical micrograph of the fabricated chip.

The cross section and the photograph of the fabricated chip is shown in Fig. 4.26. The fabrication was done in the super clean room of our laboratory by using the simplified aluminum gate technology, and the detail is explained in Ref. [46]. As shown in the inset of Fig. 4.26c the photodiode is connected to the CMOS amplifier using external resistors, R_{in} and R_f, and the photocurrent was converted to the voltage output by the inverting amplifier circuit. Here, the output voltage change is given by the input photocurrent multiplied by the feedback resistance, R_f = 100 kΩ. Figure 4.26c shows the output voltage of the Op Amp versus input optical power into the cleaved edge of the SiN waveguide together with the measured photocurrent of the photodiode [47]. As shown in the figure the output voltage of the Op Amp is almost consistent with the predicted ones, i.e., when the light input power is 15 μW, the product of photocurrent, 1.01 μA, and R_f = 100 kΩ, is 0.101 V, which well fits to the observed one (0.1 V).

4.6.2 Fluid Channel with Microvalves

As mentioned in Sections 4.2–4.5, single-item detections were successfully demonstrated. Silicon photonics technology has advantages of low-cost fabrication and high integration of small size optical device because silicon photonics technology uses CMOS compatible technology. These advantages enable an optical chip for multiple-item detection as shown in Fig. 4.1. The basic concept of a multiple-item detection system including an array of ring-resonator biosensors and a fluid channel with micro-electro-mechanical system (MEMS) microvalves. Different biomaterials are set on each biosensor by solution flow control using these microvalves. The specified optical signal from a biosensor for the target biomaterial is selected using ring-resonator wavelength selection filters. In this section we discuss about the microvalves.

In general, high operation voltage (~100 V) [48, 49] is necessary for MEMS device and it is important to reduce the operation voltage.

For this purpose, the microvalves of Fig. 4.27 is tried to be fabricated using organic material. The photoresist named as SU-8 is often used for device pattering in MEMS technology. Microvalves composed of this photoresist is considered as shown in Fig. 4.27 where a solution flows vertically at the valve area. Open/close operation is carried out by electrostatic force induced in SU-8 photoresist layers between the electrodes of a parallel circular plate. When the electrostatic force is larger than the force generated by the deformation of the valve, the solution flow is stopped by this valve. Low-voltage operation is expected, because Young's modulus of a photoresist is generally smaller than that of a nonorganic material such as silicon.

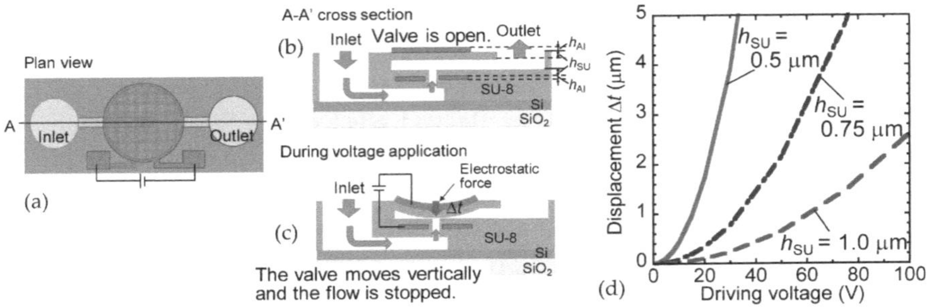

Figure 4.27 (a) Schematic image of proposed MEMS microvalve and (b), (c) driving mechanism of valve part. (d) Calculated voltage dependence of displacement of the valve Δt in Fig. (c).

Operation voltage is estimated by the voltage dependence of the maximum displacement Δt of the circular plate valve. For a clamped circular plate, the maximum displacement Δt is calculated from the force per unit area, p, and flexural rigidity, D. It is given by

$$\Delta t = (R^4 p)/(64D) \tag{4.4}$$

$$D = (E_c h_c)^3/12(1 - \nu_c^2), \tag{4.5}$$

where R, E_c, h_c, and ν_c are the radius of the circular plate, Young's modulus, thickness, and Poisson's ratio of a composite membrane, respectively. The composite membrane of the movable valve part consists of SU-8 and Al. The Young's modulus and Poisson's ratio of the composite layer are assumed to be weighted averages [50]. In this valve, the induced force p is electrostatic force and given by

$$p = 1/S \cdot \partial W/\partial d = \varepsilon V^2/2d^2, \tag{4.6}$$

where S, W, d, ε and V are the circular-plate area, the capacitive energy, the distance in electric field generated by the electrodes of the circular plate, the permittivity, and the driving voltage, respectively. In this microvalve, the permittivity ε is the permittivity of SU-8 and the distance d is two times h_{SU} because the fluid channel is filled with a solution that is generally conductive.

The maximum displacement Δt is shown in Fig. 4.27d as a parameter of the height of SU-8, h_{SU}, where the radius of the circular plate, R, and the height of the Al layer, h_{Al}, are fixed at 50 and 0.1 μm, respectively. The target distance between the electrodes of the circular-plate is <2 μm, which is the same order as the height of the fluid channel. A displacement of 3 μm is sufficient to close the valve. When h_{SU} is 0.5 μm, more than 3 μm is obtained at a driving voltage of 30 V. Generally, as the operation voltage is tried to be lower, the device size becomes larger. In proposed device, the operation voltage and device size are suppressed to be 30 V and 50 μm in radius, respectively.

4.6.3 Integration of Light-Emitting Devices

Gallium-nitride (GaN) thin film LED bonding technology was developed with the aim of integrating LEDs and different material devices. The results were reported elsewhere [51]. Until now, transfer technology for device layers has been developed by various organizations. Wafer bonding (WB) technology [52] and surface activated bonding (SAB) technology [53] have been put to practical use as direct bonding technologies. Bonding technology of gallium arsenide (GaAs) light-emitting devices on Si substrates using epitaxial lift-off [54] and advanced epitaxial film bonding (EFB) technology [55] is another promising device layer transfer technology. GaN is an important material for bio-medical applications as a light source [56]. GaN is used not only in blue LEDs but also is attracting attention as a material for next-generation power devices and high-frequency devices. Then we have applied the EFB technology to GaN devices.

An overview of the EFB process is shown in Fig. 4.28. After the GaN epitaxial layer formed on the base material (mother) substrate, (a) it is divided into multiple individual LED regions by etching. (b) The interface layer between LED and the mother substrate is selectively etched, and then the GaN-LED layer is peeled from the mother substrate. (c) The peeled GaN-LED layer is bonded onto a different material substrate (guest substrate) at room temperature and atmospheric pressure. No adhesives are used for the bonding. Bonding force is considered to be a complex force stronger than van der Waals force and weaker than covalent bond. The surface roughness of the peeled surface of the GaN-LED layer is thought to affect the bonding characteristics on the guest substrate. Therefore, the surface roughness of the peeled surface of the GaN-LED layer was measured by atomic force microscope (AFM). The resultant arithmetic average surface roughness (*R*a) was 0.7 nm. A surface roughness of *R*a <1 nm is sufficient to obtained good bonding [57].

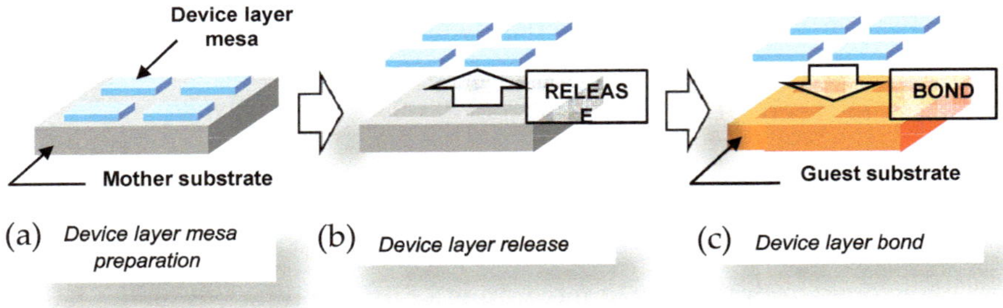

Figure 4.28 An overview of the epitaxial film bonding process (EFB).

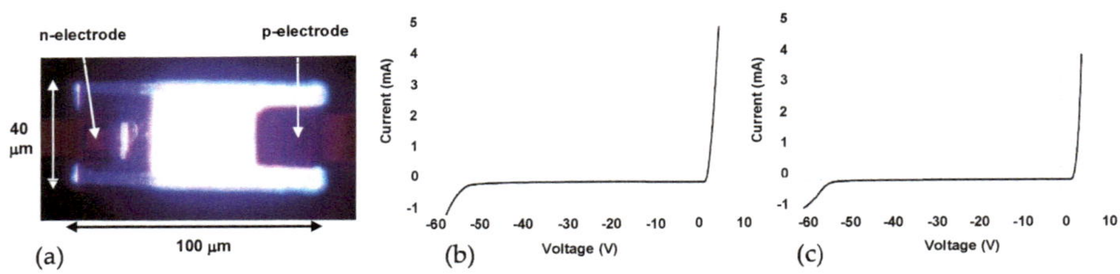

Figure 4.29 (a) Optical micrograph of a GaN thin-film LED bonded on a Si substrate when it is turned on. Typical current–voltage (*I–V*) characteristics of the GaN LED (b) before and (c) after bonding on the Si substrate.

Figure 4.29a shows an optical micrograph when the GaN thin film LED bonded on the Si substrate is turned on. It is confirmed that light is emitted almost uniformly in the light-emitting region. The peak wavelength was 430 nm. The typical current–voltage characteristics (*I–V* characteristics) of the GaN thin-film LED are shown in Fig. 4.29, in case of (b) before and (c) after bonding to Si sunstrate. The LED currents are 1 mA for both samples at the forward voltage of 4 V. It was verified that the

IV characteristics of the GaN thin film LED did not change significantly before and after bonding on the guest substrate by the EFB process.

It is also verified that the GaN thin film LEDs can be integrated on the different material substrate by the EFB process. We also succeeded in the bonding of GaN thin film LED on the grating coupler, which will introduce the light into the optical waveguide. We are verifying the light introduction from the grating coupler to the waveguide.

4.7 Summary

Our research results on optical biosensors using Si ring resonator, slot ring resonator, differential Si ring resonator, and photonic crystal resonator have been outlined. The technology for integrating optical resonators with CMOS amplifiers, photodetectors, mechanical valves and LEDs are also described. By integrating all these technologies, we would like to realize practical biosensors in near future.

Acknowledgments

The authors are deeply grateful to all co-authors of co-authored papers listed in the references. Part of the research was supported by a Grant-in-Aid for Scientific Research (B) (246360136, 2012) from the Ministry of Education, Culture, Sports, Science and Technology of Japan.

References

1. http://tumor-marker.com.
2. Pavesi, L., and Lockwood, D. J., eds. (2004). *Silicon Photonics*, Springer, ISBN 978-3-540-21022-1.
3. Wu, R., Jiang, Y., Wu, Q., Li, Q., Cheng, D. Xu, L., Zhang, C., Zhang, M., and Ye, L. (2016). Diagnostic value of microRNA-21 in the diagnosis of lung cancer: Evidence from a meta-analysis involving 11 studies, *Tumour Biol.*, **35**, pp. 8829–8836.

4. van Niel, G., D'Angelo G., and Raposo, G. (2018). Shedding light on the cell biology of extracellular vesicles, *Nat. Rev. Mol. Cell Biol.*, **19**, pp. 213–228.

5. Zheng, G., Patolsky, F., Cui, Y., Wang, W. U., Lieber, C. M. (2005). Multiplexed electrical detection of cancer markers with nanowire sensor arrays, *Nat. Biotechnol.*, **23**, pp. 1294–1301.

6. Maddalena, F., Kuiper, M. J., Poolman, B., Brouwer, F., Hummelen, J. C., de Leeuw, Dago, M., de Boer, B., Blom, and P. W. M. (2010). Organic field-effect transistor-based biosensors functionalized with protein receptors, *J. Appl. Phys.*, **108**, pp. 124501-1-4.

7. Ramachandran, A., Wang, S., Clarke, J., Ja, S. J., Goad, D., Wald, L., Flood, E. M., Knobbe E., Hryniewicz, J. V., Chu, S. T., Gill, D., Chen, W., King, O., and Little, B. E. (2008). A universal biosensing platform based on optical micro-ring resonators, *Biosens. Bioelectronics*, **23**, pp. 939–944.

8. Dostalek, J., Ladd, J., Jiang, S., and Homola, J. (2006). In: *Surface Plasmon Resonance Based Sensors*, ed., Homola, J., Springer, Berlin. p. 177.

9. Yamatogi, S., Amemiya, Y., Ikeda, T., Kuroda, A., and Yokoyama, S. (2009). Si ring optical resonators for integrated on-chip biosensing, *Jpn. J. Appl. Phys.*, **48**, pp. 04C188-1-6.

10. Zhu, H., White, I., Suter, J., Dale, P., and Fan, X. (2007). Analysis of biomolecule detection with optofluidic ring resonator sensors, *Opt. Express*, **15**, pp. 9139–9146.

11. Vollmer, F., and Arnold, S. (2008). Whispering-gallery-mode biosensing: Label-free detection down to single molecules, *Nat. Methods*, **5**, pp. 591–596.

12. Sana, A. K., Amemiya, Y., and Yokoyama, S. (2017). High-sensitivity double-cavity silicon photonic-crystal resonator for label-free biosensing, *Jpn. J. App. Phys.*, **56**, pp. 04CM06-1-5.

13. Florescu, O., Wang, K., Au, P., Tang, J., Harris, E., Beatty, P. R., and Boser, B. E. (2010). On-chip magnetic separation of superparamagnetic beads for integrated molecular analysis, *J. Appl. Phys.*, **107**, pp. 054702–054702.

14. Ogi, H., Motoshisa, K., Matsumoto, T., Hatanaka, K., and Hirao, M. (2006). Isolated electrodeless high-frequency quartz crystal microbalance for immunosensors, *Anal. Chem.*, **78**, pp. 6903–6909.

15. Gimzewski, J. K., Gerber, Ch., Meyer, E., and Schlittler, R. R. (1994). Observation of a chemical-reaction using a micromechanical sensor, *Chem. Phys. Lett.*, **217**(6) pp. 589–594.

16. Amemiya, Y., Sana, A. K., Nakashima, Y., Maeda, J., and Yokoyama, S. (2017). Silicon photonic biosensors with MEMS flow control, *Extend. Abst. Int. Conf. Solid State Devices Mater.*, pp. 366–367.

17. McCaulley, J. A., Donnelly, V. M., Vernon, M., and Taha, I. (1994). Temperature dependence of the near-infrared refractive index of silicon, gallium arsenide, and indium phosphide, *Phys. Rev. B*, **49**, pp. 7408–7417.

18. Taniguchi, K., Nomura, K., Hata, Y., Nishimura, T., Asami, Y., and Kuroda, A. (2007). The Si-tag for immobilizing proteins on a silica surface, *Biotechnol. Bioeng.*, **96**, pp. 1023–1029.

19. Ikeda, T., Hata, Y., Ninomiya, K., Ikura, Y., Takeguchi, K., Aoyagi, S., Hirota, R., Kuroda, A. (2009). Oriented immobilization of antibodies on a silicon wafer using Si-tagged protein A, *Anal. Biochem.*, **385**, pp. 132–137.

20. Fukuyama, M., Yamatogi, S., Ding, H., Nishida, M., Kawamoto, C., Amemiya, Y., Ikeda, T., Noda, T., Kawamoto, S., Ono, K., Kuroda, A., and Yokoyama, S. (2010). Selective detection of antigen-antibody reaction using Si ring optical resonators, *Jpn. J. Appl. Phys.*, **49**, pp. 04DL09-1-4.

21. Fukuyama, M., Nishida, M., Abe, Y., Nishida, M., Amemiya, Y., Ikeda, Kuroda, A., and Yokoyama, S. (2011). Detection of antigen-antibody reaction using Si ring optical resonators functionalized with an immobilized antibody-binding protein, *Jpn. J. Appl. Phys.*, **50**, pp. 04DL07-1-3.

22. Richman, D. D., Cleveland, P. H., Oxman, M. N., and Johnson, K. M. (1982). The binding of staphylococcal protein A by the sera of different animal species, *J. Immunol.*, **128**, pp. 2300–2305.

23. Taniguchi, T., Hirowatari, A., Ikeda, T., Fukuyama, M., Amemiya, Y., Kuroda, A., and Yokoyama, S. (2016). Detection of antibody-antigen reaction by silicon nitride slot-ring biosensors using protein G, *Opt. Commun.*, **365**, pp. 16–23.

24. Arbabi, A., and Goddard, L. L. (2013). Measurements of the refractive indices and thermo-optic coefficients of Si_3N_4 and SiO_x using microring resonances, *Opt. Lett.*, **38**(19), pp. 3878–3881.

25. Tu, X., Song, J., Liow, T.-Y., Park, M. K., Yiying, J. Q., Kee, J. S., Yu, M., and Lo, G.-Q. (2012). Thermal independent silicon-nitride slot waveguide biosensor with high sensitivity, *Opt. Express*, **20**, pp. 2640–2648.

26. Sjöbring, U., Bjorck, L., and Kastern, W. (1991). Streptococcal protein G. Gene structure and protein binding properties., *J. Biol. Chem.*, **266**, pp. 399–405.

27. Fukuyama, Amemiya, Y., Abe, Y., Onishi, Y., Hirowatari, A., Terao, K., Ikeda, T., Kuroda, A., and Yokoyama, S. (2011). Sensitivity improvement of biosensors using Si ring optical resonators, *Jpn. J. App. Phys.*, **50**(4), pp. 04DL11-1-5.

28. Taniguchi, T., Yokoyama, S., Amemiya, Y., Ikeda, Kuroda, A., and Yokoyama, S. (2016). Differential Si ring resonators for label free biosensing, *Jpn. J. Appl. Phys.*, **55**(4), pp. 04EM04-1-7.

29. Yokoyama, S. (2016). Study on temperature dependence of differential Si ring resonator [Japanese], *Master Thesis, Department of Semiconductor Electronics and Integration Science, Graduate School of Advanced Sciences of Matter, Hiroshima University.*

30. Taniguchi, T., Yokoyama, S., Amemiya, Y., Ikeda, T., Kuroda, A., and Yokoyama, S. (2015). Differential Si ring-resonator biosensors robust to process variations, *Extend. Abst. Int. Conf. Solid State Devices Materials*, pp. 840–841.

31. Shoji, T., Tsuchizawa, T., Watanabe, T., Yamada, K., and Morita, H. (2002). Low loss mode size converter from 0.3 μm square Si wire waveguides to singlemode fibres, *Electronics Lett.*, **38**, pp. 1669–1670.

32. Xu, Q., Schmidt, B., Pradhan, S., and Lipson, M. (2005). Micrometre-scale silicon electro-optic modulator, *Nature*, **435**, pp. 325–327.

33. Sekoguchi, H., Takahashi, Y., Asano, T., and Noda, S. (2014). Photonic crystal nanocavity with a Q-factor of ~9 million, *Opt. Express*, **22**, pp. 916–924.

34. Spencer, D. T., Tang, Y., Bauters, J. F., Heck, M. J. R., and Bowers, J. E. (2012). Integrated Si_3N_4/SiO_2 ultra high Q ring resonators, *IEEE Photonics Conference 2012*, DOI:10.1109/IPCON.2012.6358529 Corpus ID: 30720651, pp. 141–142.

35. Martiradona, L., Pisanello, F., Stomeo, T., Qualtieri, A., Vecchio, G., Sabella, S., Cigolani, R., Vittorio, M. D., and Pompa, P. P. (2010). Spectral tagging by integrated photonic crystal resonators for highly sensitive and parallel detection in biochips, *Appl. Phys. Lett.*, **96**, pp. 113702–113704.

36. Skivesen, N., Têtu, A., Kristensen, M., Kjems, J., Frandsen, L. H., and Borel, P. I. (2007). Photonic-crystal waveguide biosensor, *Opt. Express*, **15**, pp. 3169–3176.

37. Sana, A. K., Honzawa, K., Amemiya, Y., and Yokoyama, S. (2016). Silicon photonic crystal resonators for label free biosensor, *Jpn. J. Appl. Phys.*, **55**(4), pp. 04EM11-1-5.

38. Sana, A. K., Amemiya, Y., and Yokoyama, S. (2017). High-sensitivity double-cavity silicon photonic-crystal resonator for label-free biosensing, *Jpn. J. App. Phys.*, **56**(4), pp. 04CM06-1-5.

39. Kwon, S.-H., Sünner, T., Kamp, M., and Forchel, A. (2008). Ultrahigh-Q photonic crystal cavity created by modulating air hole radius of a waveguide, *Opt. Express*, **16**, pp. 4605–4614.

40. Sana, A. K., Amemiya, Y., Ikeda, T., Kuroda, A., and Yokoyama, S. (2017). Label free detection of prostate specific antigen using photonic crystal nanocavity resonator, *Extend. Abst. Int. Conf. Solid State Devices Mater.*, pp. 287–288.

41. Zlatanovic, S., Mirkarimi, L. W., Sigalas, M. M., Bynum, M. A., Chow, E., Robotti, K. M., Burr, G. W., Esener, S., and Annette Grot, A. (2009). Photonic crystal microcavity sensor for ultracompact monitoring of reaction kinetics and protein concentration, *Sens. Act. B: Chem.*, **141**(1), pp. 13–19.

42. Uruma, T., Tabei, T., Amemiya, Y., Sato, T., Yamada, S., Okada, K., and Yokoyama, S. (2018). New integration technology of optical waveguides and photodiodes with CMOS operational amplifiers, *Extend. Abst. Int. Conf. Solid State Devices Mater.*, pp. 603–604.

43. Nagata, T., Namba, T., Miyake, K., Doi, T., Miyamoto, T., Kuroda, Y., Yokoyama, S., Miyazaki, S., Koyanagi, M., and Hirose, M. (1995). Single-chip integration of light-emitting diode, waveguide and micromirrors, *Jpn. J. Appl. Phys.*, **34**, pp. 1282–1285.

44. Csutak, S. M., D-Murthy, S., and Campbell, J. C. (2002). CMOS-compatible planar silicon waveguide-grating-coupler photodetectors fabricated on silicon-on-insulator (SOI) substrates, *IEEE J. Quantum Electronics*, **38**, pp. 477–480.

45. Steyaert, M., and Sansen, W. (1987). A high-dynamic-range CMOS op amp with low-distortion output structure, *IEEE J. Solid-state Circuits*, **SC-22**(6), pp. 1204–1207.

46. Tabei, T., Sato, T., Meguro, T., Okada, K., Yamada, S., Amemiya, Y., Yokoyama, S., Nakamura, A., Murakami, H., Nishimura, S., Miyao, K., Makihira, S., Shimizu, R., Mihara, R., and Furuse, M. (2018). Simplified and disposable CMOS chip fabrication for biomedical application, *Extend. Abst. Int. Conf. Solid State Devices Mater.*, pp. 555–556.

47. Uruma, T. (2019). Development of integration technology of optical devices with silicon electronic circuits [Japanese], *Master Thesis, Department of Semiconductor Electronics and Integration Science, Graduate School of Advanced Sciences of Matter, Hiroshima University.*

48. Laser, D. J., and Santiago, J. G. (2004). A review of micropumps, *J. Micromechanics Microeng.*, **14**(6), R35.
49. Oh, K. W., and Ahn, C. H. (2006). A review of microvalves, *J. Micromechanics Microengineering*, **16**(5), R13.
50. Tabata, O., Kawahata, K., Sugiyama, S., and Igarashi, I. (1989). Mechanical property measurements of thin films using load-deflection of composite rectangular membranes, *Sens. Actuators*, **20**(1–2), pp. 135–141.
51. Ogihara, M., Yokoyama, S., and Amemiya, Y. (2018). Heterogeneous integration of nitride semiconductor device layer by epitaxial film bonding, *Technical Digest of Int. Workshop on Nitride Semiconductors (IWN 2018), Nov. 11–16, 2018, Kanazawa, Japan, TuP-OD-27*, pp. 258–2018.
52. Abe, T., Takei, T., Uchiyama, A., Yoshizawa, K., and Nakazato, Y. (1990). Silicon wafer bonding mechanism for silicon-on-insulator structure, *Jpn. J. Appl. Phys.*, **29**, pp. 2311–2314.
53. Takagi, H., Kurashima, Y., Takamizawa, A., Ikegami, T., and Yamaguchi, S. (2017). Surface activated room-temperature bonding in Ar gas ambient for MEMS encapsulation, *Jpn. J. Appl. Phys.*, **57**, pp. 02BA04-1-4.
54. Konagai, M., Sugimoto, M., and Takahashi, K. (1978). High efficiency GaAs thin film solar cells by peeled film technology, *J. Cryst. Growth*, **45**, pp. 277–280.
55. Ogihara, M., Fujiwara, H., Mutoh, M., Suzuki, T., Igari, T., Sagimori, T., Kurokawa, H., Kaneto, T., Furuta, H., Abiko, I., and Sakuta, M. (2006). LED array integrated with Si driving circuits for LED printer printhead, *Electron. Lett.*, **42**(15), pp. 881–883.
56. Takehara, H., Ohta, Y., Motoyama, M., Haruta, M., Nagasaki, M., Takehara, H., Noda, Y., Sasagawa, K., Tokuda, T., and Ohta, J. (2015). Intravital fluorescence imaging of mouse brain using implantable semiconductor devices and epi-illumination of biological tissue, *Biomed. Opt. Express*, **6**(5), pp. 1553–1564.
57. Takagi, H., Maeda, R., Chung, T. R., Hosoda, N., and Suga, T. (1998). Effect of the surface roughness on room-temperature wafer bonding, *Jpn. J. Appl. Phys.*, **37**, pp. 4197–4203.

Chapter 5

Reusable Surface Acoustic Wave Immunosensor for Enhanced Monitoring of Airborne House Dust Mite Allergens

Koji Toma, Takahiro Arakawa, and Kohji Mitsubayashi

Institute of Biomaterials and Bioengineering, Tokyo Medical and Dental University, 2-3-10 Kanda-Surugadai, Chiyoda-ku, Tokyo 101-0062, Japan

m.bdi@tmd.ac.jp

Avoiding the exposure to airborne allergens is effective in reducing the risk of experiencing allergies. This chapter describes a surface acoustic wave (SAW) immunosensor for on-site monitoring of airborne house dust mite allergens. After a short introduction to why monitoring of airborne allergens is important, recent development of mite allergen biosensors and the SAW immunosensor is introduced. At the end of the chapter, an enzymatic precipitation method enhancing the sensitivity of the SAW immunosensor is also described. It utilizes a large mass change by precipitates that are products of horse radish peroxidase (HRP)-catalyzed redox reaction. The dust mites are

Biomedical Engineering
Edited by Akihiro Miyauchi and Yuji Miyahara

ISBN 978-981-4877-63-3 (Hardcover), 978-1-003-14194-5 (eBook)
www.jennystanford.com

indirectly measured by change in mass in vicinity to the sensor surface via these precipitates.

5.1 Introduction

Allergy is a disorder of the immune system which induces rhinitis, asthma or itching [1–5]. World prevalence of allergies reaches 40% for children with rhinitis and 300 million with asthma [3, 6]. Environmental allergies are caused by surroundings such as pollens and house dust mites (HDMs). Unlikely to pollens, HDMs are difficult to avoid because they are found indoor where people usually stay without wearing a protection. Besides, they become airborne easily even by human activity such as walking or vacuum cleaning, which increases risks of inhaling them [7, 8]. Once the allergens enter the body, they remain inside the body for a long time, and the possibility of onset of allergies increases. To avoid the exposure to airborne HDMs and reduce the chance of sensitization, we have proposed a monitoring system for airborne HDMs [9]. It informs temporal change of the airborne and gives a resident warning of exposure (Fig. 5.1). The system is comprised of two parts: an airborne allergen sampler and an allergen detection part. Airborne allergens are firstly collected by the sampler in the gas phase and then transported to the detection part in the liquid phase. Through this transportation, considerable loss of allergen samples occurs at the gas-liquid interface between the sampler and the detection part. In order to compensate the loss, a sensor used in the detection part needs to be highly sensitive. Besides, it is also necessary for the sensor to be able to measure the allergens repeatedly so that people don't exchange the sensor frequently.

Immunosensor is a type of biosensor that utilizes antibodies as a recognition element to selectively capture antigens. Owing to high selectivity and sensitivity, immunosensors, such as enzyme-linked immunosorbent assays (ELISA) or lateral flow immunoassays, are widely used not only in laboratories but also in practice, including measurement of HDM allergens [10–12]. However, there is a challenge to apply immunosensors to the monitoring system because of a lack of reusability. Repeated measurement includes a regeneration process at the end of each measurement that dissociates antibody-antigen immunocomplex and removes antigens from the sensor surface to restart a measurement. Regeneration usually uses harsh chemicals with high or low pH. It potentially damages proteins and molecules building the sensor and leads to loosing functions. Therefore, almost all of the immunoassays or sensors are designed to be single-use.

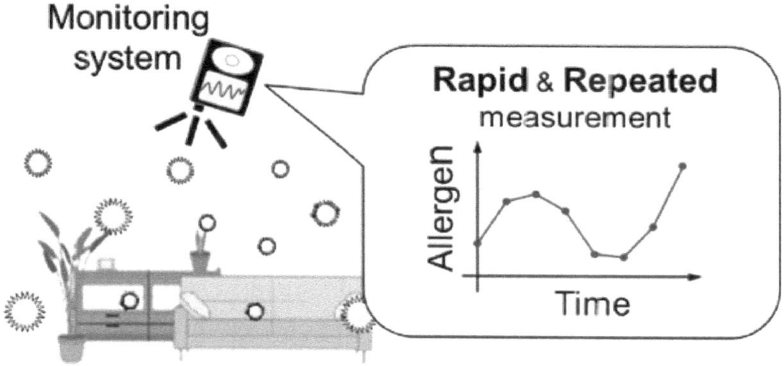

Figure 5.1 Airborne allergen monitoring system.

We have reported a reusable immunosensor for HDMs that was developed with a surface acoustic wave (SAW) device and a pH-tolerant protein scaffold for sensor surface modification. However, the sensitivity improvement was needed to compensate the huge loss of allergen samples in the monitoring system at the gas-liquid interface when they are transported from the sampler to the detection part. This chapter introduces the SAW immunosensor and "enzymatic precipitation method" to enhance the sensor's sensitivity.

5.2 Emerging Mite Allergen Biosensors

This section overviews recent studies of mite allergen biosensors. Tsai et al. reported a nanostructured biosensor for *Dermatophagoides pteronyssinus* group 2 (*Der p* 2). An electrode was made of Au nanoparticles with two different diameters of 80 nm and 10 nm [13]. The smaller Au nanoparticles were electrochemically deposited onto the larger particles to cover the surface and to increase a surface area. This electrode was used in electrochemical impedance spectroscopy (EIS) to measure *Der p* 2 and showed high sensitivity with the limit of detection of 1 pg/mL even without a detection antibody (dAb). Another effort aiming to develop an inexpensive and easy-to-use biosensor for various environmental allergens was introduced by Sarkar et al. [14], who fabricated the biosensor using screen-printing, which has a good compatibility to mass production. Rhodium-carbon mix working, silver/silver chloride reference, and carbon counter electrodes were printed on a 250 μm-thick polyester sheet. The total concentration of seven different allergens, including cockroach, cat and perennial ryegrass, is measurement by the bi-enzyme method, which utilized two kinds of enzymes, protease and amino acid oxidase. Allergens encountering protease on the electrode are hydrolysed into amino acid; then, the produced amino acid is oxidized through amino acid oxidase-catalyzed reaction. Finally, produced hydrogen peroxide is detected by amperometry to determine the total allergen concentration. Egea et al. developed a method to produce antibody used for detection of *Dermatophagoides farinae* group I (*Der f* 1) allergens [15]. They extracted IgY in chicken egg yolk laid by an immunized hen instead of IgG so that no blood sampling from an immunized animal is needed. Morris et al. used a quartz crystal microbalance to develop an immunosensor for real-time measurement of cat allergen [16].

5.3 Reusable Surface Acoustic Wave Immunosensor for Mite Allergen Monitoring

As introduced above, even recent mite allergen biosensors are mostly focused on the sensitivity or cost of sensor fabrication, and reusability of the sensor is not intensively studied. We reported a SAW immunosensor particularly focused on the reusability for monitoring purpose [17]. The SAW immunosensor was composed of a SAW device (Japan Radio) and pH-tolerant protein scaffold

(Fig. 5.2). A gold thin film with the thickness of 90 nm was deposited on a 36Y-90X quartz substrate to make an input/output electrode and a reflector. A shear-horizontal SAW, excited by applying 250 MHz AC voltage on the input electrode, propagates back and forth between the two electrodes. The SAW propagation area between the electrodes was used as a sensing region and also coated with 90 nm-thick gold film in order to make surface modification easy. Fabrication of the SAW immunosensor begins with surface modification with a self-assembled monolayer (SAM) of two mixed molecules. One is polyethylene glycol thiol that shows high anti-fouling property; the other is a membrane protein fused with protein G, ORLA85, that allows for highly ordered orientation of capture antibodies (cAbs) and robust scaffold for antibody immobilization in a broad range of pH. Afterwards, capture antibody was bound to protein G, followed by being immobilized via cross-linking using PEGylated bis(sulfosuccinimidyl)suberate.

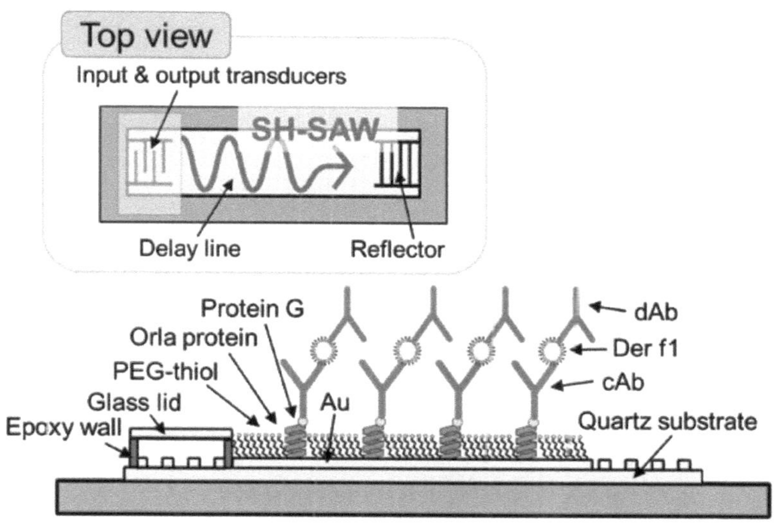

Figure 5.2 A schematic illustration of the surface acoustic wave immunosensor. Reprinted with permission from [17]. Copyright (2015) American Chemical Society.

The selectivity of the SAW immunosensor is presented in Fig. 5.3a. Various common environmental allergens including mites (*Der f* 1, *Der f* 2 and *Der p* 1), pollens (Japanese cedar pollen,

Cry j 1, and ragweed-pollen, *Amb a* 1) and fungal allergens (Alternaria alternata, *Alt a* 1) were loaded to the SAW immunosensor. Explicit sensor output is observed only for samples including a target allergen, *Der f* 1, which demonstrates high sensitivity of the sensor based on specificity of the antibody. Reusability of the SAW immunosensor was verified by 10 repeated measurement of *Der f* 1. The sensor surface was regenerated by pH 1.0 HCl at every end of the measurement. Each sensor output was reproducible as represented by the coefficient of variation of 5.6% throughout the whole measurement (Fig. 5.3b).

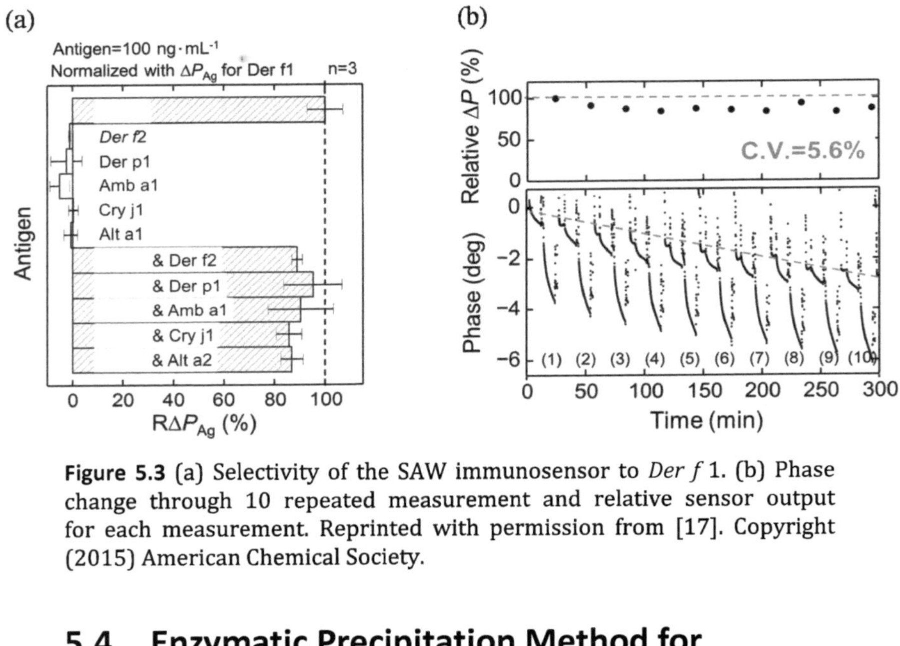

Figure 5.3 (a) Selectivity of the SAW immunosensor to *Der f* 1. (b) Phase change through 10 repeated measurement and relative sensor output for each measurement. Reprinted with permission from [17]. Copyright (2015) American Chemical Society.

5.4 Enzymatic Precipitation Method for Enhanced SAW Immunosensor

Here, we introduce a method to improve the sensitivity of the SAW immunosensor to compensate low sampling efficiency of the monitoring system. In the enzymatic precipitation method, HDMs are measured by converting the allergen concentration to mass information of precipitate that is produced through HRP-catalyzed reaction (Eq. 5.1).

$$\text{substrate} + H_2O_2 \xrightarrow{\text{HRP}} \text{product (precipitate)} + H_2O + \frac{1}{2}O_2 \quad (5.1)$$

HRP catalyzes oxidation of a substrate via hydrogen peroxide and precipitate is produced. The amount of precipitation production is dependent on HRP concentration and induces drastic mass change in vicinity to a sensor surface (Fig. 5.4). Therefore, in conjunction to a SAW device which is sensitive to mass change, highly sensitive measurement of HDM allergens is expected.

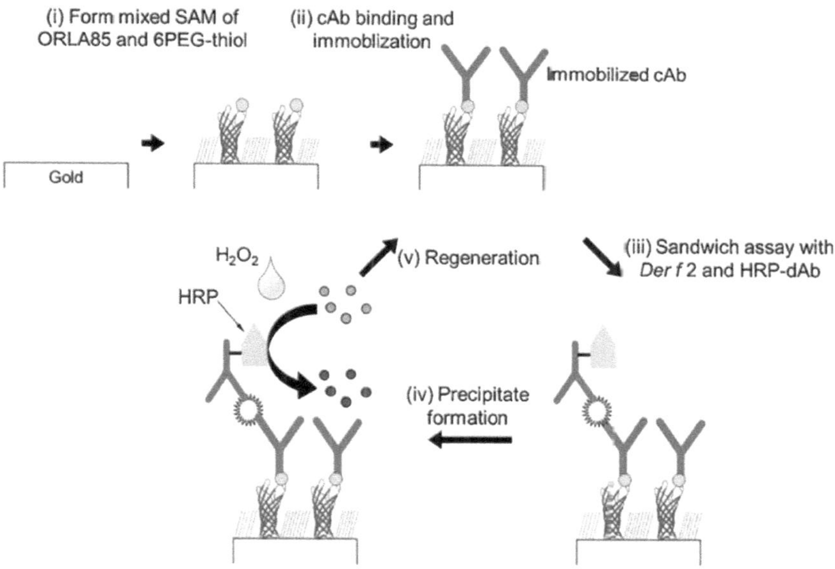

Figure 5.4 Processes of preparing the SAW immunosensor and measuring *Der f* 2 via the enzymatic precipitation method. Reprinted with permission from [18].

Three kinds of substrates, 4-chloro-1-naphthol (4CN), 3,3′,5,5′-tetramethylbenzidine (TMB) and 3,3′-diaminobenzidine (DAB), were compared in order to find a suitable substrate for sensitive and repeated measurement (Fig. 5.5). All of these substrates are oxidised by H_2O_2 under the presence of HRP labelling dAb, and precipitate and water are produced.

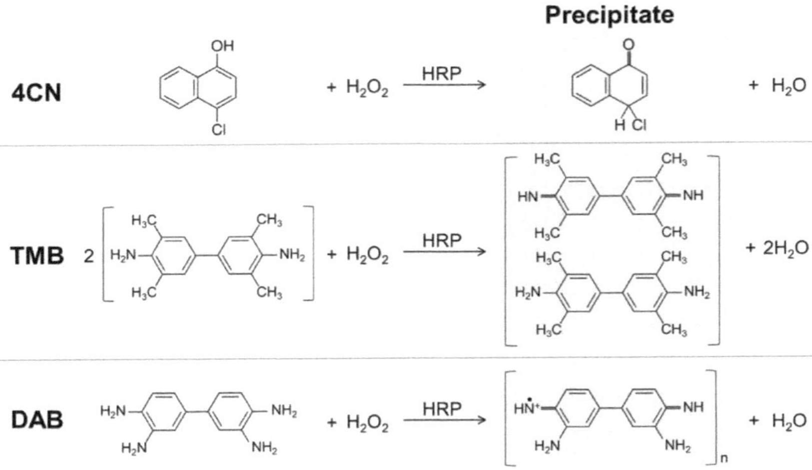

Figure 5.5 Three candidate substrates for the enzymatic precipitate method. Reprinted with permission from [18].

Typical sensorgrams are presented in Fig. 5.6a. Phase change was hardly seen when 100 ng/mL HDM allergen, *Der f* 2, was loaded because of small molecular weight of *Der f* 2. On the other hand, binding of HRP-labelled dAb to *Der f* 2 induced clear decrease in the phase due to its relatively large molecular weight. Finally, drastic phase decrease was observed when 4CN and H_2O_2 were loaded as a result of precipitate production. The sensor output was defined as a phase difference between that after rinsing of substrate solution and the baseline, $\Delta P_{\text{precipitate}}$ (precipitate: 4CN, TMB or DAB). Regeneration rate of the sensor surface was also defined as $\Delta P_{\text{Re}}/\Delta P_{\text{precipitate}}$, where ΔP_{Re} is the phase recovery through a regeneration with HCl or NaOH. Although the largest enhancement of the sensor output was obtained with DAB, the regeneration rate with DAB was poor compared to the other substrates (see Figs. 5.6b. c). Therefore, 4CN was chosen due to the second largest sensor output and the closest regeneration rate to 100%.

The sensitivity of the SAW immunosensor was evaluated by various concentrations of *Der f* 2. Sensorgrams to blank sample (0 ng/mL), 0.1 and 1.0 ng/mL *Der f* 2 are shown in Fig. 5.7a.

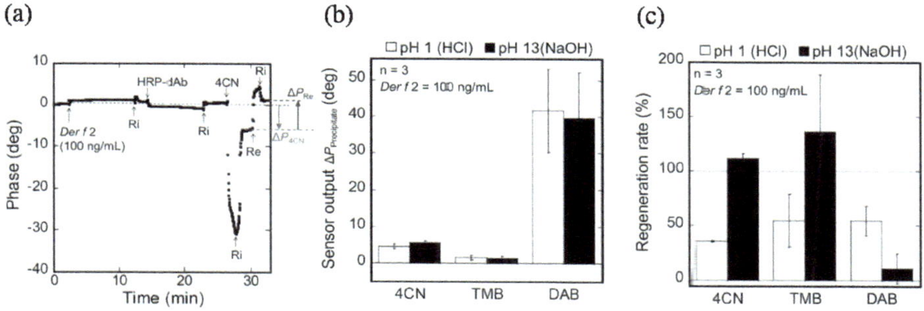

Figure 5.6 (a) Phase change in the enzymatic precipitate method with 4CN. (b) Comparison of sensor output from 4CN, TMB and DAB with regeneration using pH 1 (blank bar) and pH 13 (filled bar) reagents. (c) Comparison of surface regeneration rate with three candidate substrates using pH 1 HCl (blank bar) and pH 13 NaOH (filled bar). Reprinted with permission from [18].

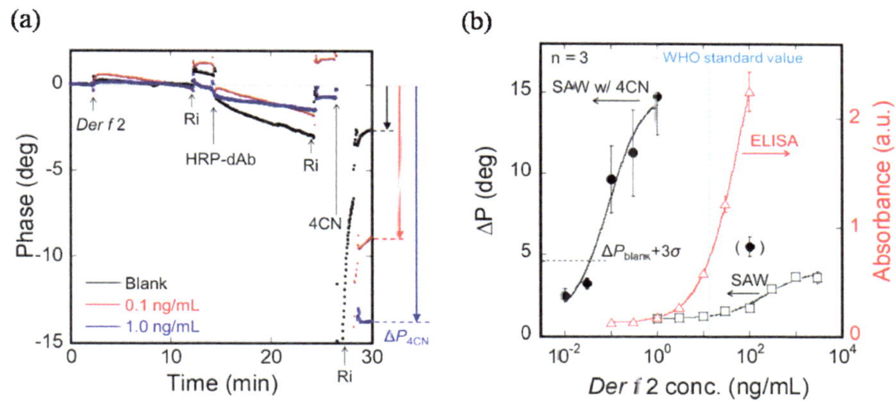

Figure 5.7 (a) Phase changes to various concentrations of *Der f* 2. Calibration curve of the SAW immunosensor using enzymatic precipitation method for *Der f* 2. Reprinted with permission from [18].

Concentration-dependent sensor output from 4CN precipitate is observed. Calibration curve summarizing the SAW immunosensor that employs the enzymatic precipitation method is shown in Fig. 5.7b. For comparisons, calibration curves of a the conventional SAW immunosensor that uses the phase shift from dAb as a sensor output and ELISA are also presented. A drastic enhancement of the sensor output is observed for 1 ng/mL of

Der f 2 by the enzymatic precipitation method, where no sensor output is obtained by the conventional SAW immunosensor. As a result, the limit of detection was 35 pg/mL for the precipitate-amplified SAW immunosensor, which is 206-fold improvement from the conventional SAW immunosensor.

5.5 Summary

This chapter has described a reusable SAW immunosensor that allows repeated measurement of HDM allergen for the airborne allergen monitoring system, and the enzymatic precipitation method to amplify the sensor output. Based on the results demonstrating unique advantages of the SAW immunosensor including high selectivity, reusability and high sensitivity, the SAW immunosensor is a potential sensor for the airborne allergen monitoring system.

References

1. Togias A. Rhinitis and asthma: Evidence for respiratory system integration. *J Allergy Clin Immunol*, 2003; 111: 1171–1183. doi:10.1067/mai.2003.1592.
2. Beasley R, Keil U, Von Mutius E, Pearce N. Worldwide variation in prevalence of symptoms of asthma, allergic rhinoconjunctivitis, and atopic eczema: ISAAC. The International Study of Asthma and Allergies in Childhood (ISAAC) Steering Committee. *Lancet (London, England)*, 1998; 351: 1225–1232. doi:10.1016/S0140-6736(97)07302-9.
3. Pawankar R, Canonica GW, Lockey RF, Holgate ST (eds). WAO White Book on Allergy 2011–2012: Executive Summary. 2011.
4. Arbes SJ, Gergen PJ, Elliott L, Zeldin DC, Park T. Prevalences of positive skin test responses to 10 common allergens in the US population: Results from the Third National Health and Nutrition Examination Survey. *J Allergy Clin Immunol*, 2005; 116: 377–383. doi:10.1016/j.jaci.2005.05.017.
5. Jackson AP, Foster AP, Hart BJ, Helps CR, Shaw SE. Prevalence of house dust mites and dermatophagoides group 1 antigens collected from bedding, skin and hair coat of dogs in south-west England. *Vet Dermatol*, 2005; 16: 32–38. doi:10.1111/j.1365-3164.2005.00427.x.

6. Wright AL, Holberg CJ, Martinez FD, Halonen M, Morgan W, Taussig LM. Epidemiology of physician-diagnosed allergic rhinitis in childhood. *Pediatrics*, 1994; 94: 895–901.

7. Knibbs LD, He C, Duchaine C, Morawska L. Vacuum cleaner emissions as a source of indoor exposure to airborne particles and bacteria. *Environ Sci Technol*, 2012; 46: 534–542. doi:10.1021/es202946w.

8. Sakaguchi M, Hashimoto M, Hospital NS, Inouye S, Sasaki R, Hashimoto M, et al. Measurement of airborne mite allergen exposure in individual subjects. *J Allergy Clin Immunol*, 1996; 97: 1040–1044. doi:10.1016/S0091-6749(96)70255-5.

9. Miyajima K, Suzuki Y, Miki D, Arai M, Arakawa T, Shimomura H, et al. Direct analysis of airborne mite allergen (Der f1) in the residential atmosphere by chemifluorescent immunoassay using bioaerosol sampler. *Talanta*, 2014; 123: 241–246. doi:10.1016/j.talanta.2013.11.033.

10. Wahn U, Lau S, Bergmann R, Kulig M, Forster J, Bergmann K, et al. Indoor allergen exposure is a risk factor for sensitization during the first three years of life. *J Allergy Clin Immunol*, 1997; 99: 763–769.

11. Tsay A, Williams L, Mitchell EB, Chapman MD. A rapid test for detection of mite allergens in homes. *Clin Exp Allergy*, 2002; 32: 1596–1601.

12. Chapman MD, Tsay A, Vailes LD. Home allergen monitoring and control–improving clinical practice and patient benefits. *Allergy*, 2001; 56: 604–610.

13. Tsai J-J, Bau I, Chen H, Lin Y, Wang G A novel nanostructured biosensor for the detection of the dust mite antigen Der p2. *Int J Nanomed*, 2011; 6: 1201–1208. doi:10.2147/IJN.S20757.

14. Sarkar P, Ghosh D, Bhattacharya D, Kataky R, Setford SJ, White SF, et al. Screen-printed biosensor for allergens. *J Chem Technol Biotechnol*, 2005; 80: 1389–1394. doi:10.1002/jctb.1340.

15. Egea E, Mendoza D, Garavito G, Saavedra S, Gómez H, Sanjuan M. Nanogold–IgY antibodies. An immunoconjugated for the detection of house dust mite (Dermatophagoides) allergens. *J Immunol Methods*, 2018; 464: 15–21. doi:10.1016/j.jim.2018.08.013.

16. Morris DRP, Fatisson J, Olsson ALJ, Tufenkji N, Ferro AR. Real-time monitoring of airborne cat allergen using a QCM-based immunosensor. *Sensors Actuators B Chem*, 2014; 190: 851–857. doi:10.1016/j.snb.2013.09.061.

17. Toma K, Miki D, Kishikawa C, Yoshimura N, Miyajima K, Arakawa T, et al. Repetitive Immunoassay with a Surface Acoustic Wave Device and a Highly Stable Protein Monolayer for On-Site Monitoring of Airborne Dust Mite Allergens. *Anal Chem*, 2015; 87: 10470–10474. doi:10.1021/acs.analchem.5b02594.
18. Toma K, Oishi K, Kato M, Kurata K, Yoshimura N, Arakawa T, et al. Precipitate-enhanced SAW immunosensor for sensitive monitoring of mite allergens. *Sensors Actuators B Chem*, 2019; 296: 126579. doi:10.1016/j.snb.2019.05.056.

Chapter 6

Development of Novel Fluorescent Sensors Based on Fluorescent Natural Compounds

Tomoya Hirano,[a,b] Hidetomo Yokoo,[a,*] Ayumi Ohsaki,[a,c] and Hiroyuki Kagechika[a]

[a]*Institute of Biomaterials and Bioengineering, Tokyo Medical and Dental University (TMDU), 2-3-10 Kanda-Surugadai, Chiyoda-ku, Tokyo 101-0062, Japan*
[b]*Faculty of Pharmacy, Osaka Medical and Pharmaceutical University, 4-20-1 Nasahara, Takatsuki, Osaka 569-1094, Japan*
[c]*College of Humanities and Sciences, Nihon University, 3-25-40 Sakurajyosui, Setagaya-ku, Tokyo 156-8550, Japan*

tomoya.hirano@ompu.ac.jp, kage.chem@tmd.ac.jp

Fluorescent molecules have been widely utilized in scientific researches, medical uses and industrial purposes. To develop those with useful and unpredictable functions, we have focused on natural compounds, and fluorescent natural compounds, Amarastelline A and Nigakinone, were identified. For the evaluation of their functions as fluorophore and the development of novel fluorescent sensors, we synthesized various derivatives of their

*Present address: *Graduate School of Medical Science, Kyoto Prefectural University of Medicine, 1-5 Shimogamohangi-cho, Sakyo-ku, Kyoto 606-0823, Japan*

Biomedical Engineering
Edited by Akihiro Miyauchi and Yuji Miyahara

ISBN 978-981-4877-63-3 (Hardcover), 978-1-003-14194-5 (eBook)
www.jennystanford.com

common structures, canthin-5,6-dione and 1,5-naphthyridin-2(1*H*)-one. Among them, novel polarity-sensitive fluorophore, which showed the shift of fluorescence maximum wavelength by the change of solvent polarity, was obtained. To apply this function to the study of biomolecule interaction, C5 peptide, that could interact calmodulin, labelled with this fluorophore, was synthesized, and its interaction with calmodulin could be detected by the ratio of the fluorescence intensities at two fluorescent maximum wavelengths. Our findings indicated the usefulness of natural compounds for the development of novel fluorescent molecules, as well as the versatility of canthin-5,6-dione and 1,5-naphthyridin-2(1*H*)-one.

6.1 Introduction

Fluorescent molecules have been widely utilized for analytical, medical and industrial purposes. They have also been utilized to develop sensors, whose fluorescence properties could be changed by binding to or reacting with each analyte such as specific ion, molecular species and enzymes, or in response to changes of microenvironment [1–3], such as pH [4] and viscosity [5, 6]. Small molecule-based fluorescent molecules are practically useful, and a number of fluorophores have been reported. To develop fluorescent molecules with desired functions, various strategies have been applied. For example, extension of conjugated system by addition of another aromatic rings would be effective for development of those with longer excitation and emission wavelengths. 6-DMN (6-*N,N*-dimethylamino-2,3-naphthalimide) derivatized from 4-DMAP (4-dimethylaminophthalimide) by introduction of one benzene ring, show longer emission wavelength [7, 8]. In some cases, replacement of atom is also effective. Tokyo Magenta [9] and POF [10] were designed by replacement of oxygen atom of TokyoGreen with silyl or phosphorus atom, respectively, which resulted in their excitation and emission wavelengths at longer region than TokyoGreen. Those strategies are thought to be useful; however, most of obtained derivatives tend to possess similar properties such as environment-dependent fluorescent change and mode of fluorescent change.

So for development of those with novel functions, other strategies yielding novel structural components are wanted.

For such purpose, construction of fluorescent compounds library and identification of compounds with desired and, in some cases, unpredictable functions have been applied [11]. We have also constructed a library of fluorescent compounds based on coumarin moiety by effective organic synthesis, and identified novel fluorescent sensors [12–14]. In addition, we also isolated fluorescent natural compounds. Amarastelline A was isolated as a novel fluorescent natural product from the bark of *Quassia amara* (Fig. 6.1) [15]. It has strong fluorescence and could stain cytoplasm of living cells. We also isolated and identified the known compound, named as Nigakinone (**1**), from the same plant, and found its solvent-dependent fluorescence properties. We considered that these structural components might be useful as novel fluorophores and fluorescent sensors, and so various derivatives of the core structure, that is, canthin-5,6-dione and 1,5-naphthyridin-2(1*H*)-one, were synthesized, and their structure-fluorescence relationship were evaluated. Further, their fluorescent properties were applied to develop novel sensors with unique function.

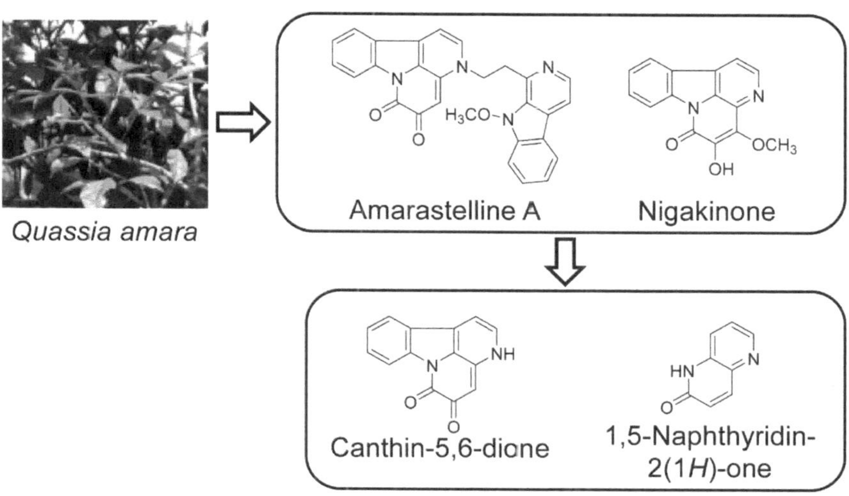

Figure 6.1 Structures of fluorescent natural compounds.

6.2 Development of Novel Fluorescent Sensors Based on Canthin-5,6-Dione Moiety

Amarastelline A and nigakinone contain a common canthin-5,6-dione structure, that is a tautomer of 5-hydroxy-canthin-6-one for the case of nigakinone (Fig. 6.2). Tautomerization is expected to alter the fluorescence properties, and could be hindered by the introduction of functional groups at the N^3-position. Functional groups on the benzene moiety linked to the tautomerizable bicyclic 1,5-naphthyridin-2-one moiety might also influence the fluorescence properties. Thus, we designed and synthesized compounds **1–10**, having a variety of substituents at the N^3-, 4- and 10-positions.

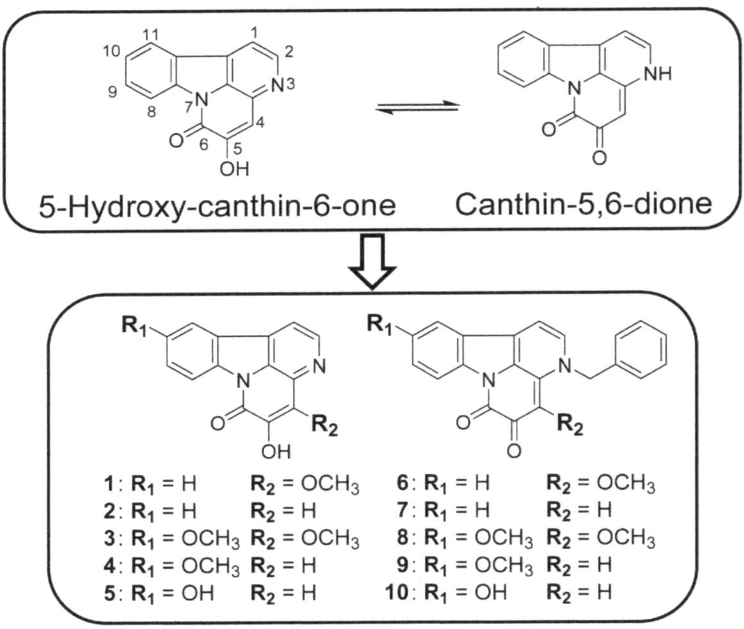

Figure 6.2 Design and structures of canthin-5,6-dione derivatives.

The fluorescence properties of compounds **1–10** were evaluated in various solvents such as chloroform, acetonitrile, DMF, DMSO, methanol and water (100 mM sodium phosphate buffer, pH 7.4), and reported in our previous paper [16]. In summary, the presence of an N^3-benzyl group greatly affected the fluorescence properties. For example, **2** showed solvent-dependent fluorescence change, that is, fluorescece maximum wavelength at around 400 and 540 nm in acetonitrile and chloroform, while only at around 500 nm in methanol and water (Fig. 6.3). On the other hand, in N^3-benzylated compound **7**, only small changes of fluorescence at about 500 nm were induced by change of solvent. Thus, the fluorescence properties of the 5,6-dione form appeared to be little affected by the solvent. On the other hand, compound **2**, that can undergo tautomerization between 5-hydroxyz-6-one and 5,6-dione forms, showed large solvent-dependent fluorescence changes.

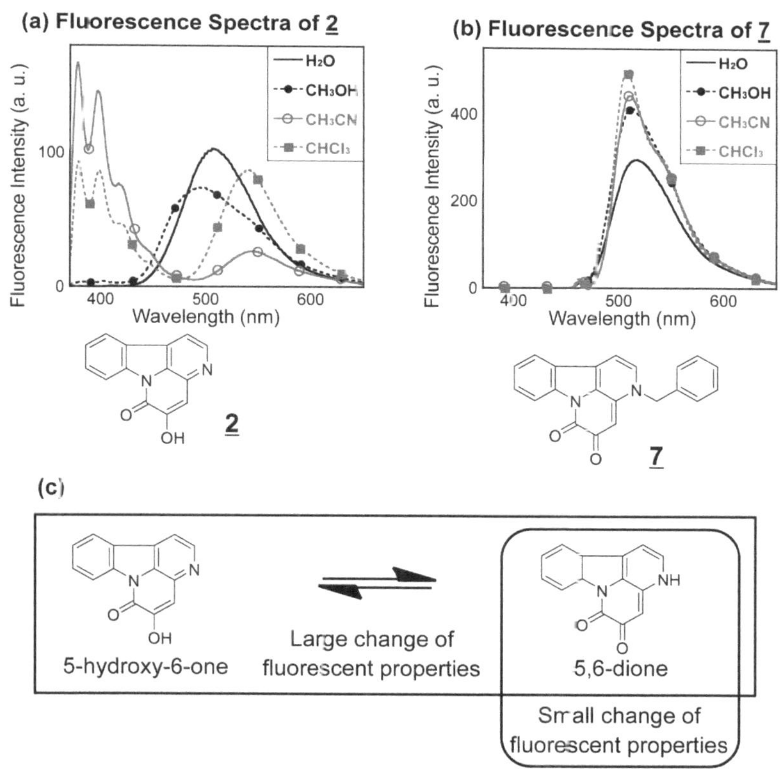

Figure 6.3 Solvent-dependent fluorescence change of canthin-5,6-dione derivatives. Fluorescence spectra of (a) **2** (e.g., 360 nm) and (b) of **7** (e.g., 460 nm) in various solvents are shown. (c) Proposed relationship of tautomerization and fluorescence change. Solvent-dependent fluorescent change of canthin-5,6-dione derivatives.

Next, the pH-dependent fluorescence changes of compounds were examined. Among them, compound **5** showed an "OFF-ON-OFF"-type fluorescence change with increase of pH apparently due to sequential deprotonations of the two hydroxyl groups. Like our previously reported sensor based on a coumarin scaffold bearing two hydroxyl groups [17, 18] and similar sensors developed by other groups [19], **5** could be utilized as a fluorescent sensor for a specific range of pH (Fig. 6.4). Such a sensor should be useful, compared with most conventional pH sensors, which sense only whether the pH is below or above a specific value.

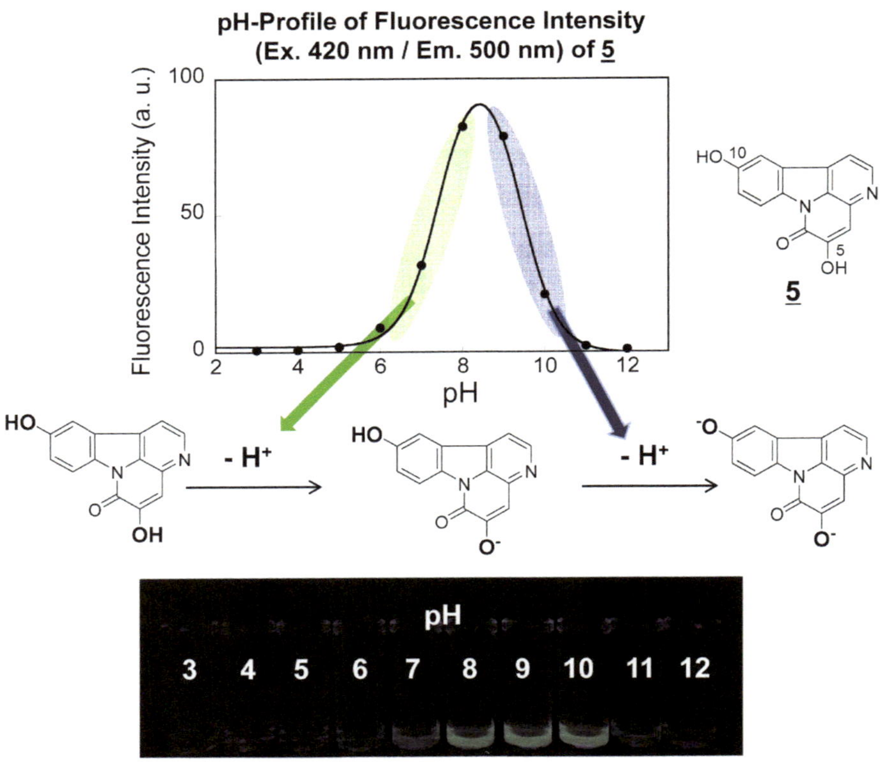

Figure 6.4 pH-dependent fluorescent change of **5**. (a) The pH profile of fluorescence intensity (excitation at 360 nm; emission at 500 nm) of **5** is shown. Those data were obtained in 100 mM sodium phosphate buffer (pH 3.0 – 12.0) containing 0.3% DMSO as a co-solvent.

6.3 Polarity-Sensitive Fluorescent Molecules Based on 1,5-Naphthyridin-2(1*H*)-One

As described in previous section, substituents at the 5-position of canthine-5,6-dione and its derivative were shown to be utilized as a fluorophore and core structure of fluorescent sensors. However, their structural divergence and versatility would be restricted, partly due to the synthetic difficulty. Therefore, we focused on the substructure of canthine-5,6-dione, that is, the bicyclic 1,5-naphthyridin-2(1*H*)-one moiety. Evaluation of the fluorescent properties of canthin-5,6-dione derivatives, tautomerization between 5,6-dione and 5-hydroxy-6-one forms would influence solvent-sensitive fluorescence properties. To characterize 1,5-naphthyridin-2(1*H*)-one, especially as the fluorophore with solvent-dependent fluorescent change, 1,5-naphthyridin-2(1*H*)-ones **11–17** with various substituents at the N^1-, 3- and 8-positions were designed and synthesized (Fig. 6.5).

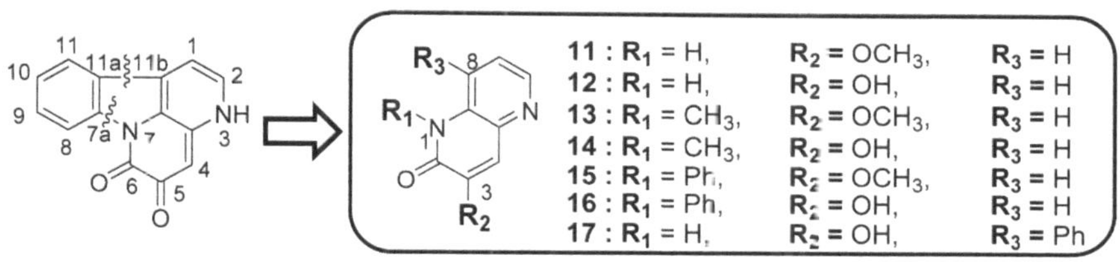

Figure 6.5 Design and structures of 1,5-naphthyridin-2(1*H*)-one derivatives.

The fluorescence properties of compounds **11–17** were evaluated in various solvents such as chloroform, acetonitrile, DMF, DMSO, methanol and water (100 mM sodium phosphate buffer, pH 7.4) [20]. In summary, the cleavage of one covalent bond of canthin-5,6-dione would not significantly affect the fluorophore. For example, the fluorescent quantum yields of 3-hydroxy derivatives (**12**, **14** and **16**) were relatively high, especially in water, that is, 0.731, 0.665 and 0.583, respectively, being larger than that of **2**. Among these compounds, **16** and **17** would be utilized as polarity-sensitive fluorescent compounds. **16** showed strong fluorescence only in polar and protic solvents, like methanol and water, and they showed stronger, bathochromically shifted fluorescence in such solvents (Fig. 6.6). Interestingly, the 8-phenyl derivative **17** showed different mode of fluorescent change from that of **16**. The characteristic stronger fluorescence and bathochromic shift of compounds **16** and **17** in polar and protic solvents are distinct from the properties of most known polarity-sensitive fluorophores, such as NBD, DANSYL and 4-DMN, which show strong fluorescence in less polar solvents. The difference in polarity-sensitivity would be helpful for developing new fluorescent probes. Compound **17** would be suitable for ratiometric measurement of microenvironmental changes of polarity, utilizing the two emission maxima.

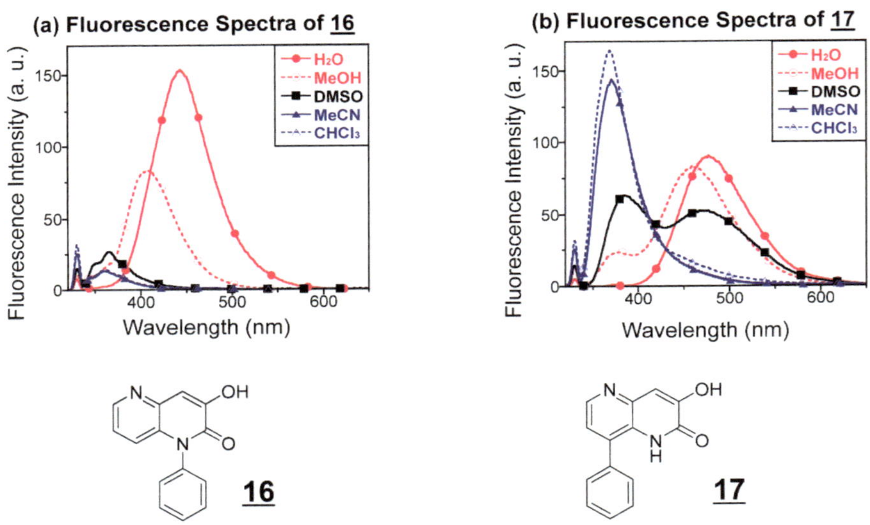

Figure 6.6 Solvent-dependent fluorescence change of 1,5-naphthyridin-2(1*H*)-one derivatives (a) **16** and (b) **17**. Excitation wavelength was 330 nm.

6.4 Application to Sensing of Biomolecular Interaction

Among the compounds based on fluorescent natural compounds, 3-hydroxy-8-phenyl-1,5-naphthyridin-2(1*H*)-one (**17**) showed a high quantum yield of fluorescence (0.34) in 100 mM phosphate buffer (pH 7.4), together with a bathochromic shift of the emission maximum wavelength in polar and protic solvents. Thus, it might be suitable for ratiometric measurements of microenvironmental polarity changes.

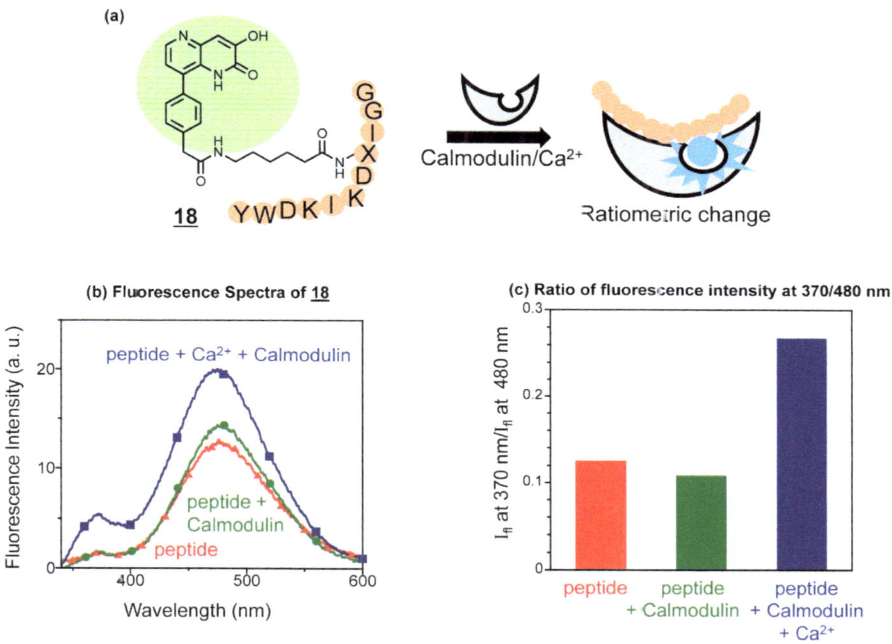

Figure 6.7 Fluorescence properties of C5 peptide derivatives containing a 1,5-naphthyridin-2(1*H*)-one fluorophore in the presence of calmodulin and Ca^{2+}. (a) Structure and proposed functions of fluorescent peptide **18**. (b) The fluorescence spectra of 5 μM of peptide **18**, 5 μM peptide and 10 μM calmodulin from bovine testes and 5 μM peptide and 10 μM calmodulin in the presence of Ca^{2+} (1 mM $CaCl_2$) in 10 mM Tris-HCl (pH 7.5) containing 1 mM magnesium acetate, 150 mM KCl and 0.5% or 1% DMSO as a cosolvent were shown. (c) Ratio of fluorescence intensities at 370/480 nm.

Calmodulin, a calcium-signal transducer protein, mediates many biological functions of Ca^{2+} in cells. Calmodulin undergoes conformational change upon Ca^{2+}-binding, exposing a hydrophobic pocket that can bind various peptides and proteins. For example, M13 peptide, one of the binding peptides of Ca^{2+}-bound calmodulin, has been utilized as a core structure of chameleon, a fluorescent indicator for Ca^{2+} [21]. The transmembrane domain of tail-anchored membrane proteins, which are delivered to the membrane of endoplasmic reticulum, binds to calmodulin for membrane insertion [22]. Tail-anchored membrane proteins are involved in many key bioprocesses, including apoptosis, lipid biosynthesis, vesicular trafficking and signal transduction [23]. Thus, fluorescent sensing of the binding of calmodulin with a partner peptide would be useful for real-time tracking of conformational changes and activation of calmodulin. So we introduced **17** to Phe8 of in C5 peptide (YWDKIKDFIGG), which is one of calmodulin-binding peptides [24], yielding fluorescence peptide **18** (Fig. 6.7).

The fluorescence change of **18** upon addition of calmodulin with or without calcium ion was shown in Fig. 6.7. Compound **18** increased the fluorescence intensity, especially at 370 nm, upon addition of both calmodulin and Ca^{2+} ion, and the ratio at 370/480 nm increased 2.4-fold. This change did not occur in the absence of Ca^{2+} ion. Thus, the fluorescent peptide **18** could sense the structural change of calmodulin induced by binding to Ca^{2+} ion. This confirms the utility of **18** as a ratiometric fluorescence probe for detecting Ca^{2+}-induced changes in the conformation of calmodulin [25].

6.5 Conclusion

Several derivatives of canthin-5,6-dione and 1,5-naphthyridin-2(1*H*)-one, which are common structural components of the fluorescent natural products amarastelline A and nigakinone, were synthesized. From the study of canthin-5,6-dione, the combination of N^3- and 10-substituted groups can regulate the fluorescence properties, and this behavior could be utilized to obtain fluorescent sensor responding to a specific range of pH. Among 1,5-naphthyridin-2(1*H*)-one derivatives, the 3-hydroxy-8-phenyl derivative **17**, has useful functions, that is, solvent-polarity-dependent change of fluorescence ratio and strong fluorescence in both aqueous solution and less polar solvents. To apply these functions to the study on the biomolecule interaction, the fluorescent amino acid **18** bearing the fluorophore of **17** was synthesized, and introduced in C5 peptide. The fluorescent peptide **18** could sense its interaction with calmodulin in the presence of calcium ion by fluorescent ratiometric measurement. Our findings indicated the usefulness of natural compounds for the development of fluorescent molecules with novel structures and functions.

Acknowledgments

The work described in this chapter was supported by Grants-in-Aid for Scientific Research from The Ministry of Education, Science, Sports and Culture, Japan (Grants No 15K08019 to TH, 26670052 to HK). TH also gratefully acknowledges funding from Terumo Life Science Foundation. This work was partially supported by Project for Development of Innovative Research on Cancer Therapeutics, JSPS Core-to-Core Program A, Advanced Research Network and Platform Project for Supporting Drug Discovery and Life Science Research funded by Japan Agency for Medical Research and Development (AMED). A part of this research is a Cooperative Research Project of the Research Center for Biomedical Engineering.

References

1. de Silva, A. P., Gunaratne, H. Q., Gunnlaugsson, T., Huxley, C. P., McCoy, A. J. M., Rademacher, J. T., and Rice, T. E. (1997). Signaling recognition events with fluorescent sensors and switches *Chem. Rev.*, **97**, pp. 1515–1566.
2. Li, X., Gao, X., Shi, W., and Ma, H. (2014). Design strategies for water-soluble small molecular chromogenic and fluorogenic probes, *Chem. Rev.*, **114**, pp. 590–659.
3. Yang, Z., Cao, J., He, Y., Yang, J. H., Kim, T., Peng, X., and Kim, S. J. (2014). Macro-/micro-environment-sensitive chemosensing and biological imaging, *Chem. Soc. Rev.*, **43**, pp. 4563–4601.
4. Han, J., and Burgessand, K. (2010). Fluorescent indicators for intracellular pH, *Chem. Rev.*, **110**, pp. 2709–2728.
5. Haidekker, A. M., Ling, T., Anglo, M., Stevens, H., Frangos, A. J., and Theodorakis, A. E. (2001). New fluorescent probes for the measurement of cell membrane viscosity, *Chem. Biol.*, **8**, pp. 123–131.

6. Haidekker, A. M., Brady, T. P., Lichlyter, D., and Theodrakis, E. A. (2006). A ratiometric fluorescent viscosity sensor, *J. Am. Chem. Soc.*, **128**, pp. 398–399.
7. Vázquez, M. E., Blanco, J. B., and Imperiali, B. (2005). Photophysics and biological applications of the environment-sensitive fluorophore 6-*N,N*-dimethylamino-2,3-naphthalimide, *J. Am. Chem. Soc.*, **127**, pp. 1300–1306.
8. Soujanya, T., Fessenden, R. W., and Samanta, A. (1996). Role of nonfluorescent twisted intramolecular charge transfer state on the photophysical behavior of aminophthalimide dyes, *J. Phys. Chem.*, **100**, pp. 3507–3512.
9. Egawa, T., Koide, Y., Hanaoka, K., Komatsu, T., Terai, T., and Nagano, T. (2011). Development of a fluorescein analogue, TokyoMagenta, as a novel scaffold for fluorescence probes in red region, *Chem. Commun.*, **47**, pp. 4162–4164.
10. Fukazawa, A., Suda, S., Taki, M., Yamaguchi, E., Grzybowski, M., Sato, Y., Higashiyama, T., and Yamaguchi, S. (2016). Phospha-fluorescein: A red-emissive fluorescein analogue with high photobleaching resistance, *Chem. Commun.*, **52**, pp. 1120–1123.
11. Vendrell, M., Zhai, D., Cheng Er, J., and Chang, Y.-T. (2012). Combinatorial strategies in fluorescent probe development, *Chem. Rev.*, **112**, pp. 4391–4420.
12. Hirano, T., Hiromoto, K., and Kagechika, H. (2007). Development of a library of 6-arylcoumarins as candidate fluorescent sensors, *Org. Lett.*, **9**, pp. 1315–1318.
13. Hirano, T., Kubo, H., Shiraishi, T., Hiromoto, K., Fujiwara, T., and Kagechika, H. (2012). Fluorescent properties of coumarins with dual functions constructed by two sequential reactions, *Tetrahedron Lett.*, **53**, pp. 5916–5919.
14. Shiraishi, T., Kagechika, H., and Hirano, T. (2015). 6-Arylcoumarins: Versatile scaffolds for fluorescent sensors, *New. J. Chem.* **39**, pp. 8389–8396.
15. Taniguchi, K., Takizawa, S., Hirano, T., Murata, S., Kagechika, H., Kishida, A., and Ohsaki, A. (2012). Amarastelline a: A fluorescent alkaloid from *Quassia amara* and its properties in living cells, *ChemPlusChem*, **77**, pp. 427–431.
16. Yokoo, H., Ohsaki, A., Kagechika, H., and Hirano, T. (2016). Structural development of canthin-5,6-dione moiety as a fluorescent dye and its application to novel fluorescent sensors, *Tetrahedron*, **72**, pp. 5872–5879.

17. Shiraishi, T., Saito, T., Kagechika, H., and Hirano, T. (2014). Development of a novel fluorescent sensor to detect a specific range of pH, *Tetrahedron Lett.*, **55**, pp. 6784–6786.

18. Hirano, T., Noji, Y., Shiraishi, T., Ishigami-Yuasa, M., and Kagechika, H. (2016). Development of an 'OFF-ON-OFF' fluorescent pH sensor suitable for the study of intracellular pH, *Tetrahedron,* **72**, pp. 4925–4930.

19. Sadhu, K. K., Mizukami, S., Yoshimura, A., and Kikuchi, K. (2013). pH induced dual "OFF-ON-OFF" switch: Influence of a suitably placed carboxylic acid, *Org. Biomol. Chem.*, **11**, pp. 563–568.

20. Yokoo, H., Ohsaki, A., Kagechika, H., and Hirano, T. (2018). Unique properties of 1,5-naphthyridin-2(1*H*)-one derivatives as environmental-polarity-sensitive fluorescent dyes, *Eur. J. Org. Chem.* pp. 679–687.

21. Miyawaki, A., Llopis, J., Heim, R., McCaffery, J. M., Adams, J. M., Ikura, M., and Tsien, R. Y. (1997). Fluorescent indicators for Ca^{2+} based on green fluorescent proteins and calmodulin, *Nature*, **388**, pp. 882–887.

22. Fry, M. Y., and Clemons, W. M. Jr. (2018). Complexity in targeting membrane proteins, *Science*, **359**, pp. 390–391.

23. Kalbfleisch, T., Cambon, A., and Wattenberg, B. J. (2007). A bioinformatics approach to identifying tail-anchored proteins in the human genome, *Traffic*, **8**, pp. 1687–1694.

24. Weng, W., Zhu, L., Hirano, Y., Marziyeh, K., Tada, S., Zhang, G., Uzawa, T., Zhang, D., Hirose, T., Taiji, M., and Ito, Y. (2016). Fluorogenic enhancement of an in vitro-selected peptide ligand by replacement of a fluorescent group, *Anal. Chem.*, **88**, pp. 7991–7997.

25. Yokoo, H., Kagechika, H., Ohsaki, A., and Hirano, T. (2019). A polarity-sensitive fluorescent amino acid and its incorporation into peptides for the ratiometric detection of biomolecular interactions, *ChemPlusChem*, **84**, pp. 1716–1719.

Chapter 7

Living-Cell Analysis by Surface Plasmon Resonance and Its Medical Application

Yuhki Yanase and Michihiro Hide

Department of Dermatology, Institute of Biomedical & Health Sciences, Hiroshima University, Hiroshima, Japan

ed1h-w1de-road@hiroshima-u.ac.jp, hiro_hide@city-hosp.naka.hiroshima.jp

Real-time and label-free monitoring of living cell conditions and functions are strongly needed in the field of basic research of cell biology and medicine. Surface plasmon resonance (SPR) sensors can sensitively detect refractive index (RI) changes on the sensor surface of sensor chip coated with gold thin film in real-time. SPR imaging (SPRI) sensors equipped with CCD or CMOS camera can monitor the distribution of RI on the area of gold thin film surface. In this chapter, we introduce techniques to analyze living cells by means of SPR and SPRI, and their applications for cell biology and medicine.

Biomedical Engineering
Edited by Akihiro Miyauchi and Yuji Miyahara

ISBN 978-981-4877-63-3 (Hardcover), 978-1-003-14194-5 (eBook)
www.jennystanford.com

7.1 SPR and SPRI Sensors

It is well known that surface plasmon resonance (SPR) sensors can sensitively measure the change of refractive index (RI) in the detection area on a sensor chip, less than 500 nm depth, in real-time without any labeling. When p-polarized, not s-polarized, collimated incident light by polarizer and collimator is reflected at the interface between glass and gold thin film (around 50 nm) at various incident angles for total reflection, (θ), the reflected light intensity is strongly attenuated at a specific incident angle which is called a resonance angle (RA). The phenomenon is induced by SPR which is due to the resonance between plasmon wave running on the gold film and the evanescent wave generated from totally reflected light at the interface of glass and gold film, which penetrates the gold film. Since, RA change is considered to be proportional to RI change in a SPR detection area on the surface of SPR sensor chip; SPR sensors can sensitively monitor the RI changes in a detection area (<500 nm) by continuous detection of RA changes in real-time [1–3] (Fig. 7.1). Generally, prism-coupling SPR sensors using Kretschmann configuration consists of a light source (Laser or LED), a p-polarizer, a collimator, a prism (RI = 1.517), and a photodiode for detection of reflected light intensity. The sensor chips were glass slides (RI = 1.517) coated with the gold thin film (1 nm Cr layer and 49 nm gold layer) by means of vapor deposition (Fig. 7.1). Figure 7.2 shows a label-free monitoring of RA changes in real-time during the measurement of antigen–antibody interaction. When SPR sensor chip treated with antibodies for specific antigen is exposed to a solution containing antigens, RA increases due to the increase of antigens in the vicinity of a sensor chip. This step is called an association step. Then RA decreases slightly, when the antigens which did not bind to the antibodies on the sensor chip are removed by washing process; this step is called a dissociation step. The amount of antigens bound to antibody is calculated from the change of RA value. The sensor chip with antigens captured by antibodies is reused by elimination of antigens by sodium hydroxide. This step is called regeneration step. Thus, SPR sensors can continuously and sensitively detect the kinetics of molecule interactions on a sensor chip [4]. Although SPR sensors can measure RI changes on the surface of sensors chip, the sensors detect only an average RI change in a sensing area of the sensor chip (light spotted area). Therefore, conventional SPR sensors cannot monitor a distribution of RI on the surface of sensor chip.

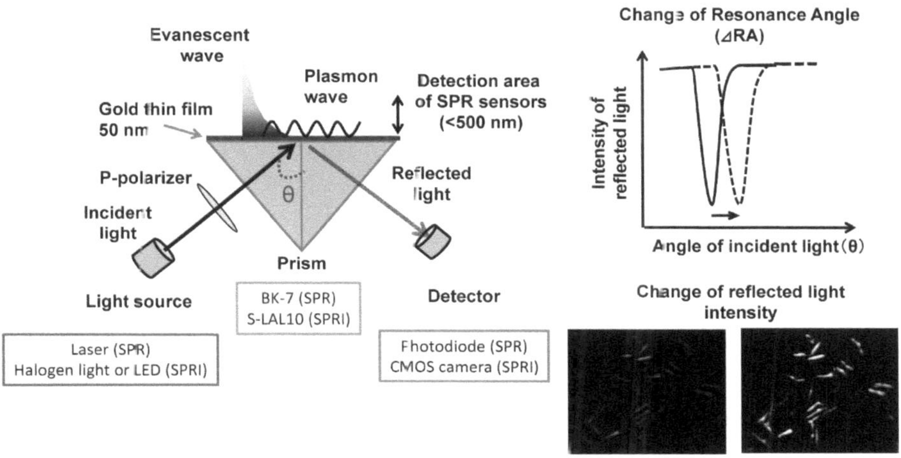

Figure 7.1 Setup of SPR and SPRI sensors. SPR sensor or SPRI sensors can detect RA changes or visualize RI distribution in detection area, respectively.

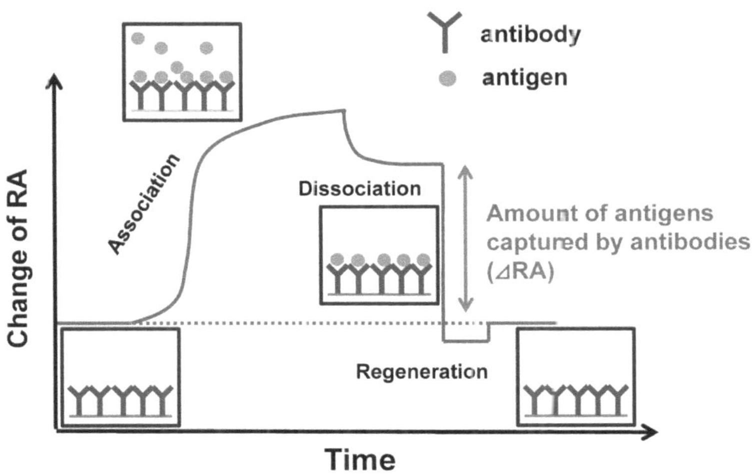

Figure 7.2 RA changes of molecular interactions monitored by SPR sensor. Adapted from [48].

To overcome this limitation of SPR sensors, SPR imaging (SPRI) systems have been developed so as to monitor RI distribution on the surface of sensor chip in an image captured by CCD or CMOS camera [5, 6]. The SPRI sensor developed by us consists of a light source (LED light), an achromatic lens for collimation of incident light, a p-polarizer, a prism (S-LAL10, RI = 1.72), a thermostat for regulation of temperature at 37°C, objective lenses (×0.5, ×2, ×4) and a CMOS camera. The sensor chips (S-LAL10, 20 mm × 20 mm × 1 mm, RI = 1.72) were coated with gold thin film (1 nm Cr layer and 49 nm gold layer) by means of vapor deposition (Fig. 7.1) [7]. Obtained images, changes of light intensity distribution, were analyzed with graphics software, such as Image-Pro (Media Cybernetics, Bethesda, MD). When the sensor surface is partitioned into multiple sensing spots, high throughput screening of molecular interactions and cell reactions on a sensor chip is also available [8].

7.2 SPR and SPRI Sensors for Living Cells Analysis

As described above, SPR sensors have great potential as sensors for non-invasive, non-label and real-time monitoring of molecule interactions and living cells behavior. In 2002, we first unveiled that SPR sensor, SPR CELLIA, (Nippon Laser & Electronics Lab.), monitored the large changes of RA in response to the activation of non-labeled RBL-2H3 cells, a rat mast cell line, in real-time [9]. Consequentially, activation of various cells, such as keratinocytes (PAM 212), human peripheral basophils and human B lymphocytes isolated from peripheral blood, cultured and/or fixed on a sensor chip were also analyzed by SPR, suggesting the potential of SPR sensors as a new technique for the evaluation of living cells using RI as a indicator of cell functions [10–12]. Mast cells and basophils express the high-affinity IgE receptors (FcεRIs), to which IgE antibodies in serum bind. When specific antigens bind to IgE ntibodies on mast cells and basophils, cells are activated and induce the degranulation of stored granules containing histamine and the morphological changes, such as ruffling and spreading [13]. RA changes detected by SPR sensors are considered to be proportional to living cells-related

RI changes on the gold surface. The binding of DNP-specific IgEs for themselves to FcεRIs expressed on the surface of RBL-2H3 cells induce only marginal or no activation of the cells. Therefore, RA is not changed (Fig. 7.3). However, when RBL-2H3 cells sensitized with dinitrophenol (DNP) specific IgE antibodies are stimulated with DNP-human serum albumin (HSA) antigens, cells are activated and RA rapidly increase for an hour (Fig. 7.3) [10]. Thus, SPR sensors can evaluate the activation of living cells cultured on the surface of SPR sensor chip in response to stimuli, rather than the binding of extracellular molecules, such as antibodies with high molecular weight (IgE = 200,000 MW), to the cell surface. To date, living cell activations- and functions-related RA changes have also been reported by several groups. Chabot et al. reported that SPR sensors can evaluate real-time adhesion and morphological changes of cells following activations by various agents [14]. Lee et al. developed a technique as a new olfactory biosensor system for selective quantitative detection of volatile compounds by combination of olfactory receptor expressing cells and SPR sensor [15]. Effects of anti-cancer drugs against cancer cells have also been evaluated [16, 17].

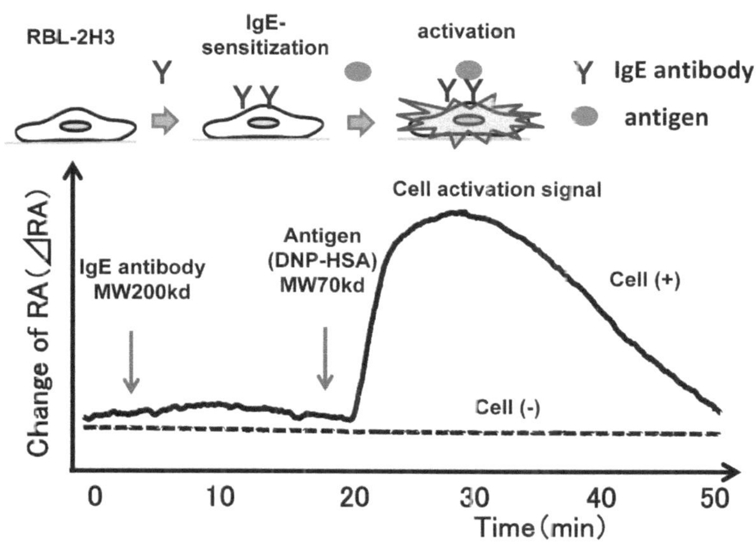

Figure 7.3 Monitoring of RA changes of RBL-2H3 cells by SPR sensors. Adapted from [48].

As described above, SPRI sensors can visualize RI pattern on the sensor chip coated with gold thin film. Figure 7.4 shows our technique for visualization of individual cells activation by SPRI. The resonance curves of assay buffer alone, cells before stimulation and cells after stimulation are plotted as (a), (b) and (c), respectively. When the incident light angle (θ) is fixed at the angle of RA of assay buffer in the absence of cells, the dark image is captured (Fig. 7.4, left image). Then, the RA shifts to higher degree in the presence of cells because the RI becomes higher than that of assay buffer. This causes the increase of the reflected light-intensity at the cell adherent area in the SPR image (Fig. 7.4, middle image). When cells are stimulated, the RA shifts further and the reflected light-intensity increases at the cell area (Fig. 7.4, right image). Using this technique, we monitored the changes of the reflected light-intensity of single RBL-2H3 cells

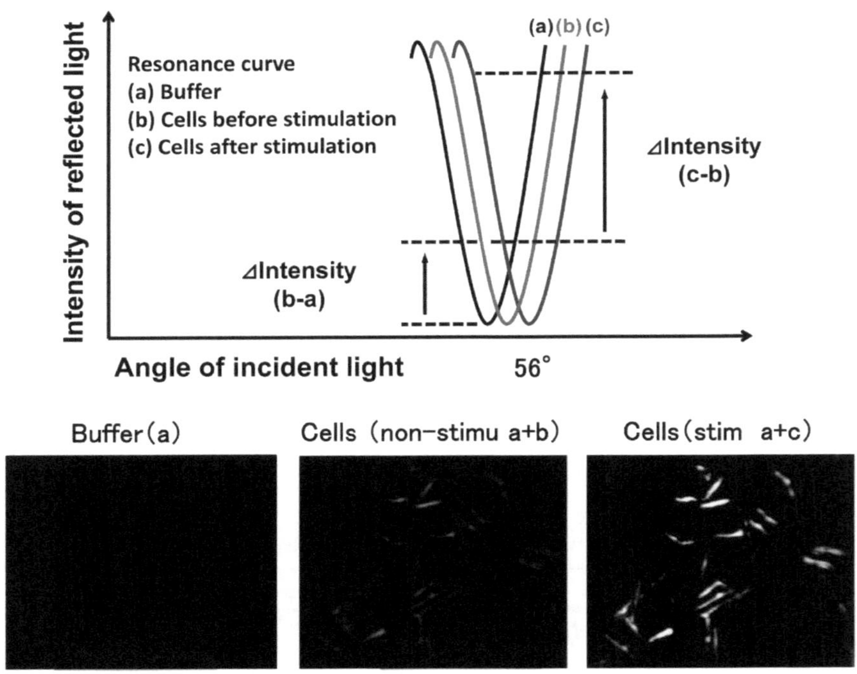

Figure 7.4 Principle of single cells visualization by means of SPRI. Adapted from [48].

(rat mast cell line), PAM212 (mouse keratinocyte line) cells and A431 cells (human epidermoid carcinoma) in response to various molecules [18]. Moreover, we also succeeded in distinguishing the reactions of activated cells from non-activated cells in continuous SPR images [18]. Several applications of SPRI sensors for living cell analysis have been reported by other groups. Real-time and non-label monitoring of activation of RBL-2H3 cells in response to stimulation by using a SPRI imaging system has also reported by Horii et al. [19]. Shinohara et al. monitored the activation of PC12 in response to stimuli, such as nerve growth factor (NGF) by means of SPRI [20]. These techniques were also reported by several groups as detecting the real-time binding of living cells, such as red blood cells and lymphocytes, using specific reactions of antibodies with antigen-coated cell surfaces [21, 22].

7.3 Application of SPR and SPRI Sensors

7.3.1 Optical Fiber SPR Sensors for Living Cell Analysis

The SPR technique is also applied for an optical fiber-type sensor which can measure the RI of liquid or gas samples [23, 24]. Several types of optical fiber SPR sensors have been developed; a hetero-core sensing structure, a D-shaped sensing structure, a tapered sensing structure, and an end-face reflected structure [25]. Among them, the end-face reflected structure has advantage in its sensor part, which may be easily inserted into objects for analysis, such as organs or even inside of the human body. We introduced a fiber optic SPR sensor with intention of medical application. The optical fiber with 200 μm core diameter and 1 cm length was coated by gold film with 50 nm thickness. A white LED was used as light-source, and attenuations of light-intensity due to an SPR phenomenon in the sensor part was analyzed using a spectrum detector. The RI changes on a gold surface were indicated by the shifts at the maximal wavelength in the absorption spectrum. Using this sensor, the difference in solvents with various RI and bindings of protein to the sensor chip was measured. Moreover, we successfully detected the reactions of RBL-2H3 mast cells adhered onto sensor part by means of the droplet method [26]. Thus, optical fiber SPR sensors can detect RI changes in solvents and also measure the continuous activations of unlabeled living cells in real-time manner. Since the sensing part of optical fiber SPR is so small and data can be collected at the other end of an optical fiber connected to a portable devise, it is feasible to embed the sensor part and fibers into an endoscope for humans to support clinical diagnosis.

7.3.2 Diagnosis of Immediate Type Allergy by SPR and SPRI Sensors

The accurate and non-invasive identification of specific allergens which induce the activation of mast cells and basophils in individuals is required to avoid symptoms of IgE antibodies-related allergic disorders, also called immediate type hypersensitivity, such as anaphylactic shock, allergic rhinitis, food allergy and asthma. The detection of allergens specific IgE antibodies in serum in each donor can predict the hypersensitivity against the allergens. Therefore, a clarification of allergen specific IgE antibodies in serum has been performed for diagnosis of IgE-related disease, especially immediate type hypersensitivity [27]. Shen et al. developed the epitope-resolved assay system for the detection of peanut-allergen specific IgE antibodies using SPRI technology [28]. The results of SPRI array and immunoCAP provided insights into the molecular epitopes involving the sensitization for peanuts. However, there are often substantial discrepancies between these serological tests and clinical symptoms [27]. In vivo tests, such as skin test and allergen challenge test, are more reliable in reflecting clinical conditions. However, these tests may be painful, and could potentially evoke anaphylactic shock when a patient is extremely sensitive to a particular antigen [29]. Moreover, the risk of sensitizing subjects who are not sensitized to the antigen by intradermal injection of an allergen cannot be fully excluded. On the other hand, mast cells and basophils are sensitized with the same repertoire of IgEs in each donor. If donors are sensitive to particular allergens, mast cells and basophils of donors release various inflammatory mediators, such as histamine, in response to the allergens. Several cell molecules, such as CD203c, CD63 and CD69, expressed the activation on cell surface, therefore these cells are used as activation markers of basophils. Thus, both in vitro histamine release test and cell surface analysis by flow cytometry for peripheral blood basophils are sensitive, safe and reliable test for allergens that cause immediate type hypersensitivity. Griese et al. reported that the histamine release test showed higher sensitivity and specificity than a skin test or serum analysis such as ImmunoCAP, based on the comparison with bronchoprovocation of extrinsic asthmatic children [30]. Moreover, the basophil activation test (BAT) based on CD203c upregulation on the surface of basophils has been validated as a reliable tool for the diagnosis of IgE-mediated allergies [31, 32]. In chronic spontaneous urticaria (CSU), responsiveness of basophils in response to anti-IgE stimulation is considered to be an indicator of disease activity in CSU [33]. Thus, evaluation of basophils activation against allergens may be a useful marker of immediate type hypersensitivity or other basophil-involved diseases. However, current techniques to detect basophil activations may require tens of milliliters of peripheral blood or not reveal any result if basophils do not response to positive control (non-responder). Therefore, we applied SPR and SPRI sensors for evaluation of basophil activation [34, 35]. Human peripheral basophils can be isolated from the fresh blood of donors by density gradient separation, followed by magnetic depletion of non-basophils by magnetic-activated cell sorting (MACS). To clarify the potential of SPRI sensor for diagnosing immediate type allergy, we examined the RI changes in basophils of healthy donors and atopic dermatitis (AD) donors in response to sweat antigen, to which patients with AD are sensitized. We observed the increase of reflected light-intensity in the basophils of AD donors, but not in the basophils of non-atopic donors, suggesting that the SPRI sensor can evaluate specific activation of basophils in response to allergens [35]. Moreover, the technique requires only few number of basophils (5–10 basophils) which is logically isolated from a few microliter of peripheral blood. We also developed a micro fluidic devise in order to isolate basophils from small blood with magnet power, transport the isolated cells to multiple SPRI-sensing area, and stimulate the basophils with various allergens for rapid and reliable diagnosis of immediate type hypersensitivity by using microfluidic device with magnetic separation techniques [36, 37].

7.3.3 High-Resolution SPRI Sensors for Living Cell Analysis

The spatial resolution of SPRI is much less than that of optical microscopy. In order to improve the spatial resolution of SPRI, several systems based on total internal reflection fluorescence microscopy (TIRFM) technique have been reported [38, 39]. The resolution of these techniques is 300 nm, which is approximately equivalent to the theoretical limit of SPRI. These techniques may allow us to obtain detailed sub-micrometer information of local RI in single cells.

7.3.4 Long-Range SPR and SPRI Sensors for Living Cell Analysis

As we described above, SPR and SPRI sensors using visible light as a light source can detect RI changes on the sensor surface with a depth of detection less than 500 nm, which is much smaller than cell height (few micrometers). Therefore, SPR sensors using visible light or conventional structure of SPR sensor chip detect RI changes only near the plasma membrane of living cells (500 nm from the surface of gold film). In order to extend the detection depth of SPR and SPRI sensors, several techniques may be applied. Fourier-transform infrared spectroscopy (FTIR-SPR) using near-infrared wavelengths can extend detection depth up to 10 μm, depending upon the IR wavelength (0.8–5 um) as a light source. Ziblat et al. monitored changes of occupancy and biochemical composition of cholesterol in plasma membrane of whole cells with FTIR-SPR [40]. Long-range SPR (LRSPR) system with multiple-layered structure for molecule interactions and living cells analysis have also been reported [41, 42]. These are based on the results that LRSPR sensors can transparent the resin, such as Cytop® by manipulating the detection depth, which is up to 1,000 nm or more by changing incident light wavelength and/or thickness of gold film. Thus, the long depth analysis of RI changes in living cells by FTIR-SPR and/or LRSPR systems may clarify detailed vertical information of RI in living cells.

7.3.5 Multi-Parametric Cell Analysis by SPR and SPRI Sensors

The information detected by using SPR and SPRI is limited to RI changes in the detection area on the gold thin film. Recently, several techniques as multi-parametric sensors have been reported. Zhang et al. proposed a method for simultaneous measurement of RI distribution and cyclic voltammetry using electrochemical-surface plasmon resonance imaging (EC-SPRI) [43]. Combining mass spectrometry (MS) with SPR sensors may identify chemical structures of the captured molecules on the surface of SPR sensor chip [44, 45]. Michaelis et al. reported a technique to detect both impedance and RI changes in living cells at the same time using electric cell substrate impedance sensing (ECIS)-SPR sensors [46]. We also developed SPRI-impedance (SPRI-IMP) sensor for simultaneous monitoring of living cell-derived RI and impedance changes on a sensor chip [47]. The SPRI-IMP sensor chips (S-LAL10, RI = 1.72) were coated with a comb-shaped gold thin film (1.0 nm Cr and 49 nm gold layer) with finger width/spacing of 20 μm by means of vapor deposition. Using this technique, we successfully monitored RI distribution and impedance which reflect the condition of RBL-2H3 cells cultured on a sensor chip without any labeling [47]. Thus, multi-parametric living cell analysis may provide complementary information regarding function and behavior of living cells.

7.4 Summary

SPR and SPRI sensors can detect and visualize living-cell reactions and conditions in real-time manner without any labeling. Long range-, high resolution- and multiparametric-SPR/SPRI sensors can clarify more detailed RI-related information of living cells. Thus, SPR- and SPRI-based techniques may be useful tools for research of cell biology and various clinical diagnoses.

Acknowledgments

We wish to thank Dr. Faiz Kermani for his manuscript review. This work was supported in part by Takeda Science Foundation, Grant-in-Aid for Scientific Research and Program for Promotion of Basic and Applied Researches for Innovation in Bio-oriented Industry.

References

1. Fivash M, Towler EM, Fisher RJ. BIAcore for macromolecular interaction. *Curr Opin Biotechnol.* 1998 Feb; 9(1): 97–101.
2. Liedberg B, Nylander C, Lundström I. Biosensing with surface plasmon resonance—how it all started. *Biosens Bioelectron.* 1995 Fall; 10(8): i–ix.
3. Homola J. Present and future of surface plasmon resonance biosensors. *Anal Bioanal Chem.* 2003 Oct; 377(3): 528–539.
4. Szabo A, Stolz L, Granzow R. Surface plasmon resonance and its use in biomolecular interaction analysis (BIA). *Curr Opin Struct Biol.* 1995 Oct; 5(5): 699–705.
5. Piliarik M, Vaisocherová H, Homola J. A new surface plasmon resonance sensor for high-throughput screening applications. *Biosens Bioelectron.* 2005 Apr 15; 20(10): 2104–2110.
6. Kodoyianni V. Label-free analysis of biomolecular interactions using SPR imaging. *Biotechniques.* 2011 Jan; 50(1): 32–40.
7. Yanase Y, Hiragun T, Kaneko S, Gould HJ, Greaves MW, Hide M. Detection of refractive index changes in individual living cells by means of surface plasmon resonance imaging. *Biosens Bioelectron.* 2010 Oct 15; 26(2): 674–681.
8. Yanase Y, Hiragun T, Yanase T, Kawaguchi T, Ishii K, Kumazaki N, Obara T, Hide M. (2014) Clinical diagnosis of type I allergy by means of SPR imaging with less than a microliter of peripheral blood. *Sens Bio-Sens Res.* 2: 43–48.
9. Hide M, Tsutsui T, Sato H, Nishimura T, Morimoto K, Yamamoto S, Yoshizato K. Real-time analysis of ligand-induced cell surface and intracellular reactions of living mast cells using a surface plasmon resonance-based biosensor. *Anal Biochem.* 2002 Mar 1; 302(1): 28–37.
10. Yanase Y, Suzuki H, Tsutsui T, Hiragun T, Kameyoshi Y, Hide M. The SPR signal in living cells reflects changes other than the area of

adhesion and the formation of cell constructions. *Biosens Bioelectron.* 2007 Jan 15; 22(6): 1081–1086.

11. Yanase Y, Suzuki H, Tsutsui T, Uechi I, Hiragun T, Mihara S, Hide M. Living cell positioning on the surface of gold film for SPR analysis. *Biosens Bioelectron.* 2007 Nov 30; 23(4): 562–567.
12. Tanaka M, Hiragun T, Tsutsui T, Yanase Y, Suzuki H, Hide M. Surface plasmon resonance biosensor detects the downstream events of active PKCbeta in antigen-stimulated mast cells. *Biosens Bioelectron.* 2008 Jun 15; 23(11): 1652–1658.
13. Varricchi G, Raap U, Rivellese F, Marone G, Gibbs BF. Human mast cells and basophils-How are they similar how are they different? *Immunol Rev.* 2018 Mar; 282(1): 8–34.
14. Chabot V, Cuerrier CM, Escher E, Aimez V, Grandbois M, Charette PG. Biosensing based on surface plasmon resonance and living cells. *Biosens Bioelectron.* 2009 Feb 15; 24(6): 1667–1673.
15. Lee SH, Ko HJ, Park TH. Real-time monitoring of odorant-induced cellular reactions using surface plasmon resonance. *Biosens Bioelectron.* 2009 Sep 15; 25(1): 55–60.
16. Kosaihira A, Ona T. Rapid and quantitative method for evaluating the personal therapeutic potential of cancer drugs. *Anal Bioanal Chem.* 2008 Jul; 391(5): 1889–1897.
17. Nishijima H, Kosaihira A, Shibata J, Ona T. Development of signaling echo method for cell-based quantitative efficacy evaluation of anti-cancer drugs in apoptosis without drug presence using high-precision surface plasmon resonance sensing. *Anal Sci.* 2010; 26(5): 529–534.
18. Yanase Y, Hiragun T, Kaneko S, Gould HJ, Greaves MW, Hide M. Detection of refractive index changes in individual living cells by means of surface plasmon resonance imaging. *Biosens Bioelectron.* 2010 Oct 15; 26(2): 674–681.
19. Horii M, Shinohara H, Iribe Y, Suzuki M. Living cell-based allergen sensing using a high resolution two-dimensional surface plasmon resonance imager. *Analyst.* 2011 Jul 7; 136(13): 2706–2711.
20. Mir TA, Shinohara H. Two-dimensional surface plasmon resonance imager: An approach to study neuronal differentiation. *Anal Biochem.* 2013 Dec 1; 443(1): 46–51.
21. Schasfoort RB, Bentlage AE, Stojanovic I, van der Kooi A, van der Schoot E, Terstappen LW, Vidarsson G. Label-free cell profiling. *Anal Biochem.* 2013 Aug 1; 439(1): 4–6.

22. Szittner Z, Bentlage AEH, van der Donk E, Ligthart PC, Lissenberg-Thunnissen S, van der Schoot CE, Vidarsson G. Multiplex blood group typing by cellular surface plasmon resonance imaging. *Transfusion*. 2019 Feb; 59(2): 754–761.

23. Nelson RW, Krone JR, Jansson O. Surface plasmon resonance biomolecular interaction analysis mass spectrometry. 2. Fiber optic-based analysis. *Anal Chem*. 1997 Nov 1; 69(21): 4369–4374.

24. Mitsushio M, Higashi S, Higo M. Theoretical analysis of gold-deposited optical fiber sensor and characterization of the gold film. *Anal Sci*. 2003 Oct; 19(10): 1421–1426.

25. Zhao Y, Tong RJ, Xia F, Peng Y. Current status of optical fiber biosensor based on surface plasmon resonance. *Biosens Bioelectron*. 2019 Oct 1; 142: 111505.

26. Yanase Y, Araki A, Suzuki H, Tsutsui T, Kimura T, Okamoto K, Nakatani T, Hiragun T, Hide M. Development of an optical fiber SPR sensor for living cell activation. *Biosens Bioelectron*. 2010 Jan 15; 25(5): 1244–1247.

27. Plebani M. Clinical value and measurement of specific IgE. *Clin Biochem*. 2003 Sep; 36(6): 453–469.

28. Shen M, Joshi AA, Vannam R, Dixit CK, Hamilton RG, Kumar CV, Rusling JF, Peczuh MW. Epitope-resolved detection of peanut-specific IgE antibodies by surface plasmon resonance imaging. *Chembiochem*. 2018 Feb 2; 19(3): 199–202.

29. Codreanu F, Morisset M, Cordebar V, Kanny G, Moneret-Vautrin DA. Risk of allergy to food proteins in topical medicinal agents and cosmetics. *Eur Ann Allergy Clin Immunol*. 2006 Apr; 38(4): 126–130.

30. Griese M, Kusenbach G, Reinhardt D. Histamine release test in comparison to standard tests in diagnosis of childhood allergic asthma. *Ann Allergy*. 1990 Jul; 65(1): 46–51.

31. Sturm EM, Kranzelbinder B, Heinemann A, Groselj-Strele A, Aberer W, Sturm GJ. CD203c-based basophil activation test in allergy diagnosis: Characteristics and differences to CD63 upregulation. *Cytometry B Clin Cytom*. 2010 Sep; 78(5): 308–318.

32. Oda Y, Washio K, Fukunaga A, et al. Clinical utility of the basophil activation test in the diagnosis of sweat allergy. *Allergol. Int*. 2020 Apr; 69(2): 261–267.

33. Oda Y, Fukunaga A, Washio K, Imamura S, Hatakeyama M, Ogura K, Nishigori C. Low responsiveness of basophils via FcεRI reflects disease activity in chronic spontaneous urticaria. *J Allergy Clin Immunol Pract*. 2019; 7(8): 2835–2844.e7. doi: 10.1016/j.jaip.2019.05.020.

34. Yanase Y, Suzuki H, Tsutsui T, Uechi I, Hiragun T, Mihara S, Hide M. Living cell positioning on the surface of gold film for SPR analysis. *Biosens Bioelectron*. 2007 Nov 30; 23(4): 562–567.

35. Yanase Y, Hiragun T, Yanase T, Kawaguchi T, Ishii K, Hide M. Evaluation of peripheral blood basophil activation by means of surface plasmon resonance imaging. *Biosens Bioelectron*. 2012 Feb 15; 32(1): 62–68.

36. Yanase Y, Sakamoto K, Kobayashi K, Hide M. Diagnosis of immediate-type allergy using surface plasmon resonance. *Opt Mater Express*. 6(4), 1339–1348.

37. Kobayashi K, Sakamoto K, Yanase Y, Hide M, Miyake R. Micro cell isolation column for allergic diagnosis. *Japanese J Appl Phys*. 55(3S2), 03DF08.

38. Peterson AW, Halter M, Tona A, Plant AL. High resolution surface plasmon resonance imaging for single cells. *BMC Cell Biol*. 2014 Dec 1; 15: 35.

39. Howe CL, Webb KF, Abayzeed SA, Anderson DJ, Denning C, Russell NA. Surface plasmon resonance imaging of excitable cells. *J Phys D Appl Phys*. 2019 Mar 6; 52(10): 104001.

40. Ziblat R, Lirtsman V, Davidov D, Aroeti B. Infrared surface plasmon resonance: A novel tool for real time sensing of variations in living cells. *Biophys J*. 2006 Apr 1; 90(7): 2592–2599.

41. Wark AW, Lee HJ, Corn RM. Long-range surface plasmon resonance imaging for bioaffinity sensors. *Anal Chem*. 2005 Jul 1; 77(13): 3904–3907.

42. Yang CT, Méjard R, Griesser HJ, Bagnaninchi PO, Thierry B. Cellular micromotion monitored by long-range surface plasmon resonance with optical fluctuation analysis. *Anal Chem*. 2015 Feb 3; 87(3): 1456–1461.

43. Zhang LL, Chen X, Wei HT, Li H, Sun JH, Cai HY, Chen JL, Cui DF. An electrochemical surface plasmon resonance imaging system targeting cell analysis. *Rev Sci Instrum*. 2013 Aug; 84(8), doi: 10.1063/1.4819027.

44. Xue J, Bai Y, Liu H. Hybrid methods of surface plasmon resonance coupled to mass spectrometry for biomolecular interaction analysis. *Anal Bioanal Chem*. 2019 Jul; 411(17): 3721–3729.

45. Madeira A, Ohman E, Nilsson A, Sjögren B, Andrén PE, Svenningsson P. Coupling surface plasmon resonance to mass spectrometry to discover novel protein-protein interactions. *Nat Protoc*. 2009; 4(7): 1023–1037.

46. Yanase, Y, Yoshizaki, K, Kimura, K, Kawaguchi, T, Hide, M, and Uno, S. (2019). Development of SPR imaging-impedance sensor for multi-parametric living cell analysis, *Int J Mol Sci.* 20(1), 45.

47. Michaelis S, Wegener J, Robelek R. Label-free monitoring of cell-based assays: Combining impedance analysis with SPR for multiparametric cell profiling. *Biosens Bioelectron.* 2013 Nov 15; 49: 63–70.

48. Yanase Y, Hiragun T, Yanase T, Kawaguchi T, Ishii K, Hide M. Application of SPR imaging sensor for detection of individual living cell reactions and clinical diagnosis of type I allergy. *Allergol Int.* 2013 Jun; 62(2): 163–169.

Chapter 8

Oximetry for Various Tissues Using Near-Infrared Spectroscopy

Masatsugu Niwayama

Research Institute of Electronics, Shizuoka University, 3-5-1 Johoku, Nakaku, Hamamatsu 432-8561, Japan

niwayama.masatsugu@shizuoka.ac.jp

Tissue oximeters using near-infrared spectroscopy (NIRS) have been applied for evaluating the viability of cerebral tissue in surgery and for monitoring muscle oxygenation in sport medicine and rehabilitation. We developed NIRS devices for muscles and the brain to measure deep and superficial tissues as well as a finger-mounted oximeter for the fetus and a neonate by miniaturizing the optical probe and analyzing light propagation in the layered tissue model. Various applications are also progressing to evaluate the flaps oxygenation and observe cerebral cortex activity. We outlined the principle of oximetry, its medical device development, and its applications.

Biomedical Engineering
Edited by Akihiro Miyauchi and Yuji Miyahara

ISBN 978-981-4877-63-3 (Hardcover), 978-1-003-14194-5 (eBook)
www.jennystanford.com

8.1 Introduction

In medical applications using spectroscopy, visible and near-infrared light (wavelengths between 650 nm and 1000 nm) is selected to focus on hemodynamics. Hemoglobin is an iron-containing protein in red blood cells. One mole of deoxygenated hemoglobin (HHb) binds with four moles of oxygen to become oxygenated hemoglobin (O_2Hb). The absorption spectra of oxygenated hemoglobin and deoxygenated hemoglobin [1] are shown in Fig. 8.1. The absorption for water is small at wavelengths between about 200 nm and about 900 nm. Considering all components related to absorption in biological tissues, measurements at wavelengths between 700 and 950 nm are particularly suitable for spectroscopy.

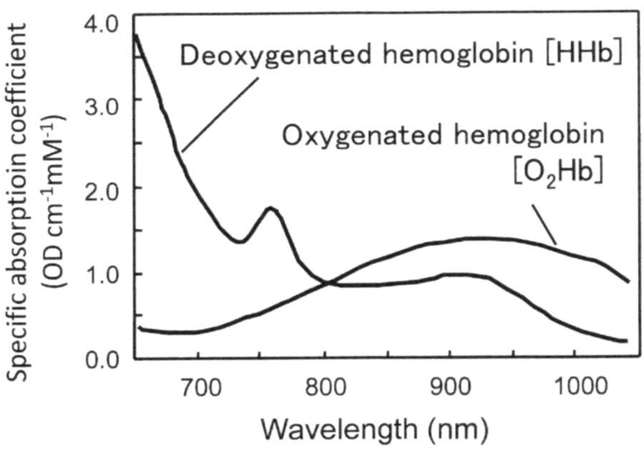

Figure 8.1 Absorption spectrum of oxygenated hemoglobin (O_2Hb) and deoxygenated hemoglobin (HHb).

Spectroscopic measurement of in vivo tissue was first studied by Nicolai et al. [2] in 1932. They examined the optical characteristics of hemoglobin. Ten years later, the first practical ear oximeter for aviation use was developed by Millikan [3]. In 1949, Wood and Geraci [4] modified this instrument to obtain absolute values of oxygen saturation of arterial blood. The basic idea of this instrument was used to manufacture ear oximeters that were used in clinical settings until the 1970s. However, ear oximeters did not have sufficient measurement stability for continuous monitoring of oxygen saturation because the calibration procedures were based on many assumptions. In 1974, Aoyagi et al. [5] presented a new idea called pulse oximetry, which utilizes the pulsation of arteries. This method allowed the accurate measurement of the oxygen saturation of arterial blood without the influence of factors other than arterial blood. Pulse oximetry is now used in clinical medicine throughout the world. As mentioned above, oxygen saturation of arterial blood mainly reflects gas exchange occurring in the lungs and is an important factor for respiratory care. However, from the viewpoint of metabolism in tissues, measurement of blood oxygenation within the capillaries of each tissue is desirable.

In 1977, Jöbsis utilized the relatively high penetration of near-infrared light and demonstrated that it was possible to measure the attenuation spectrum across the head of a cat, thereby obtaining information about tissue oxygenation [6]. In near-infrared spectroscopy (NIRS), tissue oxygenation is determined by analyzing the reflected or transmitted light intensity. However, NIRS using transmitted light is not suitable for clinical measurement because it is difficult to detect the transmitted light in adult human tissues. Therefore, reflection techniques are most commonly used nowadays. Several clinical studies on NIRS were conducted in the 1980s, including those by Ferrari et al. [7], Brazy et al. [8], Chance et al. [9], and Hoshi et al. [10]. They detected changes in concentrations of oxy and deoxyhemoglobin and in the cytochrome c oxidase redox state. They also demonstrated that NIRS is a useful, noninvasive technique for rapid detection of changes in tissue oxygenation. This chapter outlines tissue oximetry by NIRS, and also mentions NIRS devices applied to various applications by miniaturization and new calculation algorithm.

8.2 Measurement of Optical Absorption Coefficient

Four major experimental techniques exist in the field of NIR spectroscopy as shown in Fig. 8.2. The simplest one is continuous-wave spectroscopy (CWS) in which light of constant intensity is injected into the tissue, and then the attenuated light signal is measured at a distance from the light source. More elaborate approaches are spatially resolved spectroscopy (SRS), phase-modulated spectroscopy (PMS), and time-resolved spectroscopy (TRS). In TRS, temporal changes in the reflected light intensity are measured after irradiation of a picosecond pulse, thereby giving a distribution of the total path length of a photon traveling in the scattering medium. This technique can be used to determine the absorption coefficient and the reduced scattering coefficient of tissues. In SRS, an absorption coefficient is calculated from a spatial profile of light intensity. The details are described in the next section. In phase-modulated (frequency domain) measurements, pulse code or phase modulation gives mean time delay between the source and the detector. The time delay is related to light scattering and absorption, including biological signals. Table 8.1 shows a comparison of the four approaches.

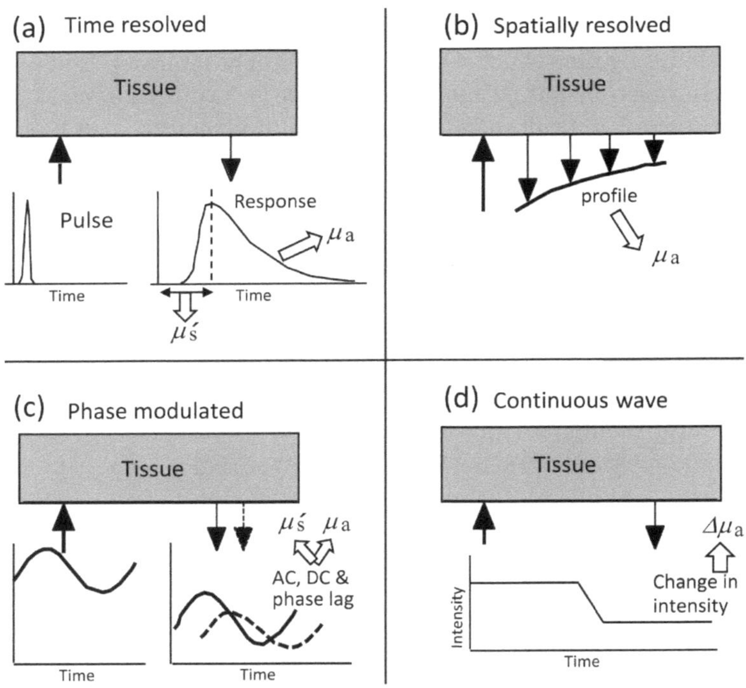

Figure 8.2 Methods for measuring optical properties using time resolved reflectance (upper left), spatially-resolved intensity profile (upper right), phase modulated wave (bottom left) and continuous wave (bottom right).

Table 8.1 Comparison of measurement methods

Method	Measured value	Light source	Detector	Size	Cost (Yen)
TRS	μ_a and μ_s'	High-speed laser	PMT	Desktop	1×10^7 to 2×10^7
PMS	μ_a and μ_s'	High-speed laser	APD	Desktop	5×10^6 to 1×10^7
SRS	μ_a	LED, Laser	PD	Wearable	5×10^5 to 2×10^6
CWS	$\Delta\mu_a$	LED, Laser	PD	Wearable	5×10^5 to 2×10^6

Abbreviations: PMT, photomultiplier tube; APD, avalanche photodiode; PD, photodiode.

In CWS, scattered light is detected at a distance from the light source, and tissue oxygenation is determined from the change in absorption coefficients of a tissue using the basic equations of conventional oximetry. Oximetry is the colorimetric measurement of the degree of oxygen saturation. Assuming that changes in light absorption are mainly due to changes in blood oxygenation or volume, $[O_2Hb]$ and $[HHb]$ can be determined as follows. Change in the absorption coefficient of a tissue a $\Delta\mu_a$ is expressed as

$$\Delta\mu = \varepsilon^{\lambda}_{O_2Hb}\Delta[O_2Hb] + \varepsilon^{\lambda}_{HHb}\Delta[HHb], \tag{8.1}$$

where $\varepsilon^{\lambda}_{O_2Hb}$ and $\varepsilon^{\lambda}_{HHb}$ are the extinction coefficients of HHb and O_2Hb, respectively, at the wavelengths λ. For example, $\varepsilon^{\lambda}_{HHb}$ at a wavelength of 760 nm is 0.1674 mM^{-1} mm^{-1} as reported by Matcher et al. [1]. In the above equations, $\varepsilon^{\lambda}_{HHb}$ of 0.385 mM^{-1} mm^{-1} (= 0.1674 × ln10) is used because the optical density is defined as the logarithm to base ten in their paper and μ_a is defined in base *e*. The two unknowns, $\Delta[O_2Hb]$ and $\Delta[HHb]$, are obtained from measurements at two wavelengths.

$$\Delta[O_2Hb] = \frac{1}{k}\left(\varepsilon^{\lambda 2}_{HHb}\Delta\mu_{a1} - \varepsilon^{\lambda 1}_{HHb}\Delta\mu_{a2}\right) \tag{8.2}$$

$$\Delta[HHb] = \frac{-1}{k}\left(\varepsilon^{\lambda 2}_{O_2Hb}\Delta\mu_{a1} - \varepsilon^{\lambda 1}_{O_2Hb}\Delta\mu_{a2}\right)O_2 \tag{8.3}$$

$$k = \varepsilon^{\lambda 1}_{\mathrm{O2Hb}}\varepsilon^{\lambda 2}_{\mathrm{HHb}} - \varepsilon^{\lambda 1}_{\mathrm{HHb}}\varepsilon^{\lambda 2}_{\mathrm{O2Hb}}. \tag{8.4}$$

The change in absorption $\Delta\mu_a$ can be determined by various NIRS techniques, such as CWS, SRS, PMS, and TRS. The CWS method, which is the simplest one, only enables determination of the change in absorption, whereas the corresponding optical properties in absolute values can be obtained by using the other techniques. However, even in these techniques, it is difficult to eliminate the effects of absorption other than that of hemoglobin, such as absorption of myoglobin. In CW-NIRS, change in the optical density, defined by $\Delta \mathrm{OD} = \ln(R_0/R)$, where R_0 and R are intensities of back-scattered light at a reference state (usually taken at the start of measurement) and during the measurement, respectively, is measured. Assuming that the scattering coefficient does not change during the measurement, we can determine $\Delta\mu_a$ using the modified Beer–Lambert law: $\Delta \mathrm{OD} = \Delta\mu_a d$, where $d = \partial \mathrm{OD}/\partial\mu_a$, which is equal to the mean optical path length. CWS systems measure only changes in OD (ΔOD), and usually, at least two different wavelengths are used to obtain spectral information. Relative changes of O_2Hb and HHb are continuously monitored utilizing Eqs. 8.2 and 8.3. Although the CW method gives only relative values, it is sufficient for many cases, such as studies of the functional activity of the brain or interventional studies for testing reactions on drugs or changes in treatment.

8.3 Principle of SRS Oximeter

Patterson et al. [11] proposed that the effective attenuation coefficient μ_{eff} of tissues can be obtained by measuring the spatial profile of the intensity of back-scattered light as a function of the distance from the light source using a large source–detector separation. They showed that the intensity of reflected light R can be expressed as follows:

$$R = \frac{\exp(-\mu_{\mathrm{eff}})}{\rho^2}, \tag{8.5}$$

where, $\mu_{\mathrm{eff}} = \sqrt{3\mu_a(\mu_a + m_s')}$.

In the case of CW spectroscopy, the local reflectance $I(\rho)$ at position ρ is expressed as an integral of $R(\rho, t)$ over time, and normalize OD is defined as the negative of the logarithm of $I(\rho)$, and is expressed by Eq. (8.6):

$$\begin{aligned} \mathrm{OD} &= -\ln I(\rho) \\ &\approx -\ln\left(\frac{z_0}{2\pi}\right) + 3\ln(\rho) - \ln(\mu_{\mathrm{eff}}\rho) + \mu_{\mathrm{eff}}\rho \end{aligned} \tag{8.6}$$

where, z_0 is depth of light propagation and is the reciprocal of reduced scattering coefficient. Differentiating OD with respect to ρ and assuming that $\mu_a << \mu_s'$ yield the following relation [12]:

$$\begin{aligned} \frac{\partial \mathrm{OD}}{\partial \rho} &= \frac{2}{\rho} + \sqrt{3(\mu_a + \mu_s')} \\ \therefore \mu_a \mu_s' &= \frac{1}{3}\left(\frac{\partial \mathrm{OD}}{\partial \rho} - \frac{2}{\rho}\right)^2, \end{aligned} \tag{8.7}$$

where is the local gradient of attenuation with respect to the source-detector separation. In the first-order approximation, μ_s' can be assumed to be constant within a narrow wavelength region in the NIR light.

The sensitivity of CWS is known to be determined by the mean optical path length L. The relationship between path length and SRS sensitivity is calculated using the voxel-based simulation model (Fig. 8.3) as follows [13]. The mean path length $\bar{L}$ of the voxel in Fig. 8.3 was calculated by $\Sigma L_i I_i / \Sigma I_i$, where L_i is the path length of i-th photon in the voxel and I_i is the final intensity of the i-th photon at a detector. To focus on the spatial sensitivities in the x-axis and z-axis directions, sensitivity values of the voxel were summed up in the y-axis direction and illustrated. The distribution of sensitivities in an x–y plane at each layer was also obtained. I_A is the light intensity detected over a short distance ρ_A from the light source, and I_B is the intensity detected over a longer distance ρ_B. As the spatial intensity slope S is the difference in light intensity per unit length, S is defined as $\ln(I_A/I_B)$. The change in S given a change in the absorption coefficient μ_a is then defined as the measurement sensitivity of SRS. The values of S are taken from optical measurements, and the unknown absorption coefficients are derived from the values of S and the theoretical curves. In Eq. (8.8), suffixes 1 and 2 denote values before and after the small change in absorption, respectively. The ΔS associated with a change in optical density ΔOD and the mean path lengths L_A and L_B is then derived as follows:

$$\begin{aligned} DS &= \ln\left(\frac{I_{2A}}{I_{2B}}\right) - \ln\left(\frac{I_{1A}}{I_{1B}}\right) \\ &= \ln\left(\frac{I_{2A}}{I_{1A}}\right) - \ln\left(\frac{I_{2B}}{I_{1B}}\right) \\ &= -\Delta \mathrm{OD_A} + \Delta \mathrm{OD_B} \\ &= \Delta \mu_a (L_B - L_A). \end{aligned} \tag{8.8}$$

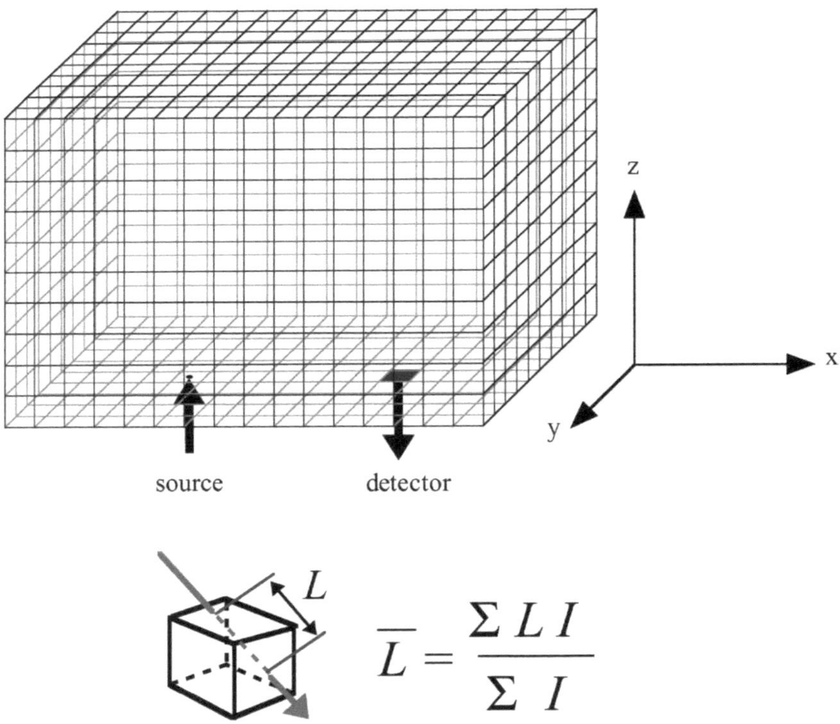

Figure 8.3 A model divided into voxels and the calculation of mean optical path length in the voxel.

In CWS, sensitivity is usually based on the mean path length, whereas in SRS the sensitivity is also influenced by the difference between L_A and L_B. On the basis of this relationship, the sensitivity of SRS for a small voxel at point (x, y, z) is given by

$$\Delta S_{x,y,z} = \Delta\mu_a^{x,y,z}(L_B^{x,y,z} - L_A^{x,y,z}). \tag{8.9}$$

By preliminary analysis to investigate the slope change due to the increase of the whole μ_a or the voxel μ_a by 1%, it was verified that Eqs. (8.8) and (8.9) held when $\Delta\mu_a$ was small and the relationship between S and μ_a could be regarded as linear. The sensitivity for each layer is derived by integrating the voxel values in the same layer. The SRS sensitivity for the surface and deep layers is derived as follows:

$$\Delta S_{\text{surface}} = \Delta\mu_a^{\text{surface}}(L_B^{\text{surface}} - L_A^{\text{surface}}), \tag{8.10}$$

$$\Delta S_{\text{deep}} = \Delta\mu_a^{\text{deep}}(L_B^{\text{deep}} - L_A^{\text{deep}}). \tag{8.11}$$

For example, L_A^{surface} denotes the intensity-weighted average path length through the surface layer that the light detected at a position A has traversed. In order to clarify the influence of the change of S on the oximetry, the absorption coefficient is calculated by the commonly used equation as follows:

$$\mu_a \approx \frac{1}{3\mu_s'}\left(\frac{S}{\rho_B - \rho_A} - \frac{2}{\frac{\rho_A + \rho_B}{2}}\right)^2. \tag{8.12}$$

The concentrations of oxyhemoglobin $[O_2Hb]$, deoxy-hemoglobin [HHb], and tissue oxygen saturation StO_2 are obtained by

$$[O_2Hb] = \frac{\varepsilon_{HHb}^{\lambda 2}\mu_a^{\lambda 1} - \varepsilon_{HHb}^{\lambda 1}\mu_a^{\lambda 2}}{\varepsilon_{O_2Hb}^{\lambda 1}\varepsilon_{HHb}^{\lambda 2} - \varepsilon_{O_2Hb}^{\lambda 2}\varepsilon_{HHb}^{\lambda 1}}, \tag{8.13}$$

$$[HHb] = -\frac{\varepsilon_{O_2Hb}^{\lambda 2}\mu_a^{\lambda 1} - \varepsilon_{O_2Hb}^{\lambda 1}\mu_a^{\lambda 2}}{\varepsilon_{O_2Hb}^{\lambda 1}\varepsilon_{HHb}^{\lambda 2} - \varepsilon_{O_2Hb}^{\lambda 2}\varepsilon_{HHb}^{\lambda 1}}, \tag{8.14}$$

$$\mathrm{StO_2} = \frac{[\mathrm{O_2Hb}]}{[\mathrm{O_2Hb}] + [\mathrm{HHb}]}, \tag{8.15}$$

where $\varepsilon_{\mathrm{O_2Hb}}^{\lambda 1,\lambda 2}$ and $\varepsilon_{\mathrm{HHb}}^{\lambda 1,\lambda 2}$ are the extinction coefficients of HHb and O_2Hb, respectively, at the wavelengths λ_1 and λ_2. Tissue oxygen saturation StO_2 is a variable that sums the concentrations of whole blood in the arteries, veins and capillaries at the measurement site.

Figure 8.4 shows our developed NIRS for the muscle and an example of the measurement result of StO_2 in the forearm. It is possible to observe in real time how the StO_2 is reduced about 50% due to the hand grip exercise. In addition, a function has been added to display the blood volume and oxygenation status of the superficial tissue together, which will help analysis of the measurement results. In order to understand the measurement sensitivity of each part of the tissue, light propagation analysis is performed based on the Monte Carlo method, and the measurement sensitivity distribution for each voxel is clarified as shown in Fig. 8.5 [14]. The optical constants of each tissue were based on literature values [15–18]. These results shows the voxel-based sensitivity $\Delta S_{\mathrm{x,y,z}}$ from two model detector combinations: ρ_{A} = 7 mm, ρ_{B} = 35 mm, and ρ_{A} = 30 mm, ρ_{B} = 35 mm. The voxel was 0.5 mm on each side. The red/yellow/green plots represent positive changes in spatial slope for a 10% increase in absorption, and the blue/cyan plots represent negative changes. In both Figs. 8.5a,b, the sensitivity of the surface layer was negative close to detector A and positive close to detector B. When blood is in the negative sensitivity area, an incorrect reverse tendency will be mixed into the calculation results of the oxygen saturation and blood volume. At a ρ_{A} of 30 mm, a strong positive sensitivity was noted within a narrow range in the deep layer, but a small negative sensitivity appeared at the side near the light source. These results suggest the following: (1) When the surface layer is heterogeneous, as is the case for veins, wounds, or inflammation, the effect on the measured value is large and can be positive or negative. (2) When both detectors A and B are distant from the light source, many sites have negative sensitivity, but information can be obtained from a narrow region of the deep layer. (3) When the gap between ρ_A and ρ_B is sufficiently long, average information can be obtained across a wide area of the deep tissue. These results are useful for interpreting the measurements more accurately.

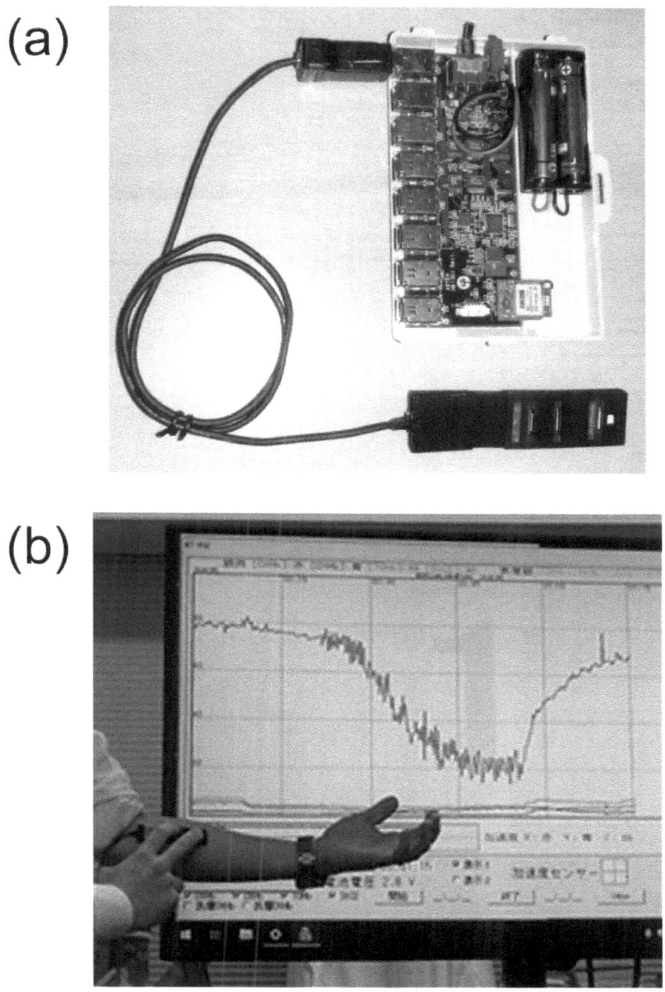

Figure 8.4 Tissue oximeter for the muscle (a) and typical trace of measurement for the forearm during grip exercise (b).

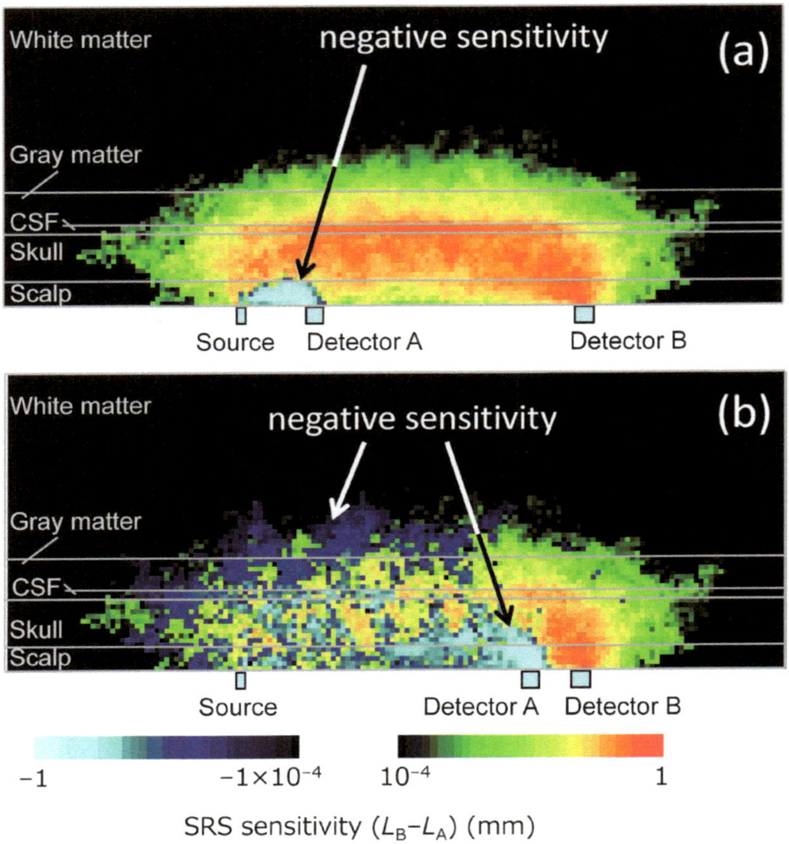

Figure 8.5 Sensitivity distribution obtained by Monte Carlo simulation from a head model: (a) ρ_A = 7 mm, ρ_B = 35 mm and (b) ρ_A = 30 mm, ρ_B = 35 mm.

8.4 Development of Oximeter for Various Tissues

In order to utilize various tissues, a calculation algorithm was developed in consideration of the multilayer structure of the tissues. Furthermore, we developed a finger-mounted NIRS that integrates the sensor with the doctor's fingertip by making the sensor probe ultra-small and thin [19, 20]. The sensor probe uses a flexible substrate made of polyimide and has a probe volume of

0.015 cm^3 (width 0.5 cm, length 1 cm, thickness 0.03 cm), which is less than one-hundredth of the conventional probe volume. Figure 8.6 shows a medical device (Astem Co., Ltd., Kawasaki, Japan, KN-15 Toccare) realized by collaborative research between the company and Hamamatsu University School of Medicine and Shizuoka University. We performed theoretical analysis of light propagation based on radiative transfer theory to produce calculation methods in a new sensor arrangement. In the case of various tissues, the sensitivity distribution was quantitatively analyzed in the same way as Fig. 8.5, namely considering the layer structure of each tissue. In this measurement, it was shown that information of about 4 to 5 mm was obtained in the depth direction.

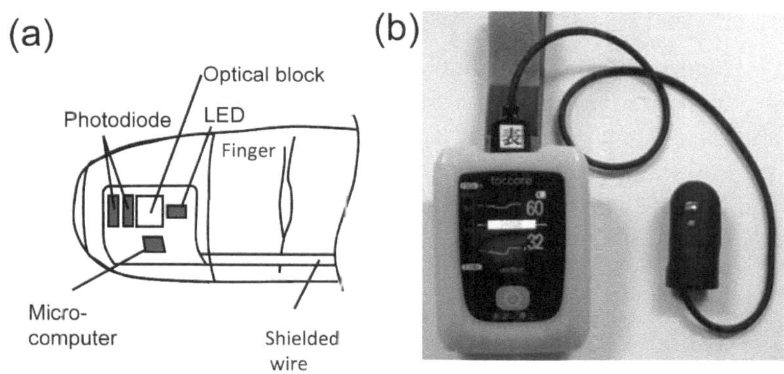

Figure 8.6 Schematic diagram of sensor unit in finger-mounted oximeter with miniaturized substrate (a) and photograph of developed NIRS instrument (b).

8.5 Application of Developed Device

Examiner's finger-mounted NIRS was first used for perinatal neonate and fetus [21, 22]. As shown in Fig. 8.7 (left), the oxygen saturation is displayed within few seconds after the doctor's finger touches the skin on the head, so it is possible to quantitatively determine whether or not the tissue is hypoxic. Thus, this NIRS device will be useful for clinical health care. Figure 8.7 (right) is a photograph when applied to measure the oxygenation state of tissue before and after operation in flap surgery. The NIRS instrument has been applied as a simple tissue oxygen monitor in the field of plastic surgery [23].

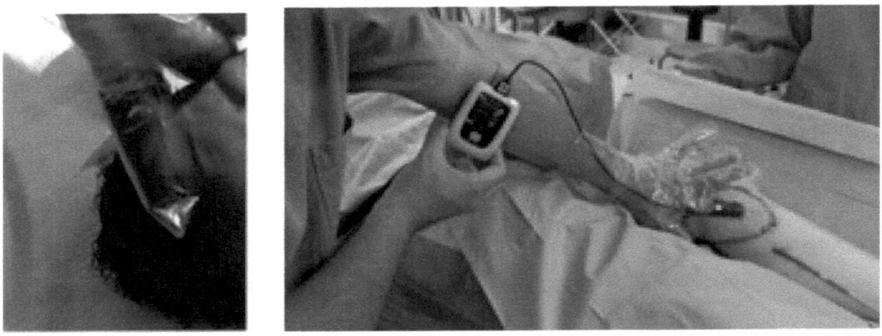

Figure 8.7 Measurement for the neonatal head after parturition (left) and the flap surgery (right) using finger-mounted oximeter.

Figure 8.8 shows an ultra-thin and flexible probe developed for implantation in the surface of the cerebral cortex [24, 25], and also shows a photograph of the probe implanted in the rat epidural. The combination of NIRS hemodynamic measurement and EEG (Electroencephalography) electrodes would contribute to more detailed analysis of cortical activity.

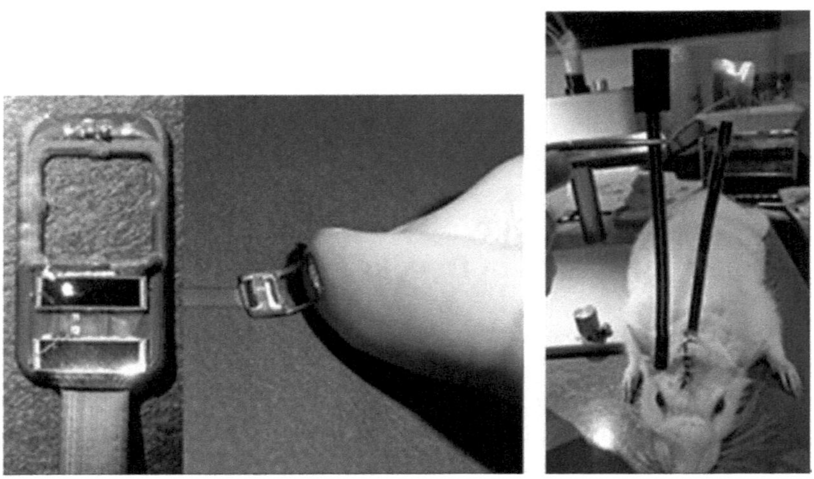

Figure 8.8 Implantable cerebral NIRS sensor (left) and animal experiments using subcutaneously embedded sensors (right).

8.6 Conclusion

An overview of tissue oximetry using near-infrared spectroscopy was given, along with the latest practical examples of tissue oximeters using spatially-resolved methods. The technology of accuracy improvement and miniaturization led to the practical application of new medical devices. Near-infrared oximetry is a non-invasive method that can determine the oxygen saturation of the tissue easily and immediately. Therefore, there will be further various needs as a method for grasping the viability of the tissues. The NIRS technology is expected to create a variety of new medical devices through collaboration between industry, medicine and engineering.

Acknowledgments

We thank Dr. Naohiro Kanayama, Dr. Naoki Unno, and Dr. Toshiyuki Uchida of Hamamatsu University School of Medicine for their valuable medical advice. We thank Mr. Hikaru Suzuki, Mr. Yutaka Yokoyama, and Mr. Yukio Chitose of Astem Co., Ltd., for their cooperation in prototype production of NIRS instruments.

References

1. Matcher, S. J., Elwell, C. E., Cooper, C. E., Cope, M., Delpy, D. T. (1995). Performance comparison of several published tissue near-infrared spectroscopy algorithms, *Anal. Biochem.*, **227**, pp. 54–68.
2. Nicolai, L. (1932). Über Sichtbarmachung, Verlauf und chemische Kinetik der Oxyhämoglobinreduktion im lebenden Gewebe, besonders in der menschlichen Haut, *Pflugers Arch.*, **229**, pp. 372–384.
3. Millikan, G. A. (1942). The oximeter, an instrument for measuring continuously the oxygen saturation of arterial blood in man, *Rev. Sci. Instrum.*, **13**, pp. 434–444.
4. Wood, E. H., Geraci, J. E. (1949). Photoelectric determination of arterial oxygen saturation in man, *J. Lab. Clin. Med.*, **34**, pp. 387–401.
5. Aoyagi, T. (1974). Improvement of the earpiece oximeter. *Abstr. Jpn. Soc. Med. Electron. Biol. Eng.*, 1974, pp. 90–91.

6. Jöbsis, F. F. (1977). Noninvasive, infrared monitoring of cerebral and myocardial oxygen sufficiency and circulatory parameters, *Science*, **198**, pp. 1264–1267.

7. Ferrari, M., Giannini, I., Sideri, G., Zanette, E. (1985). Continuous non invasive monitoring of human brain by near infrared spectroscopy, *Adv. Exp. Med. Biol.*, **191**, pp. 873–882.

8. Brazy, J. E., Lewis, D. V., Mitnick, M. H., Jöbsis vander Vliet, F. F. (1985). Noninvasive monitoring of cerebral oxygenation in preterm infants: Preliminary observations, *Pediatrics*, **75**, pp. 217–225.

9. Chance, B., Nioka, S., Kent, J., McCully, K., Fountain, M., Greenfeld, R., Holtom, G. (1988). Time-resolved spectroscopy of hemoglobin and myoglobin in resting and ischemic muscle, *Anal. Biochem.*, **174**, pp. 698–707.

10. Hoshi, Y., Tamura, M. (1993). Detection of dynamic changes in cerebral oxygenation coupled to neuronal function during mental work in man, *Neurosci. Lett.*, **150**, pp. 5–8.

11. Patterson, M. S., Chance B., Wilson B. C. (1989). Time resolved reflectance and transmittance for the non-invasive measurement of tissue optical properties, *Appl. Opt.*, **28**, pp. 2331–2336.

12. Zhang, H., Miwa, M., Urakami, T., Yamashita, Y., Tsuchiya, Y. (1998). Simple subtraction method for determining the mean path length traveled by photons in turbid media, *Jpn. J. Appl. Phys.*, **37**, pp. 700–704

13. Niwayama, M., Lin, L., Shao, J., Kudo, N., Yamamoto, K. (2000). Quantitative measurement of muscle hemoglobin oxygenation using near-infrared spectroscopy with correction for the influence of a subcutaneous fat layer, *Rev. Sci. Instrum.*, **71**, pp. 4571–4575.

14. Niwayama, M. (2018) Voxel-based measurement sensitivity of spatially resolved near-infrared spectroscopy in layered tissues, *J. Biomed. Opt.*, **23**, pp. 1–4.

15. Wan, S., Anderson, R. R., Parrish, J. A. (1981). Analytical modeling for the optical properties of the skin with in vitro and in vivo applications, *Photochem. Photobiol.*, **34**, pp. 493–499.

16. Beek, J. F. (1993). The influence of respiration on optical properties of piglet lung at 632.8 nm. Medical Optical Tomography.

17. Zaccanti, G., Taddeucci, A., Barilli, M., Bruscaglioni, P., Martelli, F. (1995). Optical properties of biological tissues. Optical Tomography, Photon Migration, and Spectroscopy of Tissue and Model Media:

Theory, Human Studies, and Instrumentation, *Proc. SPIE*, **2359**, pp. 513–521.

18. Jacques, S. L. (2013). Optical properties of biological tissues: A review, *Phys. Med. Biol.*, **58**, pp. R37–R61.
19. Kanayama, N., Niwayama, M. (2014) Examiner's finger-mounted fetal tissue oximetry, *J. Biomed. Opt.*, **19**, pp. 067008 1–5.
20. Uchida, T., Kanayama, N., Mukai, M., Furuta, N., Itoh, H., Suzuki, H., Niwayama, M. (2016). Examiner's finger-mounted fetal tissue oximetry: A preliminary report on 30 cases, *J. Perinat. Med.*, **44**, pp. 745–749.
21. Uchida, T., Kanayama, N., Kawai, K., Mukai, M., Suzuki, K., Itoh, H., Niwayama, M. (2018). Reevaluation of intrapartum fetal monitoring using fetal oximetry: A review, *J. Obstet. Gynaecol. Res.*, **44**, pp. 2127–2134.
22. Mukai, M., Uchida, T., Itoh, H., Suzuki, H., Niwayama, M., Kanayama, N. (2017). Tissue oxygen saturation levels from fetus to neonate, *J. Obstet. Gynaecol. Res.*, **43**, pp. 855–859.
23. Tsuge, I., Enoshiri, T., Saito, S., Suzuki, S. (2017). A quick evaluation of TRAM flap viability using fingerstall-type tissue oximetry, *Plast. Reconstr. Surg. Glob. Open*, **5**, e1494.
24. Niwayama, M., Yamakawa, T. (2014). Implantable thin NIRS probe design and sensitivity distribution analysis, *Electron. Lett.*, **50**, pp. 346–347.
25. Yamakawa, T., Inoue, T., He, Y., Fujii, M., Suzuki, M., Niwayama, M. (2014): Development of an implantable flexible probe for simultaneous near-infrared spectroscopy and electrocorticography, *IEEE Trans. Biomed. Eng.*, **61**, pp. 388–395.

Chapter 9

Development of THz Laser Spectrometer and Its Application for Pharmaceutical Inspection

Tetsuo Sasaki,[a,b] Tomoaki, Sakamoto,[b,c] and Makoto Otsuka[d]

[a]*Graduate School of Medical Photonics, Shizuoka University,*
3-5-1 Johoku, Naka-ku, Hamamatsu, Shizuoka 432-8011, Japan
[b]*Research Institute of Electronics, Shizuoka University,*
3-5-1 Johoku, Naka-ku, Hamamatsu, Shizuoka 432-8011, Japan
[c]*Division of Drugs, National Institute of Health Sciences,*
3-25-26 Tonomachi, Kawasaki-ku, Kawasaki, Kanagawa 210-9501 Japan
[d]*Research Institute of Pharmaceutical Sciences, Musashino University,*
Nishi-Tokyo, Tokyo 202-8585, Japan

sasaki.tetsuo@shizuoka.ac.jp

Terahertz (THz) frequencies are particularly sensitive to crystal structures, and thus can be used to examine small concentrations of defects within crystals, such as impurity molecules. In contrast to direct observation, the influence of the defect/impurity is evident in the response of the crystal to THz frequencies. Thus, THz spectroscopy provides the means to identify and control the defect concentration or impurity amount. For example, in pharmaceutical manufacturing applications, THz spectroscopy

Biomedical Engineering
Edited by Akihiro Miyauchi and Yuji Miyahara

ISBN 978-981-4877-63-3 (Hardcover), 978-1-003-14194-5 (eBook)
www.jennystanford.com

of solid molecular crystals provides high sensitivity and a low detection limit for pharmaceutical inspection.

In this chapter, we introduce our originally developed high-frequency-accuracy, high-frequency-resolution THz laser spectrometer. Using this spectrometer, we constructed a THz spectral database for pharmaceuticals, for use in drug material and crystal polymorph identification and quantification. Temperature-dependent THz spectra are useful for assigning absorption lines to molecular vibrations in the THz range. We also demonstrate trace impurity detection in pharmaceuticals and show that our approach is suitable for middle molecular weight pharmaceuticals, which are expected to become mainstream in the near future.

9.1 Introduction: Terahertz Waves and Terahertz Spectroscopy

Terahertz (THz) waves are electromagnetic waves with frequencies that between those of microwaves and infrared (IR) light. Initially, developments of THz wave applications were slow pace due to a lack of availability of a good light source. Following remarkable progress over the past three decades, however, the range of THz wave applications has advanced rapidly, as evidenced by THz developments in various fields including high-speed, high-capacity wireless communications [1] and screening of people, luggage, and packages for security purposes [2].

At present, IR spectroscopy is the most commonly used spectroscopic technique for identification and quantitative analysis of materials. The absorption lines observed in the mid-IR range generally correspond to the vibrational modes of molecular functional groups. In contrast, absorption lines in the THz range correspond to skeletal mode vibrations of the molecule or intermolecular mode vibration of the crystal, which are unique to the molecule, crystal, or crystal polymorph [3]. Probing these vibration modes using THz waves allows for in-depth analysis of the crystal structure and defects within the crystal [4, 5].

THz-time domain spectroscopy (THz-TDS) [6] uses a high-speed photoconductive switch to generate a short electromagnetic pulse with a femtosecond laser as the light source. This is the most commonly used configuration in THz spectroscopy research. However, the THz light source used for THz-TDS is not monochromatic; thus, the frequency resolution of the system is low.

Our group developed a wide frequency range, high-power THz-wave signal generator (THz-SG) using a gallium phosphide (GaP) crystal [7–9]. By applying the GaP THz-SG as the light source, we successfully identified organic materials, such as amino acids, DNA bases, and pharmaceuticals [10]. Since its conception, the original GaP THz-SG has been modified for continuous wave (CW) operation as a CW-THz SG, based on the same principle [11–15].

When using the CW-THz SG as the light source, the THz spectrometer attains much higher accuracy and resolution; as such, we refer to it as the THz laser spectrometer. Recently, we used the THz laser spectrometer to detect trace amounts of impurities via precise measurement of the absorption peak shift [16]. This technique is especially useful for detecting trace impurities in active pharmaceutical ingredients (APIs) during production. Moreover, THz laser spectroscopy can be used to evaluate the crystal quality of middle molecular weight (MMW) pharmaceuticals, which show very sharp absorption lines.

In this chapter, we describe the development of the THz laser spectrometer and discuss its application to pharmaceutical inspection.

9.2 Development of the THz Laser Spectrometer

A monochromatic, coherent THz wave can be generated according to the principle of difference frequency generation (DFG) of IR laser beams in a GaP crystal. A wide frequency range and high power are realized, based on the high transparency of GaP for both IR and THz waves. Two IR beams enter the GaP crystal at a small angle to satisfy the phase-matching condition, as shown in Fig. 9.1. When the energy and momentum conservation laws are fulfilled at the same time, coherent lattice vibration of the crystal generates THz waves. The THz frequency can be tuned by controlling the wavelength of the IR beams and the angle between the two beams at each frequency. A nanosecond-pulse THz-SG was realized as a first step, with frequency-variable pulse lasers excited by flash lamps. The pulse-type spectrometer did not obtain high frequency resolution due to the Fourier transform limit. Additionally, it did not have long-term stability due to the laser fluctuations resulting from flash lamp degradation. Recently, we realized a CW-THz SG using a fiber laser or fiber amplifier system as pump beams for the spectrometer [14, 15].

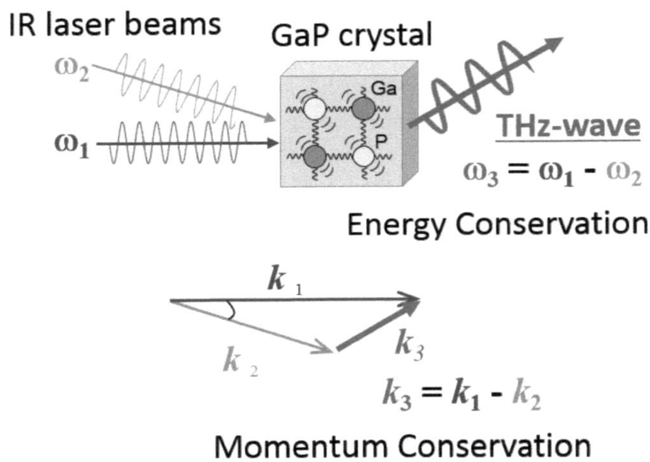

Figure 9.1 Terahertz (THz) wave generation based on difference frequency generation (DFG) under small-angle phase-matching conditions in a GaP crystal.

Monochromatic CW-THz emission has been achieved using low-temperature-grown gallium arsenide as a photoconductive switch [17–20] and two semiconductor lasers; despite the high resolution of this THz spectroscopy system, the frequency range was limited to 1.5 THz, as it showed exponential attenuation with increasing frequency. In this case, the difference frequency THz wave overlapped the large thermal radiation generated by pump beam absorption and Joule heating via the photocurrent.

Figure 9.2 shows a schematic diagram of our CW GaP THz spectrometer. A monochromatic, coherent THz beam is generated in the GaP crystal via DFG. Two IR beams are delivered from a distributed feedback laser (DFB; DL-DFB; Toptica Photonics AG, Munich, Germany) and a mode-hop-free external cavity diode laser (ECDL; λ-master 1040; Spectra Quest Lab, Inc., Chiba, Japan). Each beam can be amplified to a constant power of 10 W at any wavelength using polarization-maintained ytterbium (Yb)-doped optical fiber amplifiers (YbFAs; CYFAPB series; Keopsys, Lannion, France). The wavelength of the DFB laser ranges from 1,071.7 to 1,074.4 nm (279.0–279.7 THz), whereas that of the ECDL is continuously tunable from 1,000 to 1,080 nm (277.6–299.8 THz) but limited to between 1,050 and 1,075 nm (278.9–285.5 THz) in our system by the available range of the YbFAs. The wavelengths of the beams are monitored and controlled by a two-channel frequency meter (WS-7; HighFinesse GmbH, Tubingen, Germany) for simultaneous high frequency accuracy at any frequency. Laser power is monitored by thermal power meters and maintained by feedback control at each frequency. Absolute accuracy of the wave meter is guaranteed to 60 MHz, with frequent calibration using a standard wavelength. However, the accuracy of the generated THz frequency depends not on the "absolute accuracy," but rather on the "relative accuracy," for measurement of the wavelengths of the two IR beams, which were estimated to be a few MHz. The polarization of each beam is adjusted to be perpendicular with respect to the other beam by tilting the fiber output. The beams are then combined with a planar polarizer. To satisfy nonlinear phase-matching conditions, precise controls of the beam overlap, as well as of the small angle between the two beams inside the GaP crystal, are required at each frequency. The optimum phase-matching condition is established using a lens and a linear stage. In the system configuration, the GaP crystal can be tilted using a rotary stage to prevent total reflection of generated THz waves at the back surface. The THz output beam is then collected by parabolic mirrors and focused onto a niobium (Nb) transition edge superconductor (TES) bolometer, cooled by a low vibration pulse tube cooler (QNbB/PTC; QMC Instruments, Ltd., Cardiff, UK) after passing through the sample pellet set in a cryostat (Microstat He2; Oxford Instruments, Abingdon, UK) cooled by liquid helium/nitrogen. A black polyethylene (PE) sheet is used as an IR cut filter.

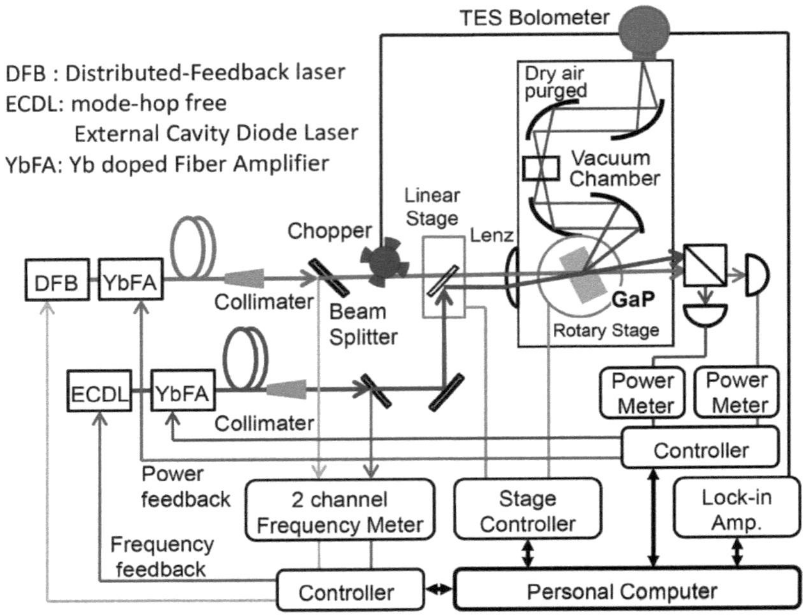

Figure 9.2 Schematic diagram of the THz spectrometer using a GaP continuous wave (CW)-THz signal generator (SG). The frequency and power of the pump beams are monitored by a frequency meter and a power meter, respectively, and are feedback controlled.

The sample temperature was controlled between 4 and 400 K, with better than ±0.05 K stability. The entire THz-wave path was purged with dry air to a dew point of less than −60°C, to avoid water vapor absorption effects. Lock-in detection of the THz wave with a chopping frequency of approximately 700 Hz afforded high sensitivity and long-term signal stability. The resulting spectra were highly reproducible, and the highest absolute frequency accuracy and resolution were 3.0 and 8.0 MHz, respectively [15]. Measurement sequences were controlled using software developed in our laboratory with a personal computer.

We confirmed THz power generation from 0.1 to 6.2 THz. The lowest frequency is limited by the reduction in THz output power, to close to the noise level. The highest frequency (6.2 THz) is limited by the tunable range of the ECLD. With respect to the maximum power and the noise floor level, the maximum signal-to-noise (S/N) ratio exceeded 1,000. We were able to observe

THz power, even with a low-sensitivity pyroelectric deuterated L-alanine triglycine sulfate detector operating without a cooler; however, this detector is not optimal for practical use, because the maximum S/N ratio does not exceed 10.

9.3 Typical THz Spectrum of Pharmaceuticals

Pharmaceutical development is one area in which THz spectroscopy can play an important role, as this technique is especially sensitive to quality degradation, e.g., during the manufacturing process and with respect to the shelf life. For example, polymorphs and pseudo-polymorphs of organic crystals, including pharmaceuticals, can easily be distinguished using THz spectroscopy, as they have unique spectra in this frequency regime [3, 21–23]. This suggests that THz spectroscopy can be used as a nondestructive analytical tool in pharmaceutical quality control testing or process analysis.

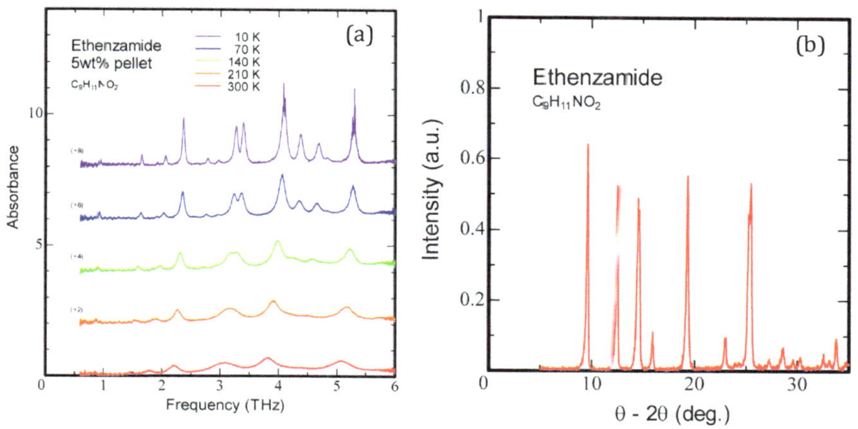

Figure 9.3 Temperature dependence of the THz absorption spectra of ethenzamide in the form of a 5 wt% pellet (a). Powder X-ray diffraction spectrum of the same sample (b).

However, absorption spectral data for pharmaceuticals in the THz frequency range have tended to be insufficient; this prompted us to create a THz spectral database for pharmaceuticals, as presented in [10]. Figure 9.3 (left) shows the temperature dependence of THz absorbance spectra for an ethenzamide 5 wt% powder pellet, as a typical example. The measurement temperature was 10, 70, 140, 210, and 300 K. The measurement time was almost 1 day for one sample. With decreasing temperature, sharp absorption lines appeared due to the suppression of thermal energy, which caused dispersion in the molecular vibration frequency. A low-temperature spectrum is also useful for comparison with quantum calculation results. Figure 9.3 (right) shows powder X-ray diffraction (XRD) spectra of the same sample. As the polymorph shows a different spectrum, it is important to confirm the crystal structure of the sample.

9.4 Vibrational Mode Assignments in the Terahertz Frequency Region

Many API materials in powder form show unique absorption lines in the THz frequency range. However, most of the absorption lines have not been assigned to the molecular vibrations of a particular crystal until now. Quantum chemical calculation facilitates a mode assignment, by comparing the vibrational frequencies and intensities of normal mode peaks with those obtained by absorption peak measurements. However, the calculation is complicated because very weak forces, such as intermolecular forces, are effective in the low-energy range (THz frequency range). Density functional theory (DFT) provides a compromise whereby the necessary accuracy can be obtained with a relatively small time cost.

A simple comparison between measurement and calculation results is not sufficient for vibrational mode assignment. For the APIs of typical pharmaceutical products, many absorption lines appear in the THz range and overlap each other. To resolve overlapping lines, spectral measurement at low temperatures is often effective. From the standpoint of calculations, normal modes are analyzed at 0 K; thus, it is preferable to compare these with absorption modes at low temperature. Exploiting the effect of an isotope shift (typically deuterium exchange) is one solution to achieve a precise comparison [24, 25]; the other involves using THz polarization spectroscopy. Accurate assignment is made possible by using THz polarization spectroscopy to compare crystal axis-dependent vibration (dipole moment) with the polarization-dependent spectra of a single crystal [26, 27].

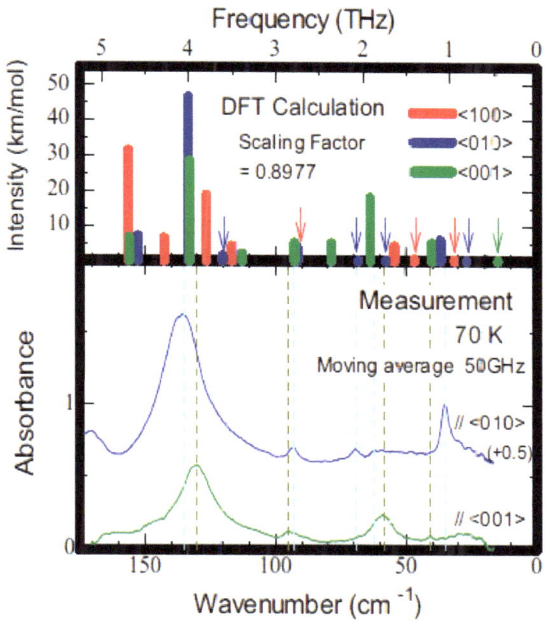

Figure 9.4 The top graph shows DFT calculated results of vibrational frequencies for theophylline crystal scaled with 0.8977 and intensities of each normal mode. The color indicates direction of the vibration. The graph below is the polarization dependent spectra for theophylline single crystal. Spectra for the polarization direction of THz wave parallel to <010> and <001> directions are blue and green lines, respectively.

As an example, single-crystal theophylline anhydrous (TPAH) was successfully fabricated by the temperature difference method in an aqueous solution. The crystal structure of the grown crystals was confirmed by powder XRD measurements, and the crystal orientation was verified in pole figure measurements. THz polarization spectroscopy measurements were performed on TPAH crystal samples at 70 K. Assignment of the absorption peaks was carried out by comparing the measurement results with those derived from DFT calculations under periodic boundary conditions. The top part of Fig. 9.4 shows the DFT-calculated results of vibrational frequencies and intensities of each normal mode; the bottom part of the figure shows the polarization THz spectra of the TPAH single crystal for the crystal angle parallel to the <010> and <001> directions [28]. Almost all of the calculated modes could be assigned to the measured absorption lines in each direction.

9.5 Sharp Absorption Spectra of Middle Molecular Weight Pharmaceuticals in the Terahertz Frequency Region

Producing novel pharmaceuticals based on conventional small molecular weight (SMW) chemical substances is becoming increasingly difficult, while the number of diseases requiring treatment is increasing. SMW pharmaceuticals generally have low target selectivity, which may be attributed to their molecular size. Large molecular weight (LMW) pharmaceuticals, such as antibody pharmaceuticals, have attracted much attention and constitute the majority of the new pharmaceutical products [29]. LMW pharmaceuticals have superior bioavailability and cause few side effects compared with conventional SMW pharmaceuticals due to their high target specificity and selectivity [30]. However, the use of LMW pharmaceuticals is limited because they must be administered by injection. Furthermore, they are relatively expensive because they are produced via cell culture.

MMW pharmaceuticals (MW: 400–4,000) are of interest for possible use in new medications [31, 32]. MMW pharmaceuticals have potentially superior bioavailability and few side effects due to their high target selectivity, and are less expensive to produce. Supplying MMW pharmaceuticals in crystal form, as is done for conventional SMW pharmaceuticals, is important for quality uniformity during manufacturing and long-term stability during storage [33].

We found that MMW pharmaceuticals show sharp absorption peaks at low temperatures, based on measurements obtained with a high-frequency resolution THz laser spectrometer [34, 35]; as examples, α-cyclodextrin hexahydrate, amoxicillin trihydrate, atorvastatin calcium trihydrate, probucol, and α, β, γ, δ-tetrakis(1-

methylpyridinium-4-yl)porphyrin p-toluenesulfonate (TMPyP) show sharp absorption peaks at 10 K. Typically, the observed full width at half maximum (FWHM) values are on the order of a few GHz. Such narrow absorption peaks enable inspection of MMW pharmaceuticals, especially for the evaluation of crystal quality, and trace amount of impurity detection described later in Section 9.6.

XRD is normally used to evaluate crystal quality. However, accurate analysis of crystal quality via XRD is difficult, due to the presence of many overlapping reflection lines from the numerous atoms in the unit cell. Measurements at low temperatures can reduce the linewidths and render the lines distinguishable; however, XRD measurement at cryogenic temperatures is cumbersome. On the other hand, transmittance spectroscopy can easily be carried out, even at cryogenic temperatures.

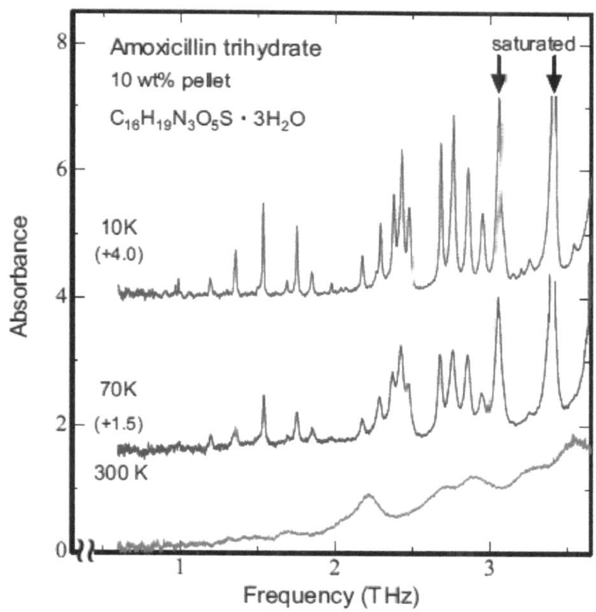

Figure 9.5 Temperature dependence of THz absorption spectra for the 10 wt% pellet of amoxicillin tryhydrate.

Figure 9.5 shows the temperature dependence of THz absorption spectra of a 10 wt% pellet of amoxicillin trihydrate.

The frequency range was limited to 0.6–3.65 THz, because the full peak of strong and sharp absorptions was difficult to detect at higher frequencies. The frequency step was 1 GHz, with accuracy better than 100 MHz. Sharp peaks were visible only at low temperatures; at room temperature, it was difficult to resolve these peaks.

There are still large differences between the spectra at 10 and 70 K. Figure 9.6 shows detailed absorption spectra of amoxicillin trihydrate of a 30 wt% diluted pellet in the range of 0.95–1.00 THz, with a 100 MHz step at 10 K. Twin sharp peaks, not observable by 1 GHz frequency step measurement at 70 K, were partially observable at 10 K. Least squares fitting of the Lorentz function revealed peak frequencies at 0.96492 and 0.98450 THz, and FWHM values of 5.639 and 6.180 GHz. Fitting by a Lorentz function instead of a Gaussian function implies that the crystal is nearly perfect.

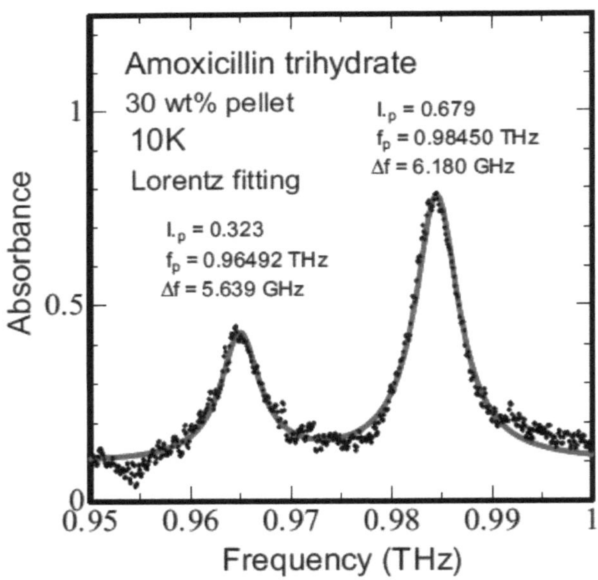

Figure 9.6 Details of THz absorption spectra for the 30 wt% pellet of amoxicillin tryhydrate measured at 10 K.

MMW crystals seem to provide sharper spectra than smaller crystals; this may be attributable to an ambiguity in the crystal structure, due to a larger degree of freedom in the molecular arrangement of SMW molecules. Crystalline MMW molecules seem to readily crystallize into high-quality crystals.

9.6 Detection of Trace Amounts of Impurities in Pharmaceuticals with High-Accuracy Terahertz Spectroscopy

As with IR spectroscopy, quantitative analyses are possible in the THz region by comparing the relative intensity of absorption peaks. Generally, such analyses require a standard curve that correlates material content with absorption peak intensity or integrated peak area. Therefore, the limit of detection (LOD) depends strongly on the S/N ratio of the spectroscopic measurement and the degree of peak separation. Pharmaceuticals, for example, contain several ingredients, resulting in spectra with multiple peaks. For accurate quantitation, these peaks should be resolved separately.

We originally proposed and demonstrated that defects in organic crystals can be detected as slight peak frequency shifts in the absorption lines of THz spectra, and that the magnitudes of these shifts are dependent on the defect concentration [36–38]. Sensitivity and detection limits depend strongly on frequency measurement accuracy. We applied our THz laser spectrometer to check the LOD for trace amounts of impurities in pharmaceuticals.

During pharmaceutical production, the levels of impurities are strictly controlled based on the International Council for Harmonization (ICH) of Technical Requirements for Pharmaceuticals for Human Use guidelines. Possible impurities in drugs are described in ICH guideline Q3A [39] and can be classified into three types: organic impurities, inorganic impurities, and residual solvents. Liquid chromatography (LC) is commonly used for high-sensitivity detection of impurities in pharmaceuticals. LC separates impurities from APIs based on the transit-time differences that arise due to differences in the degree of interaction as the APIs pass through the column. If the molecular species have similar molecular structures and weights, it may be difficult for LC to resolve individual constituents. The organic impurities in pharmaceuticals include starting materials, by products, intermediates, and degradation products, etc., and are similar to those of API molecules in terms of species, structure, and molecular weight. Enantiomers are especially difficult to detect with LC, as they are of the same molecular weight and species. The highly sensitive impurity detection technique proposed here does not depend on molecular weight or species, thereby overcoming a weakness of LC.

As an example, L-asparagine (L-Asn; $C_4H_8N_2O_3$) aqueous solution was contaminated with L-Asp ($C_4H_7NO_4$) at doping levels ranging from 0 to 12.5 wt% at 40°C in a beaker. It is known crystals of L-Asn monohydrate maintained their crystal form (orthogonal, space group $P2_12_12_1$) at L-Asp doping levels below 15 mol%, with L-Asp being substituted for L-Asn [40, 41]. The beaker was kept in a clean draft chamber until crystallization, and the crystals were dried completely. Whole, needle-shaped crystals were collected and ground into a powder with an agate mortar and pestle. The samples were mixed with PE powder and pressed into 3.0 wt% pellets weighing 300 mg, with a diameter of 20 mm and an approximate thickness of 1 mm. We found three absorption peaks that exhibited decreasing intensity, broadening line width, and frequency shifts with increasing L-Asp content.

Figure 9.7 (left) shows a typical spectrum (one of three THz absorption spectra) of L-Asn monohydrate doped with L-Asp, measured at 10 K in 200 MHz steps. Purple, red, and black lines denote spectra with a 0, 1, and 12.5% doping level, respectively. The peak frequency shift is attributable to the L-Asp molecule; as an impurity, it affects the host lattice vibrations of the L-Asn crystal. Figure 9.7 (right) shows the doping dependence of this absorption peak frequency within 1%. A linear fit is possible in this range; the sensitivity was 4.51 GHz/%. As the frequency accuracy of our THz laser spectrometer is better than 3 MHz, an LOD of better than 10 ppm is possible under ideal conditions. However, peak frequency instability via temperature fluctuation limits the LOD to about 52 ppm. Highly sensitive detection is made possible by detecting impurity molecules indirectly, according to their effect on the mother crystal, rather than by detecting the impurity molecule directly. Additionally, THz spectroscopy frequency measurements eliminate the need for precise density measurements, which are prone to error due to differences in concentration and spatial dispersion among samples, particularly diluted samples.

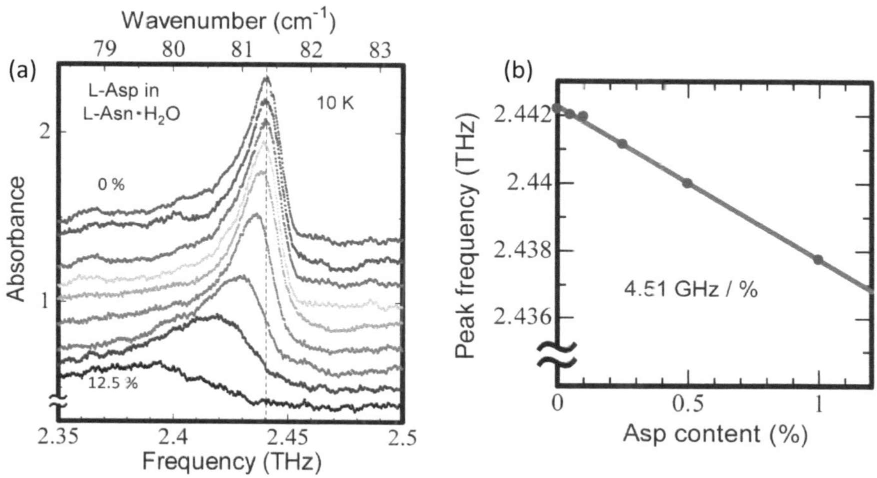

Figure 9.7 THz absorption peaks of L-Asn monohydrate at 10 K near 2.43 THz (left). L-Asp content dependence of peak frequencies (right).

9.7 Conclusion

The presence of trace amounts of impurities is inevitable, and monitoring and control thereof is very important in pharmaceutical production. We proposed and demonstrated a novel technique to detect trace amounts of impurities in pharmaceuticals using our originally developed THz laser spectrometer, which offers high accuracy and high resolution. The technique is suitable for crystal quality evaluation and detection of ultralow-level impurities in MMW pharmaceuticals, which are expected to become mainstream in the near future.

Acknowledgments

We are grateful to Dr. Jun-ichi Nishizawa for his guidance regarding impurity detection using THz spectroscopy. This work was partly supported by the Cooperative Research Project of

Research Center for Biomedical Engineering, the Japan Agency for Medical Research and Development (AMED), and Grants-in-Aid for Scientific Research (B) (Grant No. 16H03882) from the Japan Society for the Promotion of Science.

References

1. J. Federici and L. Moeller, Review of terahertz and subterahertz wireless communications, *J. Appl. Phys.*, 107, 2010, 111101.
2. M. C. Kemp, P. F. Taday, B. E. Cole, J. A. Cluff, A. J. Fitzgerald, and W. R. Tribe, Security applications of terahertz technology, *Proc. SPIE*, 5070, 2003, 44.
3. P. F. Taday, I. V. Bradley, D. D. Arnone, and M. Pepper, Using terahertz pulse spectroscopy to study the crystalline structure of a drug: A case study of the poly-morphs of ranitidine hydrochloride, *J. Pharm. Sci.*, 92(4), 2003, 831–838.
4. J. Nishizawa, K. Suto, T. Sasaki, T. Tanabe, T. Tanno, Y. Oyama, and F. Sato, GaP Raman terahertz high accuracy spectrometer and its application to detect organic and inorganic crystalline defects, *Proc. Japan Acad. Ser. B*, 82(9), 2006, 353–358.
5. J. Nishizawa, T. Sasaki, K. Suto, M. Ito, T. Yoshida, and T. Tanabe, High-resolution GaP terahertz spectrometer and its application to detect defects in gamma-irradiated glucose crystal, *Int. J. Infrared Millimeter Waves*, 29(3), 2008, 291–297.
6. D. A. Auston, K. P. Cheung, and P. R. Smith, Picosecond photoconducting Hertzian dipoles, *Appl. Phys. Lett.*, 45, 1984, 284.
7. T. Tanabe, K. Suto, J. Nishizawa, T. Kimura, and K. Saito, Frequency-tunable high-power terahertz wave generation from GaP, *J. Appl. Phys.*, 93(8), 2003, 4610–4615.
8. T. Tanabe, K. Suto, J. Nishizawa, K. Saito, and T. Kimura, Frequency-tunable terahertz wave generation via excitation of phonon-polaritons in GaP, *J. Phys. D: Appl. Phys.*, 36(8), 2003, 953–957.
9. T. Tanabe, K. Suto, J. Nishizawa, K. Saito, and T. Kimura, Tunable terahertz wave generation in the 3- to 7-THz region from GaP, *Appl. Phys. Lett.*, 83(2), 2003, 237–239.
10. https://www.rie.shizuoka.ac.jp/~thz/database/.
11. J. Nishizawa, T. Tanabe, K. Suto, Y. Watanabe, T. Sasaki, and Y. Oyama, Continuous-wave frequency-tunable terahertz-wave generation from GaP, *IEEE Photonics Technol. Lett.*, 18(19), 2006, 2008–2010.

12. S. Ragam, T. Tanabe, K. Saito, Y. Oyama, and J. Nishi-zawa. Enhancement of CW THz wave power under non collinear phase-matching conditions in DFG, *J. Lightwave Technol.*, 27(15), 2009, 3057–3061.

13. T. Tanabe, S. Ragam, and Y. Oyama, CW THz wave spectrometer based on diode laser pumping: Potential applications in high resolution spectroscopy, *Rev. Sci. Instrum.*, 80, 2009, 113105.

14. T. Sasaki, T. Tanabe, and J.-I. Nishizawa, Frequency stabilized GaP continuous-wave terahertz signal generator for high-resolution spectroscopy, *Opt. Photonics J.*, 4, 2014, 8–13

15. T. Sasaki, T. Tanabe, and J.-I. Nishizawa, Development of continuous wave terahertz signal generator based on difference frequency generation in gallium phosphide crystal, *J. Jpn. Soc. Infrared Sci. Technol.*, 26, 2016, 74–81.

16. T. Sasaki, T. Sakamoto, and M. Otsuka, Detection of impurities in organic crystals by high-accuracy terahertz absorption spectroscopy, *Anal. Chem.*, 90, 2018, 1677.

17. E. R. Brown, K. A. McIntosh, K. B. Nichols, and C. L. Dennis, Photomixing up to 3.8 THz in low-temperature grown, *Appl. Phys. Lett.*, 66(3), 1995, 285–287.

18. K. A. McIntosh, E. R. Brown, K. B. Nichols, O. B. McMahon, W. F. DiNatale, and T. M. Lyszczarz, Terahertz photomixing with diode lasers in low-temperature-grown GaAs, *Appl. Phys. Lett.*, 67(26), 1995, 3844–3846.

19. S. Matsuura, M. Tani, and K. Sakai, Generation of coherent terahertz radiation by photomixing in dipole photoconductive antennas, *Appl. Phys. Lett.*, 70(5), 1997, 559–561.

20. A. J. Deninger, T. Göbel, D. Schönherr, T. Kinder, A. Roggenbuck, M. Köberle, F. Lison, T. Müller-Wirts, and P. Meissner, Precisely tunable continuous-wave terahertz source with interferometric frequency control, *Rev. Sci. Instrum.*, 79(4), 2008, 0447020.

21. M. Walther, B. M. Fischer, and P. U. Jepsen, Noncovalent intermolecular forces in polycrystalline and amorphous saccharides in the far infrared, *Chem. Phys.*, 288, 2003, 261–268.

22. J. Zeitler, D. Newnham, P. Taday, T. Threlfall, R. Lancaster, R. Berg, C. Strachan, M. Pepper, K. Gordon, and T. Rades, *J. Pharm. Sci.*, 95, 2006, 2486–2498.

23. G. Day, J. Zeitler, W. Jones, T. Rades, and P. Taday, Characterization of temperature-induced phase transitions in five polymorphic forms of sulfathiazole by terahertz pulsed spectroscopy and differential scanning calorimetry, *J. Phys. Chem. B*, 110, 2006, 447–456.

24. F. Zhang, H.-W. Wang, K. Tominaga, M. Hayashi, and T. Sasaki, High-resolution THz spectroscopy and solid-state density functional theory calculations of polycyclic aromatic hydrocarbons, *J Infrared Milli Terahz Waves*, 41, 2019, 1378–1392.

25. F. Zhang, O. Kambara, K. Tominaga, J. I. Nishizawa, T. Sasaki, H. W. Wang, and M. Hayashi, Analysis of vibrational spectra of solid-state adenine and adenosine in the terahertz region, *RSC Adv.*, 4, 2014, 269–278.

26. M. Takahashi, Y. Kawazoe, Y. Ishikawa, and H. Ito, Low-frequency vibrations of crystalline α,α-trehalose dehydrate, *Chem. Phys. Lett.*, 429, 2006, 371–377.

27. R. Rungsawang, Y. Ueno, I. Tomita, and K. Ajito, Angle-dependent terahertz time-domain spectroscopy of amino acid single crystals, *J. Phys. Chem. B*, 110, 2006, 21259–21263.

28. T. Sasaki, O. Kambara, T. Sakamoto, and M. Otsuka, J. Nishizawa, Single crystal growth and polarization absorption spectroscopy of theophylline anhydrous for terahertz vibrational mode assignment, *Vibrational Spectrosc.*, 85, 2016, 91–96.

29. B. Torre, F. Albericio, The Pharmaceutical Industry in 2016. An analysis of FDA drug approvals from a perspective of the molecules, *Molecules*, 22, 2017, 368.

30. P. Declerck, Biologicals and biosimilars: a review of the science and its implications, *Generics Biosimilars Initiat. J.*, 1, 2012, 13.

31. T. Kimura, Screening techniques using the periplasmic expression of peptide libraries and target molecules, *J. Bioanal. Biomed.*, 9, 2017, 263.

32. H. Tamamura, T. Kobayakawa, and N. Ohashi, *Mid-Size Drugs Based on Peptides and Peptidomimetics: A New Drug Category*, in Springer Briefs in Pharmaceutical Science & Drug Development book series, Springer, 2018.

33. N. Blagden, M. de Matas, P. T. Gavan, and P. York, Crystal engineering of active pharmaceutical ingredients to improve solubility and dissolution rates, *Adv. Drug Deliv. Rev.*, 59, 2007, 617.

34. T. Sasaki, K. Itatani, T. Sakamoto, and J. Nishizawa, Nondestructive sample preparation of pharmaceutical samples for wide frequency range THz spectroscopy, *Proc. IRMMW-THz 2012*, Australia, 2012.

35. T. Sasaki, T. Sakamoto, and M. Otsuka, Sharp absorption peaks in THz spectra valuable for crystal quality evaluation of middle molecular weight pharmaceuticals, *J. Infrared Millimeter Terahz Waves*, 39, 2018, 828–839.

36. J. Nishizawa, K. Suto, T. Sasaki, T. Tanabe, T. Tanno, Y. Oyama, F. Sato, GaP Raman Terahertz high accuracy spectrometer and its application to detect organic and inorganic crystalline defects, *Proc. Jpn. Acad. Ser. B*, 82, 2006, 353–358.

37. J. Nishizawa, T. Sasaki, K. Suto, M. Ito, T. Yoshida, T. Tanabe, High-resolution GaP terahertz spectrometer and its application to detect defects in γ-irradiated glucose crystal, *Int. J. Infrared Millimeter Waves*, 2008, 29, 291–297.

38. J. Nishizawa, T. Tanno, T. Yoshida, K. Suto, Consequence of a defect on the terahertz spectra of L-Asparagine monohydrate, *Chem. Lett.*, 36, 2007, 134–135.

39. International Conference on Harmonization; Impurities in New Drug Substances, 1995 (https://database.ich.org/sites/default/files/Q3A%28R2%29%20Guideline.pdf).

40. L. Addadi, Z. Berkovitch-Yellin, N. Domb, E. Gati, M. Lahav, L. Leiserowitz, Resolution of conglomerates by stereoselective habit modifications, *Nature*, 296, 1982, 21–26.

41. L. Wang, Z. Berkovitch-Yellin, L. Leiserowitz, Location of 'tailor-made' additives in the crystal and their effect on crystal habit. A study on the host-additive system L-asparagine-L-aspartic acid monohydrate, *Acta Crystallogr. Sect. B: Struct. Sci.*, 41, 1985, 341–348.

Chapter 10

Microwave Imaging for Breast Cancer Screening

Takamaro Kikkawa,[a] Hang Song,[a] Koji Arihiro,[b] and Shinsuke Sasada[c]

[a]*Research Institute for Nanodevice and Bio Systems, Hiroshima University, 1-4-2 Kagamiyama, Higashi-Hiroshima, Hiroshima 739-8527, Japan*
[b]*Department of Pathology, Hiroshima University Hospital, 1-2-3 Kasumi, Minami-ku, Hiroshima 734-8551, Japan*
[c]*Department of Breast Surgery, Hiroshima University Hospital, 1-2-3 Kasumi, Minami-ku, Hiroshima 734-8551, Japan*

kikkawat@hiroshima-u.ac.jp

Microwave imaging has been developed as a new diagnostic modality for breast cancer screening. The principle is based on the fact that the dielectric properties of breast cancer tissues are different from those of normal tissues. The microwave imaging has shown the potential of the imaging of breast cancers as an alternative to X-ray mammography. However, there are remaining challenges to be solved. In this chapter, dielectric characteristics of breast cancer tissues and confocal microwave imaging for breast cancer detection are described.

Biomedical Engineering
Edited by Akihiro Miyauchi and Yuji Miyahara

ISBN 978-981-4877-63-3 (Hardcover), 978-1-003-14194-5 (eBook)
www.jennystanford.com

10.1 Introduction

The advantages of microwave imaging are non-invasive, no-radiation exposure, no-pain and possible frequent-examinations. The physical basis for microwave breast imaging is the fact that the dielectric constants of breast cancers tissues are higher than those of normal tissues [1–12]. The microwave imaging methods have been reviewed in the literatures [13–21], which are referred to in this chapter.

The current standard modality for breast cancer screening is X-ray mammography. The X-ray mammogram provides a map of the density of the breast tissue, which is equivalent to weight per volume. The advantage of the X-ray is high resolution; however, there are limitations in terms of sensitivity and specificity in a dense glandular breast [22, 23], the high false positive rate that leads to unnecessary biopsy [24], the high false negative rate that causes delays in diagnosis and treatment [25], and radiation induced cancer due to high radiation doses from frequent scans [26]. In addition, many women find X-ray mammography uncomfortable and painful due to exposure to ionizing radiation and compressing their breasts [13, 14].

10.2 Histopathological and Dielectric Characteristics of Breast Cancer

Dielectric characteristics of breast cancer tissues have shown significant variability. Although it has been attributed to the variability of individual patients, it is found that the histopathological classification of cancers plays an important role. Most of the published papers did not clearly report what classifications of cancers were measured, but only a few papers have described the histology of measured breast tissues. In this section, histopathological and dielectric characteristics of breast cancers are discussed.

10.2.1 Histopathology of Breast Cancer

World Health Organization (WHO) Classification of Tumors of the Breast [27] classifies breast cancers as ductal carcinoma in situ (DCIS) and invasive carcinoma of no special type (ICNST) or invasive ductal carcinoma, not otherwise specified (IDC NOS). On the other hand, the morphological classification code for clinical diagnoses in Japan is different from that of WHO [28, 29], probably due to degree of differentiation, differences in lymph node metastasis, prognosis, infiltration type, etc. Based on the histological type code in Japan, the invasive ductal carcinoma, which accounts for 80–85% of total breast cancers, is classified as papillo-tubular carcinoma, solid-tubular carcinoma and scirrhous carcinoma, whereas WHO classifies as invasive carcinoma, not otherwise specified.

Figure 10.1 shows comparative photomicrographs of DCIS, papillo-tubular carcinoma, solid-tubular carcinoma, scirrhous carcinoma and mucinous carcinoma [30]. DCIS is known as non-invasive intra-ductal carcinoma. DCIS appears as clustered micro-calcifications as shown in Fig. 10.1a. The morphology of DCIS is not uniform but heterogeneous: 62% of DCIS had calcification, 22% had soft tissues and 16% had no mammographic (X-ray) findings [29].

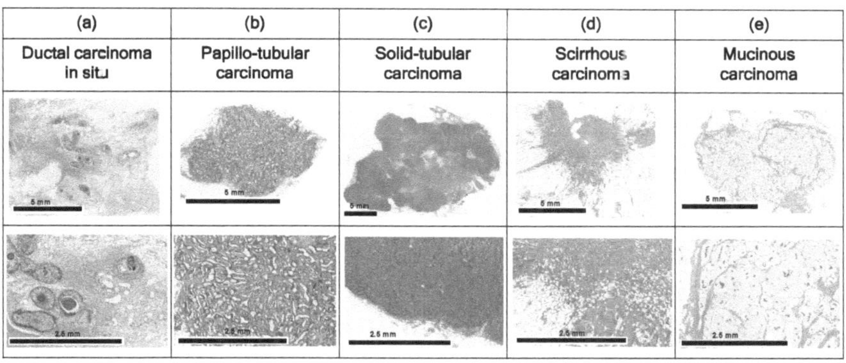

Figure 10.1 Photomicrographs of DCIS, papillo-tubular carcinoma, solid-tubular carcinoma, scirrhous carcinoma and mucinous carcinoma. © 2021 IEEE. Reprinted, with permission, from [30].

Invasive ductal carcinomas (IDC) constitute a heterogeneous group of lesions, which have different clinical presentation and pathological features [29]. The microscopic appearance of IDC is highly heterogeneous with respect to growth pattern, cytologic features, mitotic activity, abnormal desmoplasia and extent of the associated DCIS component. Variability in histologic features may be seen within a single case. Among IDC, papillo-tubular carcinomas are characterized by a proliferation of well-formed glands as shown in Fig. 10.1b. Papillo-tubular carcinomas are in association with DCIS. These tubules tend to be ovoid in shape and sharply angular contours. Solid-tubular carcinomas have well-defined solid-mass, central necrosis and expansion in the peripheral regions as shown in Fig. 10.1c. A rock-hard mass that has a gray-white gritty surface on the cut section characterizes scirrhous carcinomas. Scirrhous carcinomas have stellate or spiculated contours with irregular peripheral margins as shown in Fig. 10.1d. Mucinous carcinomas are known as colloid carcinoma and are the result of extracellular mucin production. Mucinous carcinomas are circumscribed by a variably soft and gelatinous consistency as shown in Fig. 10.1e.

Figure 10.2 shows an enlarged photomicrograph of scirrhous carcinoma shown in Fig. 10.1d. It is found that non-uniform distributions of cancer cells, adipose cells and stroma cells of a glandular tissue were observed in the cancer tissue. It means that the complex permittivity of the cancer tissue is not constant but may have large variability due to the volume fractions of the cancer cells, the stroma cells and adipose cells.

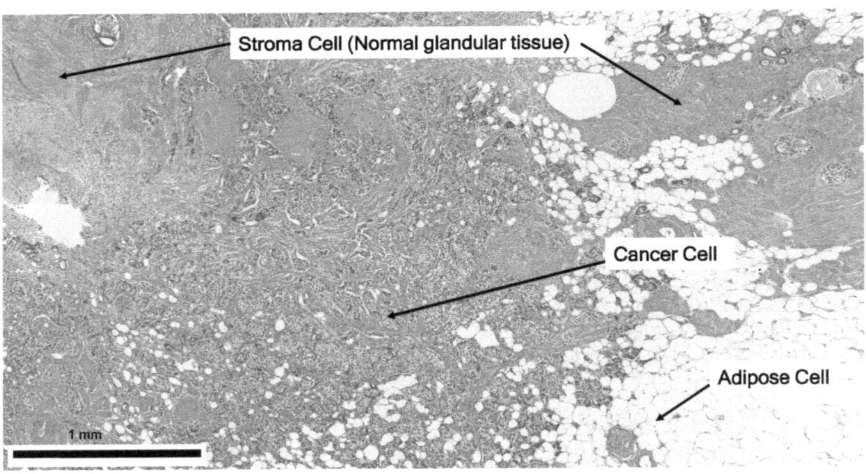

Figure 10.2 Enlarged photomicrograph of scirrhous carcinoma which shows heterogeneous distributions of cancer cells, adipose cells and stroma (glandular) cells.

10.2.2 Dielectric Models of Breast Cancer

The dielectric spectrum of a biological tissue is characterized by three main relaxation regions such as in low, medium and high frequencies of microwave. Each of these relaxation regions corresponds to a polarization mechanism characterized by a single time constant t, which gives the complex relative permittivity e* as a function of angular frequency (w) as Eq. (10.1) [7].

$$\varepsilon^*(\omega) = \varepsilon'(\omega) - j\varepsilon''(\omega) = \varepsilon_\infty + \frac{\varepsilon_s - \varepsilon_\infty}{1 + j\omega\tau} \tag{10.1}$$

This equation is known as Debye model, where ε_∞ is the permittivity at frequencies $\omega\tau >> 1$, and ε_s is the permittivity at $\omega\tau << 1$. The magnitude of the frequency dispersion is described as $\Delta\varepsilon = \varepsilon_s - \varepsilon_\infty$.

The summation of Debye dispersions in addition to a conductivity term is proposed [31], where σ_s is the static ionic conductivity and ε_0 is the permittivity of free space as Eq. (10.2),

$$\varepsilon^*(\omega) = \varepsilon'^{(\omega)} - j\varepsilon''(\omega) = \varepsilon_\infty + \sum_{n=1}^{N} \frac{\Delta\varepsilon_n}{1 + j\omega\tau_n} + \frac{\sigma_s}{j\omega\varepsilon_0}, \tag{10.2}$$

where τ_n and $\Delta\varepsilon_n$ are relaxation time and frequency dispersion in low, medium and high frequencies of microwave.

However, each dispersion region may be broadened due to the complexity of biological tissues. The broadening of the dispersion could be empirically expressed by introducing a distribution parameter, α, so that the Debye equation is modified as the Cole–Cole Eq. (10.3).

$$\varepsilon^*(\omega) = \varepsilon'(\omega) - j\varepsilon''(\omega) = \varepsilon_\infty + \frac{\Delta\varepsilon}{1 + (j\omega\tau)^{1-\alpha}} \tag{10.3}$$

The spectrum of a tissue can be expressed in terms of multiple Cole–Cole dispersion as Eq. (10.4).

$$\varepsilon^*(\omega) = \varepsilon'^{(\omega)} - j\varepsilon''(\omega) = \varepsilon_\infty + \sum_{n=1}^{N} \frac{\Delta\varepsilon_n}{1 + (j\omega\tau_n)^{(1-\alpha_n)}} + \frac{\sigma_s}{j\omega\varepsilon_0}, \tag{10.4}$$

where α_n is the parameter of broadening of the dispersion in low, medium and high frequencies of microwave.

10.2.3 Dielectric Measurement of Breast Cancer

The dielectric properties of ex vivo normal and malignant breast tissues in microwave frequencies between 3 MHz and 3 GHz were measured in 1984 [1]. Significant differences in the dielectric properties between normal and malignant tissues were observed. The Cole–Cole models of complex permittivity for the center of the tumor, the surrounding tissue and peripheral tissue were reported [2]. Although significant dielectric contrasts between normal and tumor tissues were observed [3], the difficulty for distinguishing the tumor from normal tissues was suggested due to the similarity in dielectric properties of malignant and benign tumors. The dielectric properties of normal and malignant breast tissues were measured from 50 to 900 MHz and the average difference in permittivity and conductivity of malignant breast tissues to normal ones were 233 and 577%, respectively [4]. The dielectric properties of normal and cancerous tissue of various human organs have been studied extensively by Gabriel et al. [5–7]. The most comprehensive examinations of the dielectric properties of normal and malignant breast tissues were conducted by Lazebnik et al. [9, 10, 32].

To measure the dielectric properties of breast tissues, the tissues were obtained from breast reduction surgeries at hospitals [9]. The tissue handling protocol is as follows [9, 10, 11]. When the tissue was transported from an operating room to a pathology suite, a pathologist paged one of the engineers to conduct measurements. The time between excision and measurements was as little as 5 min, or as much as 30 min. The sizes of each sample were approximately from 5 to 30 cm. The pathologist cut the desired tissue samples from the bulk specimens for diagnosis either prior to or after measurements, depending on emergency. The measurement of dielectric properties of breast tissues using a precision open-ended coaxial probe technique were reported [33]. The measurements were taken in the frequency band of 0.5–20 GHz for adipose, fibroconnective/glandular and tumor tissues as shown in Fig. 10.3a [11].

Figure 10.3a shows a photograph of electromagnetic measurement using an open-ended coaxial probe with the outer diameter of 2.2 mm on the tumor region of ill-defined and grayish-white on the cut surface. Yellowish regions and a brown-colored region are adipose tissues and skin, respectively. A cross section of a tissue sample was prepared for making a histology slide. Gross histology of the tumor tissue was conducted based on visual inspection under the microscope. A digital photomicrograph image of the malignant tumor tissue with hematoxylin-eosin stain is shown in Fig. 10.3b. It should be noted that a block of the cancer tissue shown in Fig. 10.3a is not filled with cancer cells but there are stroma cells and carcinoma associated fibroblasts as well as adipose cells within the cancer tissue. Therefore, the measured dielectric constant of the cancer tissue may not be always constant but has large variability due to the heterogeneous distribution of the cancer, stroma and adipose cells.

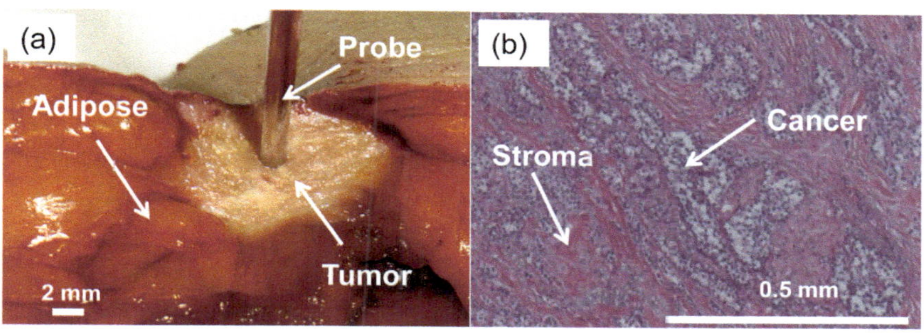

Figure 10.3 Photographs of electromagnetic measurement and digital photomicrographic image. (a) A picture of electromagnetic measurement using an open-ended coaxial probe with the outer diameter of 2.2 mm on the tumor region of ill-defined and grayish-white on the cut surface. (b) A digital photomicrograph image of the tumor tissue with hematoxylin-eosin stain. Reproduced from [11], with the permission of AIP Publishing.

Stainless steel and borosilicate glass, hermetically sealed precision probes were custom-designed. The probes were flange-free to ensure good contact with the tissue across the entire aperture; the outer diameter and the length of the probe aperture were 2.2 and 200 mm, respectively, as shown in Fig. 10.4. Agilent

85070 dielectric probe kit was used in conjunction with an Agilent E5071C vector network analyzer (VNA). A high-quality flexible cable connected the probe to the VNA.

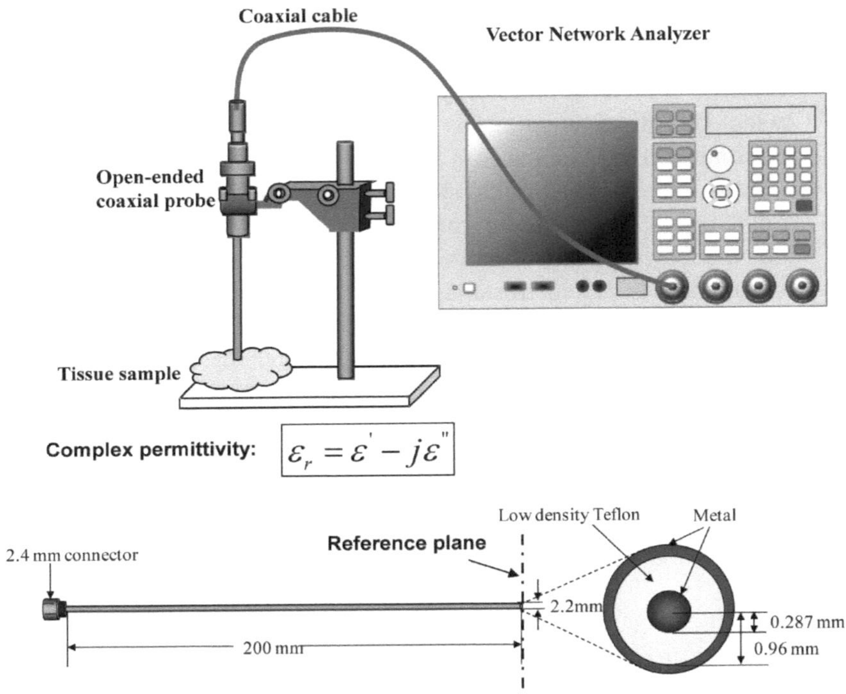

Figure 10.4 Measurement setup for electromagnetic properties of breast tissues and open-ended coaxial probe. Reproduced from [11], with the permission of AIP Publishing.

The tissue samples were placed on a stand, and the cable and probe were held firmly in place in a mechanical jig connected to the stand. For every measurement, the jig was manually lowered until the entire probe aperture made firm contact with the tissue sample. The VNA was calibrated at the reference plane of the coaxial probe tip using calibration standards such as an open circuit in air, a short circuit with a metal, and load in liquids. The probe was immersed in the water and ethanol by moving the liquids to the probe for calibration.

10.2.4 Dielectric Characteristics of Breast Cancer

To investigate the dielectric dispersion of the breast tissues, the frequency dependency of the complex permittivity was measured as shown in Fig. 10.5. It is found that measured dielectric constants and the conductivities of cancer tissues overlapped with those of stroma (glandular) tissues. Furthermore, the variabilities of the dielectric constant and conductivity for cancer and stroma (glandular) tissues were significant.

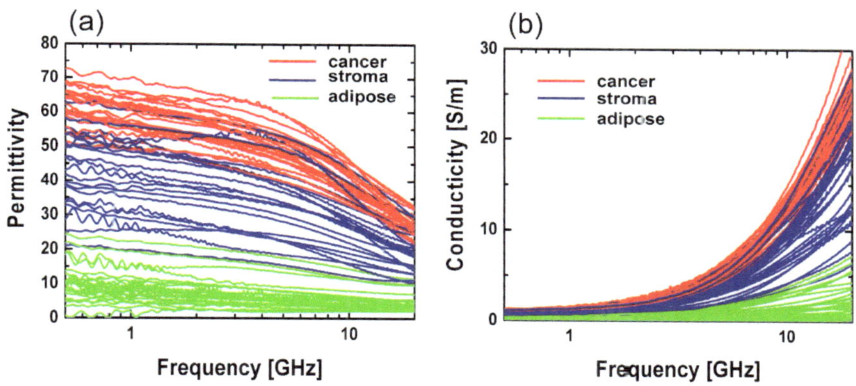

Figure 10.5 Frequency spectra of dielectric constants and conductivities of freshly excised breast cancer, stroma, and adipose tissues. (a) Dielectric constant versus frequency. (b) Conductivity versus frequency. Reproduced from [11], with the permission of AIP Publishing.

Some of the dielectric constants of the stroma (glandular) tissues were close to those of cancer tissues probably because some of them were located in the vicinity of the cancer tissues as shown in Fig. 10.2, which might be carcinoma associated fibroblasts. On the other hand, the others of the stroma (glandular) tissues were close to those of adipose tissues probably because they have more adipose cells distributed in the stroma (glandular) tissues as shown in Fig. 10.2.

In order to analyze the characteristics quantitatively, a modified two-pole Cole–Cole model was developed to fit the measurement results of complex permittivity versus frequency in 0.5–20 GHz as Eq. (10.5) [11]:

$$\varepsilon^*(\omega) = \varepsilon'^{(\omega)} - j\varepsilon''(\omega) = \varepsilon_\infty + \frac{\varepsilon_m - \varepsilon_\infty}{1+(j\omega\tau_Q)^{(1-\beta)}} + \frac{\varepsilon_s - \varepsilon_m}{1+(j\omega\tau_P)} + \frac{\sigma_s}{j\omega\varepsilon_0} \quad (10.5)$$

In the model, β is a measure of the broadening of the dispersion. τ_P is the relaxation time of low frequency and τ_Q is the relaxation time of high frequency.

Measured results of dielectric properties of cancer, glandular and adipose tissues and the fitted data are shown in Fig. 10.6. The dielectric constant versus frequency, conductivity versus frequency and the Cole–Cole plot are shown in Figs. 10.6a-c, respectively. All the measured data were fitted in the entire frequency range from 0.5 to 20 GHz.

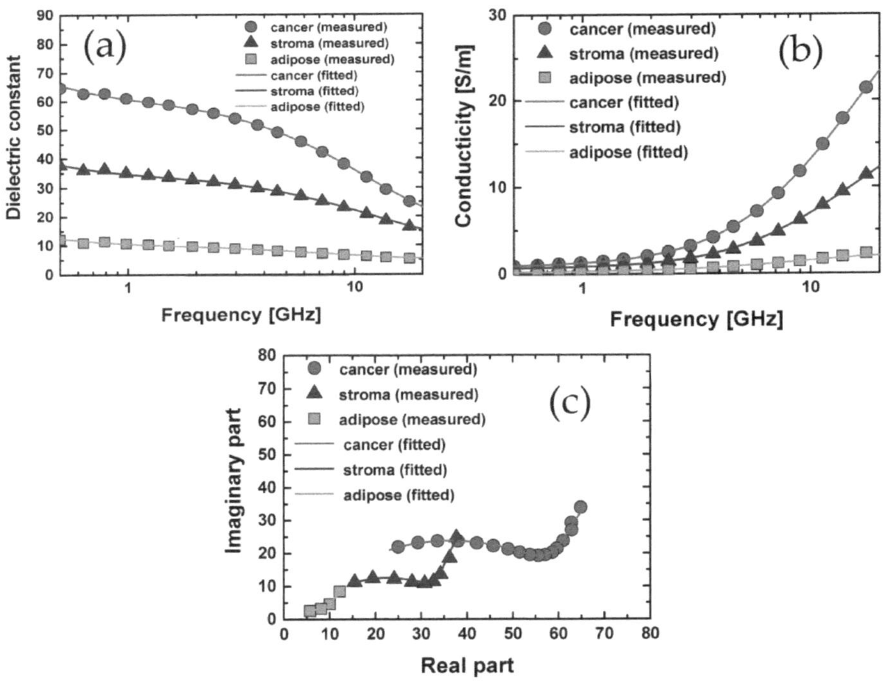

Figure 10.6 Data fitting by use of modified two-pole Cole–Cole model. (a) Dielectric constant versus frequency. (b) Conductivity versus frequency. (c) Cole–Cole plot. Reproduced from [11], with the permission of AIP Publishing.

Table 10.1 shows the median dielectric properties of the cancer, stroma (glandular), and adipose tissues derived from the modified Cole–Cole model for 102 samples. The median values of the permittivity ε_m at the intermediate frequency for cancer, stroma (glandular), and adipose tissues were approximately 59.5, 33.2, and 9.3, respectively. The intermediate frequency is defined as the frequency at which the Cole–Cole plot has an inflection point as shown in Fig. 10.6c. The median values of the conductivities σ_S for cancer, stroma (glandular), and adipose tissues were approximately 0.76, 0.55, and 0.18 [S/m], respectively.

Table 10.1 Extracted parameters of the dielectric properties of the cancer, glandular and adipose tissues obtained from the modified Cole–Cole plot Eq. (10.5)

Coefficients	Cancer	Stroma (Glandular)	Adipose
ε_∞	7.2	7.9	4.3
ε_m	59.5	33.2	9.3
ε_s	68.0	40.3	12.6
τ_P (ns)	0.21	0.23	0.16
τ_Q (ps)	13.9	13.7	18.3
β	0.11	0.074	0.062
σ_S (S/m)	0.76	0.55	0.18

Source: Reproduced from Ref. [11] with permission of AIP Publishing.

Although it is difficult to distinguish some of the cancers from the normal tissues with respect to dielectric constants statistically, the difference between cancer and stroma tissues was more significant for an individual patient as shown in Fig. 10.7. Figure 10.7a shows dielectric constants of cancer, stroma (glandular) and adipose tissues measured at 6 GHz for the 35 individual patients. The median values of dielectric constants of cancer, stroma and adipose tissues are shown as red circle, blue triangle and green square, respectively. The absolute values of the dielectric constants of the individual breast tissues varied depending on the patients and temperatures. The dielectric constants of the cancer tissues were approximately 4 times higher than those of the adipose tissues. The dielectric constants of the cancer tissues were distributed from approximately 35 to 65 at 6 GHz, whereas those of stroma tissues were from 15 to 50.

The standard deviation of the dielectric constants for cancer, stroma (glandular) and adipose tissues were approximately 5.1, 9.2 and 4.5, respectively. The reason why the standard deviation of the stroma (glandular) tissues was larger than other tissues is associated with the fact that the adipose cells were distributed in the stroma (glandular) tissues more significantly than those in cancer cells as shown in Fig. 10.2.

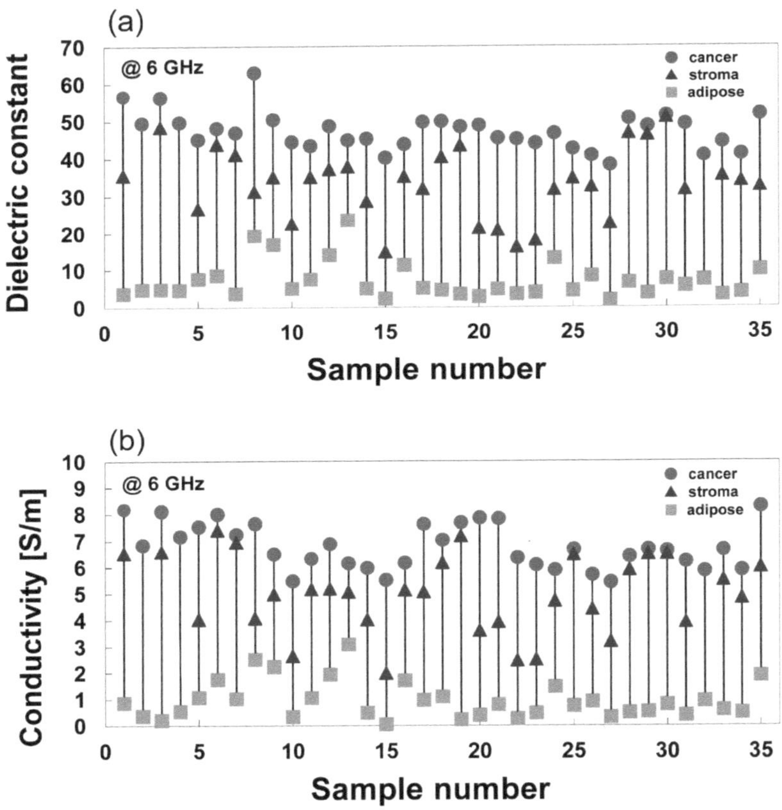

Figure 10.7 Distribution of dielectric constant and conductivity of cancer, stroma and adipose tissues for individual patients. Red circle, blue triangle and green square are cancer, stroma and adipose tissues, respectively. (a) Dielectric constant. (b) Conductivity. Reproduced from [11], with the permission of AIP Publishing.

Median values of conductivities of cancer, stroma and adipose tissues for the 35 individual patients are shown in Fig. 10.7b. The conductivities of the cancer tissues were distributed from approximately 5 to 8 S/m at 6 GHz, whereas those of stroma tissues were from 2 to 7 S/m. The standard deviation of the conductivities of cancer tissues, stroma tissues and adipose tissues were 0.79, 1.40 and 0.67 S/m, respectively. It could be attributed to the fact that there are adipose cells distributed in the stroma (glandular) tissues more significantly as shown in Fig. 10.2.

In order to investigate the variability of dielectric constant and conductivity of cancer tissues quantitatively, Bruggeman's effective medium approximation theory was applied to inhomogeneous tumor tissues as dielectric materials [34]. The effective permittivity of a cancer tissue was calculated as an inhomogeneous dielectric material which was a mixture of the cells with high and low dielectric constants. The effective medium approximations for permittivity and conductivity are expressed as Eqs. (10.6), (10.7) and (10.8), respectively,

$$\sum_{i}^{n} \phi_i \frac{\varepsilon_i - \varepsilon_e}{\varepsilon_i + 2\varepsilon_e} = 0 \tag{10.6}$$

$$\sum_{i}^{n} \phi_i \frac{\sigma_i - \sigma_e}{\sigma_i + 2\sigma_e} = 0 \tag{10.7}$$

$$\sum_{i}^{n} \phi_i = 1 \tag{10.8}$$

When $n = 3$, ε_1, ε_2 and ε_3 are the permittivities of cancer cells, stromal cells and adipose cells, respectively. ε_e is the effective permittivity of the measured tumor tissue. σ_1, σ_2 and σ_3 the conductivities of cancer cells, stromal cells and adipose cells, respectively. σ_e is the effective conductivity of the measured tumor tissue. ϕ_1, ϕ_2 and ϕ_3 are the volume fractions of cancer cells, stromal cells and adipose cells, respectively.

Correlation between the measured dielectric constant and the measured volume fraction of cancer cells is shown in Fig. 10.8a.

The dielectric constants of the excised cancer tissues varied from approximately 38 to 62 at 6 GHz. Equation (10.6) is plotted with ε_1 = 66.5 and ε_2 = 33, assuming that ϕ_3 is negligible in the measured specimens. Correlation between the measured conductivity and the measured volume fraction of cancer cells is shown in Fig. 10.8b. The conductivities of the excised cancer tissues varied from approximately 5.5 to 8.4 S/m at 6 GHz. Equation (10.7) is plotted with σ_1 = 10.5 and σ_2 = 4.3, assuming that ϕ_3 is negligible in the measured specimens.

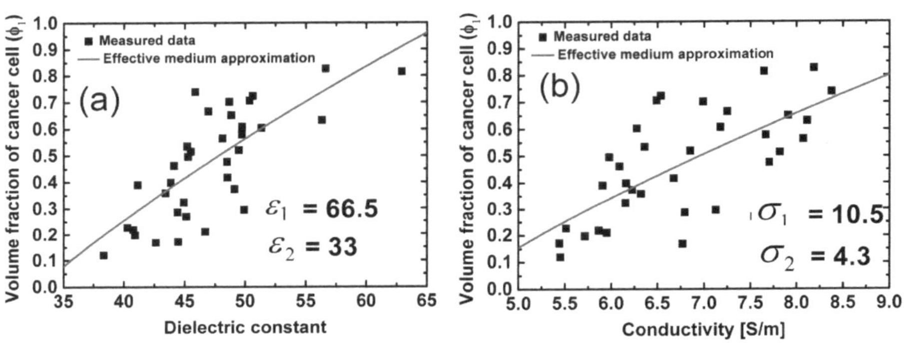

Figure 10.8 Volume fraction of cancer cell versus dielectric constant and conductivity. (a) Dielectric constant. (b) Conductivity. Reproduced from [11], with the permission of AIP Publishing.

It was also found that significant dielectric heterogeneity in normal breast tissue were observed [9]. The reason for heterogeneity was explained as the location from which samples of normal tissue were taken. The glandular tissues in the vicinity of tumors have less adipose contents, whereas the normal glandular tissues have a higher adipose content compared to the glandular tissue surrounding the tumor. It was reported that 50 of the 60 cancer samples (83%) contained 0–20% adipose tissue and all 60 cancer samples contained 10% or less glandular tissue [10]. The dielectric properties of breast tissue were primarily a function of the adipose content of the tissue. Adjusting for adipose content, it is found that the difference between the conductivity of normal tissue and malignant tissue was only 10% and that the difference in permittivity is approximately 8% at 5 GHz.

On the contrary, it was also reported that the cancer tissues contained approximately 10–80% stroma (glandular) cells including carcinoma associated fibroblasts as shown in Figs. 10.2 and 10.3 [11, 30]. It was found that the volume fraction of the adipose cells was negligible in the measured cancer specimens except peripherals [11], which could correspond to the fact that 65% of the cancer samples contain only 10% adipose tissues [10]. According to Bruggeman's effective medium approximation theory, the effective permittivity of a cancer tissue is a function of volume fractions of cancer cells and stroma (glandular) cells including carcinoma associated fibroblasts in the cancer tissues.

The higher permittivity of the dissected cancer specimen could be attributed to the higher density of cancer cells in comparison with the stroma (glandular) cells, while the lower permittivity could be due to the adipose contents. The higher permittivity of the stroma (glandular) tissues in the dissected breast specimen might be attributed to the higher density of carcinoma associated fibroblasts in the vicinity of cancer tissues.

In conclusion, the causes for the variability of the complex permittivity of the cancer and stroma (glandular) tissues could be attributed to the variability of the volume fractions of cancer cells, stroma cells and adipose cells in the dissected tissues.

10.3 Confocal Microwave Imaging

Based on the fact that the complex permittivities of breast cancer tissues are different from those of normal breast tissues, the amount of scattered electromagnetic energy from the breast interior can be either calculated to reconstruct an energy map of the highly scattering object, or it can be used to reconstruct quantitative distributions of the dielectric constants and the conductivities within the whole breast. The former approach is called as a radar-based imaging, while the latter is referred to microwave tomography. The radar-based imaging is widely adopted for its computation simplicity and robustness, whereas microwave tomography requires more computational power.

One of the earliest radar-based imaging methods for breast cancer detection was developed in 1998. It was often referred to as confocal microwave imaging [13, 14, 35]. Synthetic focusing was performed under the assumption that the dielectric constant of breast was homogeneous. The homogeneous dielectric properties of normal adipose tissues allow coherent addition of the backscattered signals. The measured signal was normalized and time shifted to create a synthetic focus at a spatial position. The time delay for each spatial position was calculated based on the signal path between the transmitter and the receiver antennas and the average propagation speed of the microwave, which was inversely proportional to square root of the dielectric constant.

The time-shifting of the measured signals and summing to achieve a synthetic focus were referred to delay and sum (DAS) beamforming. A tissue sensing adaptive radar (TSAR) was developed by extending the idea of synthetic focusing [36, 37]. It could suppress background clutters and enabling coherence in the measured signals. The electromagnetic signals scattered from the target location could be added coherently after time-shifting. The coherence factor was calculated either independently or adaptively based on the measured data.

An additional weighting factor was introduced to enable coherence in the delayed signals, resulting in suppression of incoherent clutters. It was called as the improved delay and sum (IDAS) beamformer [38]. The IDAS method was validated on simulated and phantom data [39, 40], and applied to clinical data for tumor detection. The delay-multiply-and-sum (DMAS) beamformer was based on the multiplication of time-shifted signals to enable coherence [41]. It was used in breast imaging studies [42].

An adaptive ultra-wide-band (UWB) beamforming method was developed. It demonstrated the efficacy by comparing it with a data-independent beamformer on experimental and clinical data [43]. Other radar-based imaging methods include filtered delay and sum (FDAS) [44], multi-static adaptive microwave imaging (MAMI) [45], microwave imaging via space time (MIST) beamformer [46], and quasi-multi-static MIST beamformer [47] have been applied to synthetic and experimental microwave data.

Radar-based imaging methods are computationally simple and have shown encouraging results for the detection of cancer tissues in moderately dense breasts [48–50]. These methods reconstruct an energy map, which shows the qualitative position of the highest intensity of the confocal image of the scattered signals. Clinical examinations were conducted using prototypes of breast cancer detectors [48–51].

10.3.1 System Design for Confocal Imaging

The architecture of a breast cancer detector for confocal imaging is depicted in Fig. 10.9 [51]. Technical details were described in the literatures [52, 53]. The total size of the detector is 19.1 cm × 17.7 cm × 18.8 cm. This detector consists of a step-motor, a control module, a radio-frequency (RF) module and a dome antenna array. The block diagram of the circuits is shown in Fig. 10.9a. The dome antenna array is connected with the

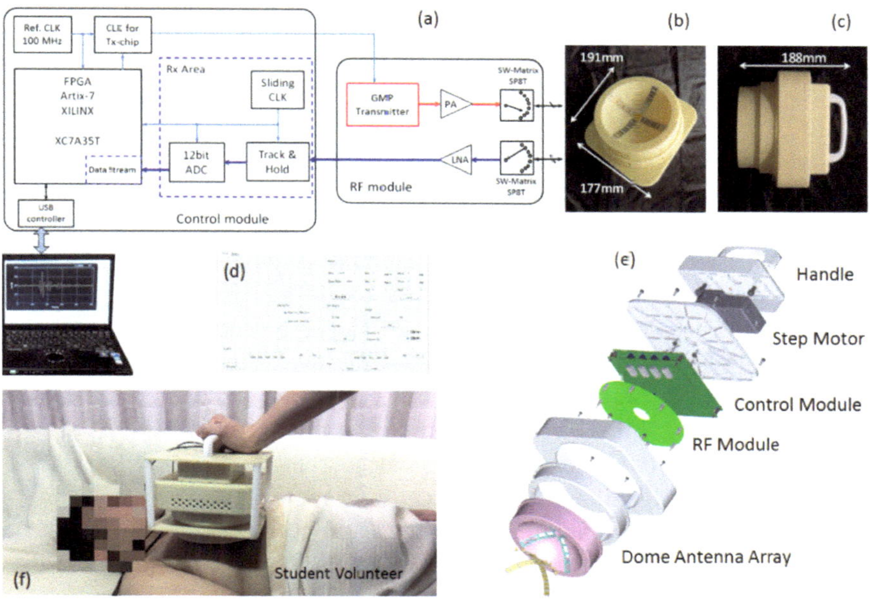

Figure 10.9 The architecture of the breast cancer detector. (a) The block diagram of the circuits. (b) Photograph of the bottom view showing the dome antenna array. (c) Photograph of the side view. (d) The control software graphic interface. (e) The breakdown diagram of the system. (f) The hand-held microwave breast cancer detector system in position for radar-based imaging [51].

circuits through the two single-pole-8-throw (SP8T) switching matrix. The antenna configuration is shown in Fig. 10.9b, in which cross-shape 4×4 antennas are formed. The step motor is mounted on the top of the detector as shown in Fig. 10.9e. The step-motor can rotate with 1°/step. The detector is connected to a laptop computer by a universal serial bus (USB) cable for exchanging data and sending command. Customized software is developed to control the operation of the detector. The graphic interface of the software is shown in Fig. 10.9d. In the clinical applications, a plastic cover is formed on the antenna dome to protect patient breast under test from friction movement. Figure 10.9f shows a hand-held microwave breast cancer detector system in position for radar-based imaging on a breast of a male student for demonstration.

10.3.2 Averaging Method for Confocal Imaging

The direct wave from a transmitter antenna to a receiver antenna and reflections from the breast skin compose the dominant part of the received signal of early arrival. Therefore, the amplitude of the target reflection from the interior of the breast becomes much weaker in comparison with the artifacts in terms of the dynamic range. To extract the weaker target signal from the larger raw signal, an averaging method is developed to make the reference signal which is used to be subtracted from the original received signal. Figure 10.10 shows a schematic diagram of the averaging method for artifact removal. Since the antenna of the breast cancer detector rotates 360° around the breast as shown in Fig. 10.9, each received signal contains both the direct wave and the target signal at every step of rotation angles. The target signal arrives at the different delay time for the different rotation angle. The reference signal can be obtained by averaging all the received signals at all angles so that it does not contain the target signals. Then, the target signal can be extracted by subtracting the reference signal from the raw received signal at every rotation angle as shown in Fig. 10.10.

All received signals are defined as Eq. (10.9),

$$\mathbf{S} = \{\mathbf{S}_1, \ldots, \mathbf{S}_i, \ldots \mathbf{S}_N\}, \tag{10.9}$$

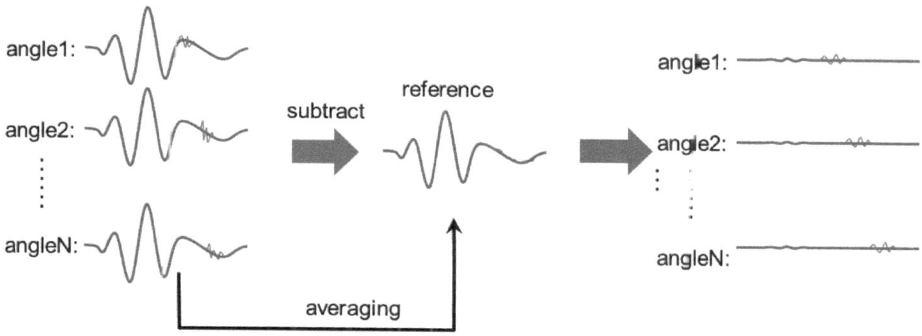

Figure 10.10 Schematic diagram of the averaging method for artifact removal [51].

where N is the number of channel which is the transmitter (Tx)-receiver (Rx) antenna pair. $\mathbf{S}_i$ is composed of the signals from channel i at all angels as Eq. (10.10),

$$\mathbf{S}_i = \{S_{i1}[n], ..., S_{ij}[n], ..., S_{iM}[n]\}, \tag{10.10}$$

where M is the number of the angles rotated. Because of the jitter existing in the system, the received signals have phase difference between each other which will introduce a big noise residual in the dominant part after subtraction. Therefore, the alignment based on least square method is applied to suppress the phase error which can be depicted as Eq. (10.11),

$$\min_{\Delta n} \sum_{n=t_s}^{t_e} \left| S_{i1}[n] - S_{ij}[n + \Delta n_{ij}] \right|^2 . \tag{10.11}$$

where Δn_{ij} is the amount of time offset to compensate the phase shift between signals; t_s and t_e are the start time and end time of the range, respectively, for calculating the optimal Δn_{ij}. Since the dominant parts of the signals from the same channel are similar, by averaging the signals, a reference signal can be obtained as Eq. (10.12),

$$S_{i,\text{ave}} = (S_{i1}[n] + \cdots + S_{iM}[n + \Delta n_{iM}])/M . \tag{10.12}$$

Then the target information can be extracted by subtracting the reference signal from the original ones. The subtracted signal from i-th channel and j-th rotation angle is denoted as $D_{ij}[n]$. The finite impulse response band-pass filter is applied to the subtracted signals for suppressing noise as Eq. (10.13),

$$y_{ij}[n] = \sum_{k=0}^{L} h[n] \cdot D_{ij}[n-k], \tag{10.13}$$

where h is the filter coefficients and L is the filter order. The processed data $\{y_{ij}[n]\}$ are used for the image generation.

The DAS method is adopted in the system for its robustness and less computation consuming. For any focal point $\mathbf{r}$, the length of the propagation path $L(\mathbf{r})$ corresponding to a certain channel can be calculated by Eq. (10.14),

$$L(\mathbf{r}) = \left|\mathbf{r}_{Tx} - \mathbf{r}\right| + \left|\mathbf{r}_{Rx} - \mathbf{r}\right|, \tag{10.14}$$

where $\mathbf{r}_{\mathrm{Tx}}$ and $\mathbf{r}_{\mathrm{Rx}}$ are the positions of the Tx and Rx antenna. The x and y coordinates of antenna at j-th rotation angle besides the initial one can be calculated by Eq. (10.15),

$$\begin{aligned} x_j &= x_{\text{center}} + \sqrt{\left(x_1 - x_{\text{center}}\right)^2 + \left(y_1 - y_{\text{center}}\right)^2} \cdot \cos\left(\arctan\left(\frac{x_1 - x_{\text{center}}}{y_1 - y_{\text{center}}}\right) - (j-1)\cdot\theta\right) \\ y_j &= y_{\text{center}} + \sqrt{\left(x_1 - x_{\text{center}}\right)^2 + \left(y_1 - y_{\text{center}}\right)^2} \cdot \sin\left(\arctan\left(\frac{x_1 - x_{\text{center}}}{y_1 - y_{\text{center}}}\right) - (j-1)\cdot\theta\right), \end{aligned} \tag{10.15}$$

where x_{center} and y_{center} are the position of the dome center in x–y plane. θ is the rotation step. Since the rotation is parallel to the x–y plane, the z coordinate is constant. Then the delay time of the reflection from the selected focal point can be calculated by Eq. (10.16),

$$\tau_r = L(\mathbf{r}) \cdot \sqrt{\varepsilon_r} / c, \tag{10.16}$$

where c is the speed of light, ε_r is the effective permittivity of the breast interior. Here it is assumed to be constant. Finally, the intensity of the focal point $\boldsymbol{I}(r)$ is calculated by adding the contribution of all the channels and all the rotation angles as Eq. (10.17),

$$I(\mathbf{r}) = \sum_{i=1}^{N}\sum_{j=1}^{M} y_{ij}(T_c + \tau_r), \tag{10.17}$$

where T_c is the system calibration time. Define the area under the dome as the imaging area. By calculating the intensities of all focal point inside the imaging area, the reflection energy distribution can be obtained. From the imaging results, the position of the target can be estimated.

10.3.3 Artifact Removal for Confocal Imaging

One of the most important challenges is the removal of artifacts for confocal imaging. There are several possibilities for the causes of artifacts: scattering either at the interface between antennas and breast skins or in air-gaps between the antenna radome and the breast skin or at the interface between breast skin and breast fat layers.

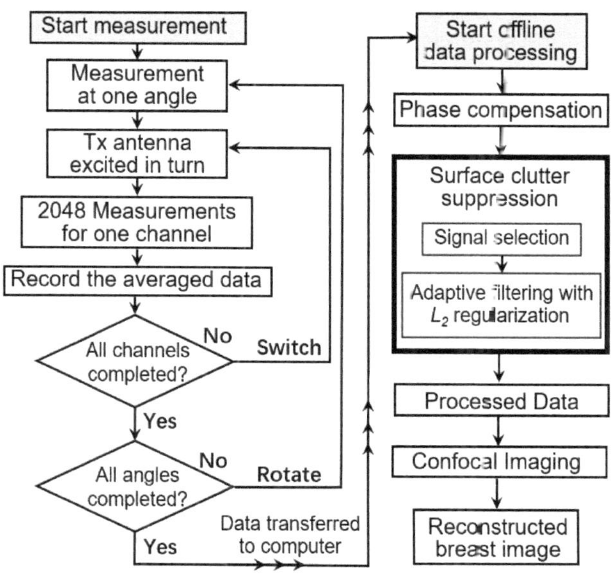

Figure 10.11 Flowchart of confocal microwave imaging. © 2021 IEEE. Reprinted, with permission, from [54].

Figure 10.11 shows a flowchart of confocal microwave imaging [54]. In order to remove the artifacts for confocal imaging, a two-stage rotational surface clutter suppression method is developed. The first stage is a signal selection by correlation coefficient and the second stage is the adaptive filtering with a prior constraint using L_2 regularization.

As pre-processing, all the raw received signals were normalized to the maximum peak. The normalized signal is calculated as Eq. (10.18),

$$s_{\text{norm}} = \frac{s - LSB_0}{\max\{s - LSB_0\}}, \tag{10.18}$$

where s is the raw received signal and s_{norm} is the normalized signal. LSB_0 is the output least significant bits (LSB) of the analog-to-digital converter (ADC) when the amplitude of the analog signal is 0 V. To suppress the surface clutter from a certain channel at a certain rotation angle, signals with high similarity are selected from the same channel at all rotation angles. In the signal selection stage, the degree of similarity is assessed using the correlation coefficient.

For the rotational configuration shown in Fig. 10.9, the correlation coefficient is calculated as Eq. (10.19),

$$\rho_{k,i,j} = \frac{\sum (s_{k,i}[n] - \overline{s}_{k,i})(s_{k,j}[n] - \overline{s}_{k,j})}{\sqrt{\sum (s_{k,i}[n] - \overline{s}_{k,i})^2} \sqrt{\sum (s_{k,j}[n] - \overline{s}_{k,j})^2}}, \tag{10.19}$$

where $\rho_{k,i,j}$ is the correlation coefficient between the signals from k-th channel at i-th and j-th rotation angles. $s_{k,i}[n]$ is the signal received by the k-th channel at the i-th rotation angle. $s_{k,i}[n]$ is the object signal which is to be processed for clutter suppression. $\overline{s}_{k,i}$ and $\overline{s}_{k,j}$ are the temporal averages of the $s_{k,i}[n]$ and $s_{k,j}[n]$.

The correlation coefficients are calculated between $s_{k,i}[n]$ and signals from all other angles. A threshold ρ_{th} is set to choose the possible candidate signals for adaptive filtering. Signals from adjacent angles are excluded since the reflections from breast interior in these signals may appear at the same timing as that in the object signal.

Figures 10.12a and 10.12b show the correlation coefficient map of the signals and counts of the selected angles when the correlation coefficient is ρ = 0.98, respectively. It can be seen that the signals around 0–40° and 330–360° have relative low similarity to the signals at other angles, while the signals from 40° to 330° have high similarity. In order to remove the artifact of the object signal at a certain angle, the signals from angles with large ρ are selected. Here, a threshold ρ_{th} is set to limit the possible candidate signals to ensure the similarity of the signal.

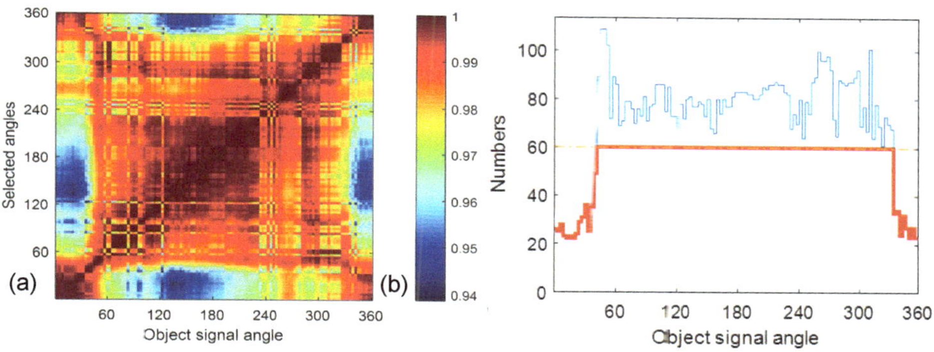

Figure 10.12 (a) The correlation map of the signals. (b) Counts of the selected angles when the correlation coefficient is ρ = 0.98.

After the exclusion of signals having low similarity and adjacent signals, the possible signals are sorted from highest correlation coefficient to lowest one. Then the top M signals are chosen as the entries for removing the artifact of the object signal. If the number of the possible signals is less than M, then all the possible signals are used. If there is no signal whose similarity is larger than ρ_{th}, then $s_{k,i}[n]$ is excluded in the imaging process.

After signal selection, the adaptive filtering is employed to remove the artifact of object signal $s_{k,i}[n]$. In this stage, a prior constraint is introduced using L_2 regularization to facilitate the filtering process. The prior constraint is chosen based on the fact that the selected signals are with high similarity.

Figure 10.13 shows the schematic diagram of the adaptive filter for artifact removal. In order to remove the artifact of the object signal at a certain angle, the chosen signals at other angles in the former selection step are employed to approximate the artifact in the object angle with a linear combination. The weight vector is $[w_1, w_2, \ldots \ldots, w_M]^T$, where M is the number of selected signals for the object signal. Using the linear combination of the other signals, an approximated signal is generated and subtracted from the object signal for artifact removal. In fact, the averaging method is a special case of the adaptive filter, where the weight factor is $\mathbf{w} = [1, 1, \ldots \ldots, 1]^T/M$.

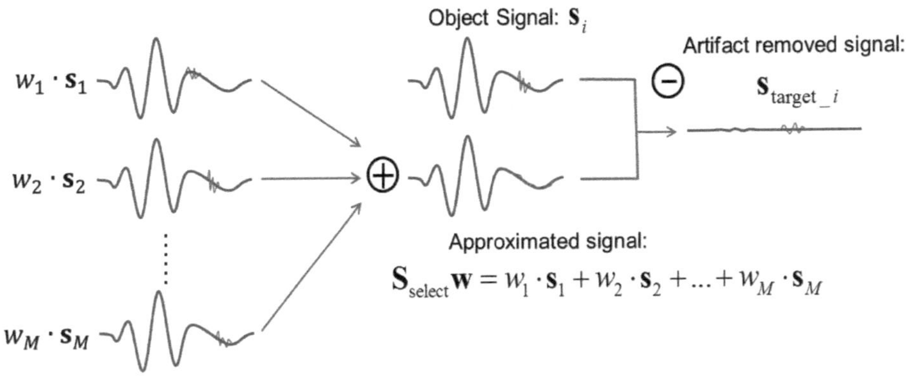

Figure 10.13 The schematic diagram of the adaptive filter for artifact removal [20].

Figure 10.14 shows the schematic diagram of the received signal waveforms versus time at different rotation angles for adaptive filtering. Time interval $(n_0 + 1, n_0 + L)$ with respect to analog-to-digital sampling timing includes the artifacts such as surface scattering or antenna coupling.

To get rid of the artifact in the time scale of L, the approximated signal at every rotation angle is generated as a linear combination of $\boldsymbol{S}_{\mathbf{select}} \cdot \mathbf{w}$.

The selected signals for $s_{k,i}[n]$ from the previous stage are defined as $\mathbf{S}_{\text{select}} = \{\mathbf{s}_{ki,1}, \ldots, \mathbf{s}_{ki,j}, \ldots, \mathbf{s}_{ki,m}\}$, where $s_{ki,j}$ is the vector form of $s_{ki,j}[n]$. The notation ki,j stands for the j-th selected signal for $s_{k,i}[n]$ and m is the total number of the selected signals.

Similar to the wiener filter method [46], the selected signals are employed to estimate the artifact and then subtracted from the object signal as Eq. (10.20),

$$\mathbf{S}_{\mathrm{cs},k,i} = \mathbf{S}_{k,i} - \mathbf{S}_{\mathbf{select}} \cdot \mathbf{w}, \tag{10.20}$$

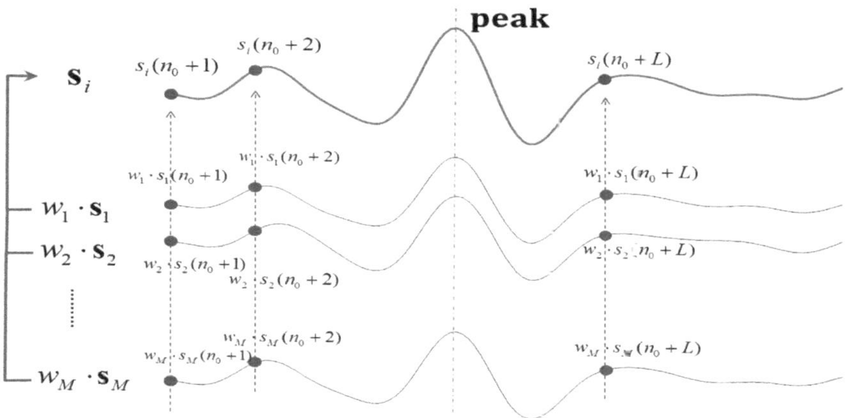

Figure 10.14 The schematic diagram of the received waveforms at different rotation angles for adaptive filtering [20].

where $\mathbf{s}_{\mathrm{cs},k,i}$ is the clutter suppressed signal for $s_{k,i}[n]$ and $\mathbf{w}$ is the filter weight vector. The task is to find an optimal weight vector, by which the clutters can be suppressed and the reflections from the breast interior can be preserved. A column vector of L is defined as the number of time samples for $s_{k,i}[n]$ as Eq. (10.21),

$$\mathbf{b}_{k,i} = [s_{k,i}[n_0 + 1], \ldots, s_{k,i}[n_0 + L]]^T, \tag{10.21}$$

where n_0 is the start of the signal. Time interval $(n_0 + 1, n_0 + L)$ only includes the surface scattering or antenna coupling. Let the $L \times m$ matrix $\mathbf{H} = [\mathbf{b}_{ki,1},\ldots,\mathbf{b}_{ki,j},\ldots,\mathbf{b}_{ki,m}]$ be the counterparts from the selected m signals within the same time interval.

To estimate the artifact, the weight vector is expected to satisfy $\mathbf{Hw} = \mathbf{b}_{k,i}$. For this linear equation, the number of equations should be larger than the number of the unknown weight vector. Otherwise, the problem will be underdetermined, resulting in infinite solutions or no solution. Therefore, the number of the selected signal, which is m, should be smaller than L. Conventionally, the optimal weight vector is obtained in a least square sense by minimizing $||\mathbf{b}_{k,i} - \mathbf{Hw}||^2$. However, the similarity of the signals may lead to large norm of the weight which amplifies the noise. Instead, in an improved adaptive filtering method, the similarity is regarded as beneficial information for filtering.

A prior constraint is introduced to regularize the least square using L_2 regularization as Eq. (10.22),

$$\min_{\mathbf{w}}\left[\left\|\mathbf{b}_{k,i}-\mathbf{Hw}\right\|^2+\lambda\left\|\mathbf{w}-\bar{\mathbf{w}}\right\|^2\right], \tag{10.22}$$

where λ is the constraint parameter and $\bar{\mathbf{w}}$ = $[1, 1, \ldots\ldots, 1^T]/m$; $\bar{\mathbf{w}}$ is chosen based on the fact that the selected signals are with high degree of similarity to the object signal. The optimization problem (10.22) is equivalently seeking the optimal solution around $\bar{\mathbf{w}}$ to solve Eq. (10.22), two variables are introduced as $\mathbf{x} = \mathbf{w} - \bar{\mathbf{w}}$ and $\mathbf{y} = \mathbf{b}_{k,i} - \mathbf{H}\bar{\mathbf{w}}$. Inserting $\mathbf{x}$ and $\mathbf{y}$ in Eq. (10.22), the problem can be rewritten as

$$\min_{\mathbf{x}}\left\|\begin{pmatrix}\mathbf{H}\\ \sqrt{\lambda}\cdot\mathbf{I}\end{pmatrix}\mathbf{x}-\begin{pmatrix}\mathbf{y}\\ \mathbf{0}\end{pmatrix}\right\|^2. \tag{10.23}$$

The normal equation for Eq. (10.23) is given by

$$\begin{pmatrix}\mathbf{H}\\ \sqrt{\lambda}\cdot\mathbf{I}\end{pmatrix}^T\begin{pmatrix}\mathbf{H}\\ \sqrt{\lambda}\cdot\mathbf{I}\end{pmatrix}\hat{\mathbf{x}}=\begin{pmatrix}\mathbf{H}\\ \sqrt{\lambda}\cdot\mathbf{I}\end{pmatrix}^T\begin{pmatrix}\mathbf{y}\\ \mathbf{0}\end{pmatrix}, \tag{10.24}$$

which is also written as

$$(\mathbf{H}^T\mathbf{H}+\lambda\mathbf{I})\hat{\mathbf{x}}=\mathbf{H}^T\mathbf{y}, \tag{10.25}$$

where $\hat{\mathbf{x}}$ is the solution for Eq. (10.23). Solve Eq. (10.25) and substitute $\hat{\mathbf{x}}$ and $\mathbf{y}$ with $\hat{\mathbf{w}} - \bar{\mathbf{w}}$ and $\mathbf{b}_{k,i} - \mathbf{H}\bar{\mathbf{w}}$.

The optimal solution $\hat{\mathbf{w}}$ for Eq. (10.22) is

$$\hat{\mathbf{w}}=\bar{\mathbf{w}}+(\mathbf{H}^T\mathbf{H}+\lambda\mathbf{I})^{-1}\mathbf{H}^T(\mathbf{b}_{k,i}-\mathbf{H}\bar{\mathbf{w}}). \tag{10.26}$$

10.3.4 Clinical Tests for Breast Cancer Screening

In order to develop the breast cancer detector and the imaging algorithm, the sensitivity is evaluated by the use of the breast phantom first, then excised breast tissues after mastectomy, and finally pilot clinical tests for patients are conducted at the hospital. The performed pilot clinical tests are conducted by the guidelines and protocols of the Japan Clinical Oncology Group protocol manual ver. 2.6, which approved the breast cancer detector and its measurement procedure.

First, the evaluation using a breast phantom is conducted. A silicone breast prosthesis is used as a normal breast tissue phantom as shown in Fig. 10.15a. This prosthesis is originally used for breast reconstruction after mastectomy. The dielectric constant of the silicone is 4 at 6 GHz, which is close to that of an adipose tissue. The detector rotates in clockwise around the breast as shown in Fig. 10.15b. A 1 cm^3-size target whose dielectric constant is 45 at 6 GHz is inserted into the phantom. Received signal waveforms are obtained from 120 angles as shown in Fig. 10.15c.

Since the signal intensity of a target reflection is very weak compared with the direct wave, it cannot be observed explicitly in the raw signals shown in Fig. 10.15c. In order to extract the signal from a target, a reference signal is formed by averaging all received signals from all the angles so that the target reflection can be extracted in the subtracted signals after subtracting the reference signal from the original raw signal. The subtracted waveforms for 0–360° rotation (120 angles) are shown in Fig. 10.15d. Please note that the amplitude is 100 LSB (least significant bit) after analog-to-digital conversion due to the loss in the phantom in comparison with the maximum peak of 2300 LSB corresponding to the 12-bit for the received signals. The reconstructed confocal images of the breast are generated using the subtracted signals as shown in Fig. 10.15e When the target size is $0.5 \times 0.5 \times 0.5$ cm^3, corresponding images are shown in Fig. 10.15f. The successful detection demonstrates the detection ability of targets with the size as small as $0.5 \times 0.5 \times 0.5$ cm^3.

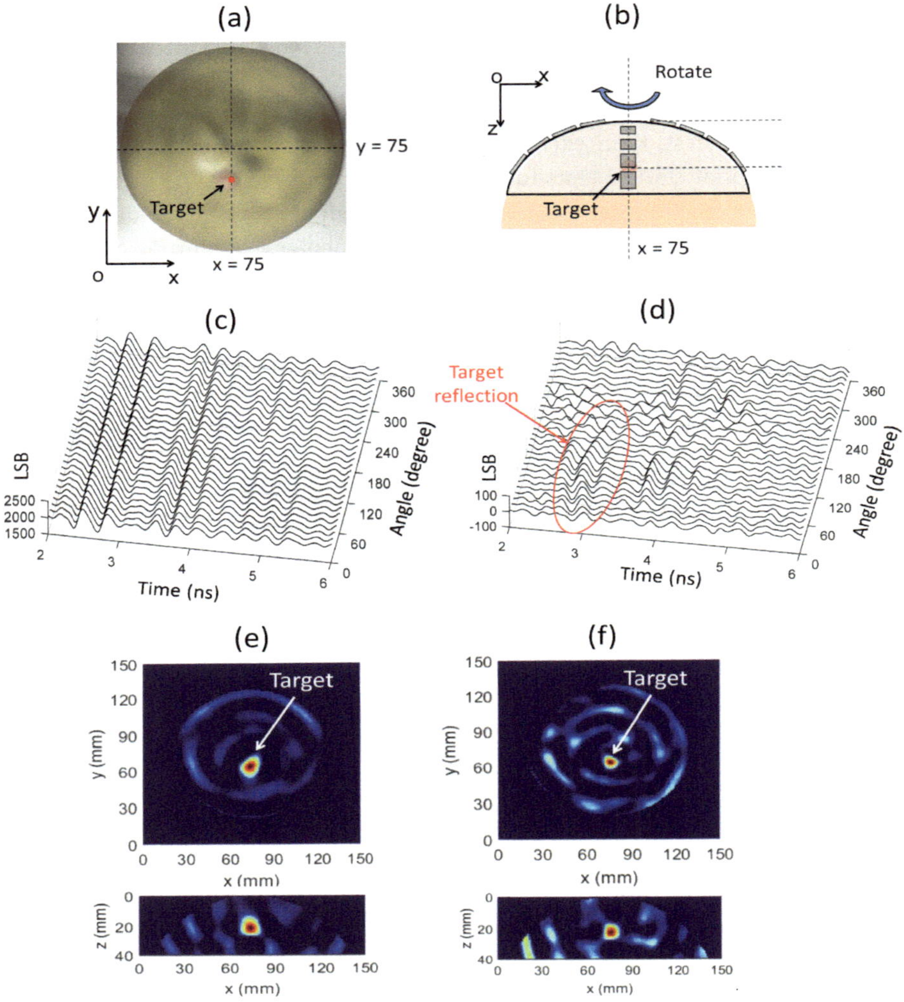

Figure 10.15 (a) Plan-view photograph of breast phantom. (b) Cross-sectional view of breast phantom showing the target position and rotation of antennas. (c) Received signal waveforms corresponding to the rotation angles. (d) Subtracted signal waveforms where the target reflection is shown. (e) Reconstructed confocal image of the target with the size of 1 cm^3 in x–y plane and x–z plane. (f) Reconstructed confocal image of the target with the size of $0.5 \times 0.5 \times 0.5$ cm^3 in x–y plane and x–z plane [51].

Next, the system is applied to the excised breast tissues after mastectomy of the cancer surgery at the hospital. After the mastectomy cancer surgery operation is over, the breast is first dissected by the pathologist doctor to confirm the position of the tumor and take tumor samples as shown in Figs. 10.16a,b. Then the breast is covered with polyethylene film to isolate the blood and fold the cut incision, then, the detector is placed on the cut breast to conduct the detection experiment as shown in Fig. 10.16c. After the experiment, the electrical properties of the tissues are measured using a 2.2 mm-radius coaxial probe. Dielectric constants and conductivity versus frequency for tumor, glandular and adipose tissues are shown in Figs. 10.16d,e. Cole–Cole plot for the breast tissues is shown in Fig. 10.16f. The measurement results show that the difference between tumor tissue and normal tissues are apparent. The confocal imaging results are shown in Figs. 10.16g,h, corresponding to Figs. 10.16a,b, respectively.

From the reconstructed breast images, the tumor is successfully recognized and the position is almost consistent with the tumor physical position. Compared with the phantom results, the signal-to-noise ratio becomes worse in the excised breast case. This is caused by the inhomogeneous feature of the real breast tissues. The detectability of malignant tumors is demonstrated for excised breast tissues after mastectomy of the cancer surgery. The three-dimensional positions of the tumors are consistent with the results of the histopathology analysis. The successful detection of the tumor in the excised breast demonstrates the robustness of the system and the imaging algorithm.

In the clinical examination five volunteer patients were recruited, who have been diagnosed to have breast cancers. The malignant tumors include invasive ductal carcinoma (IDC) and ductal carcinoma in situ (DCIS). The patients were informed the total process of the detection and signed the consent. Before the test, the clinical doctors were trained how to use the detector. The clinical tests were conducted at the hospital by the oncologists without any engineers on the spot. After the tests, the raw data were sent and the information of the cancer details was not notified. Then, the imaging process was conducted and the results were sent to the doctors for evaluation. By comparing the imaging results with the MRI, X-ray and PET (position emission tomography), the conclusion was made.

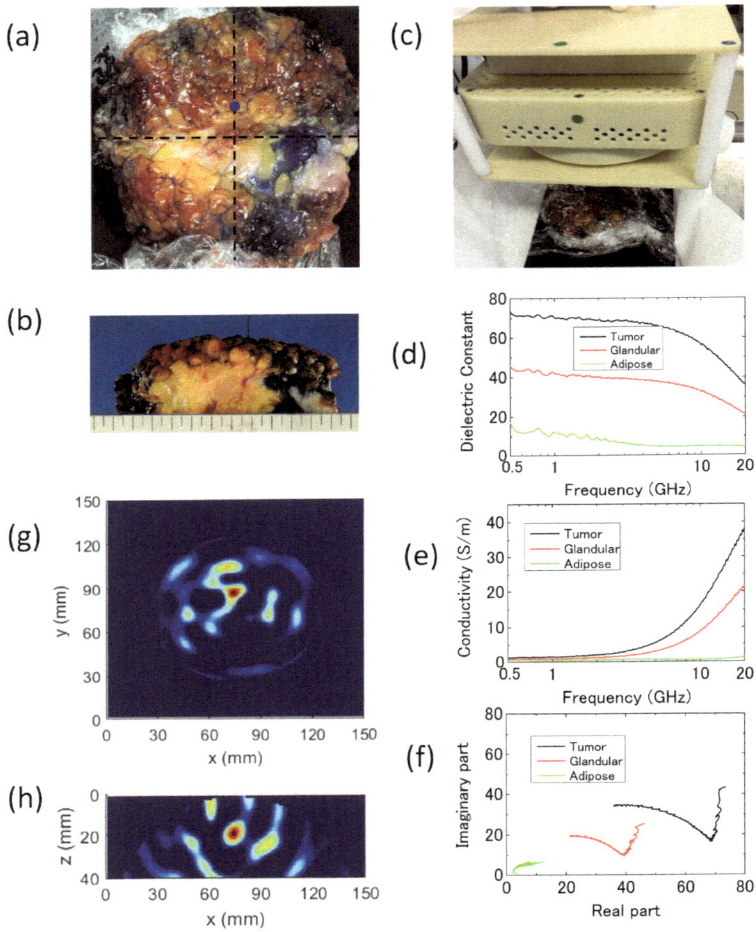

Figure 10.16 (a) Plan-view photograph of excised breast tissue after mastectomy. (b) Cross-sectional view photograph of excised breast tissue after mastectomy. (c) Photograph of breast cancer detector on the cut breast being covered with a poly-ethylene film. (d) Dielectric constant versus frequency for tumor, glandular and adipose tissues. (e) Conductivity versus frequency for tumor, glandular and adipose tissues. (f) Cole–Cole plot of the breast tissues. (g) Reconstructed plan-view image of the breast corresponding to Fig. 10.16a. (h) Reconstructed cross-section-view image of the breast corresponding to Fig. 10.16b [51].

During the test, the patients were asked to lie on the supine position and the detector is put on the breast as shown in Figs. 10.17a,b. The rotation is clockwise. The confocal imaging results of one patient breast scan are shown in Figs. 10.17c,d. The 3-D display area shown in Fig. 10.17e is created by the threshold of 0.7 of the maximum. The grey cover is the profile of the dome antenna and the white squares are the antenna positions. The MRI scan is shown in Fig. 10.17f. There is a good agreement in both methods, demonstrating the detectability of the breast tumor using the breast cancer detector.

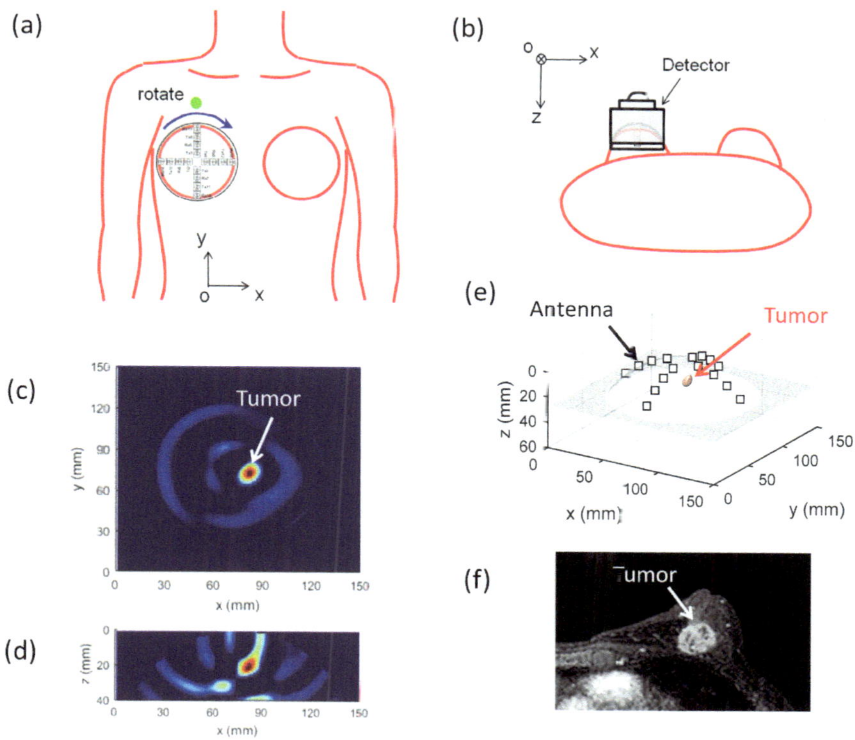

Figure 10.17 Results of pilot clinical test. (a) Plan-view illustration of clinical test for the right breast. (b) Cross-sectional view illustration of patient with supine position. (c) Reconstructed plan-view of confocal image. (d) Reconstructed cross-sectional view of confocal image. (e) Three-dimensional view of confocal image showing the location of a tumor with respect to antenna positions. (f) MRI scan of corresponding breast [51].

In conclusion, the detectability of a hand-held impulse-radar breast tumor detector is demonstrated. The successful detection of the tumor in the cut breast after mastectomy shows the feasibility of the hand-held impulse-radar detector system in real inhomogeneous scenario. The pilot clinical test is conducted on malignant breast tumors of IDC and DCIS for five patients at the hospital. The imaging results show a good agreement with those of MRI. These promising results show the possibility of hand-held breast tumor detection and monitoring system for easy access to everyone.

10.4 Challenges to Microwave Imaging

Since many clinical investigations of microwave breast imaging have been published, the results have indicated the potential of microwave imaging to detect breast cancer with sensitivity results reported from women with dense breasts. The remaining challenges of clinical trials will include specificity with no breast abnormalities or benign breast diseases. Performance comparison of microwave imaging systems and issues were reviewed in the literature [55, 56].

The radar-based confocal imaging approach cannot provide quantitative dielectric properties of a target object, whereas microwave tomography can determine the quantitative distribution of the constitutive dielectric properties of the target object. The tomography algorithms can be categorized as frequency domain or time domain techniques. Frequency domain methods use single or multiple frequency measurements to iteratively solve the microwave inverse problem. Time domain methods use UWB impulse signals to iteratively solve the microwave inverse problem. The inverse scattering problem for tomography is solved from the scattered electromagnetic energy although it is inherently ill-posed.

The first clinical prototype of microwave tomography for breast imaging was developed in 2000 [57]. It was a frequency domain microwave tomography method called the log-magnitude unwrapped-phase technique [58]. This method was based on the iterative Gauss–Newton approach to reconstruct the dielectric properties of experimental phantoms [59, 60].

The effect of tomography on the evaluation of neoadjuvant chemotherapy for breast cancer was examined for eight patients [61]. The microwave tomography reconstructed images of the distribution of dielectric properties and demonstrated changes with the degree of treatment response with respect to pathology [62, 63]. The water content distribution in fibro-glandular tissue was also analyzed for 43 women, resulting in the distribution of the permittivity [64]. Several nonlinear iterative algorithms [65–68] were developed to reconstruct the quantitative dielectric distributions of the breast.

In terms of frequency domain, various tomography methods such as distorted born iterative method [69–72], variations of Gauss–Newton iterative method [57, 65], wavelet-based iterative method [70], and the iterative contrast source inversion technique [71, 73, 74] were developed. Multiple-frequency tomography methods were also developed to estimate the average dielectric properties of the breast [75–78]. The qualitative properties, such as shape, size, and location could be calculated by either linear or nonlinear methods [79–82]. Linear approximations (mainly Born and Rytov) were used to estimate the qualitative properties of the target.

Time domain microwave tomography methods were developed by the use of UWB microwave to iteratively solve the microwave inverse problem. A gradient-based approach, conjugate gradient, was used to update the dielectric properties at each iterative step of the inversion process. A time domain tomography method, called forward-backward time stepping, was developed to reconstruct dielectric properties using UWB microwave measurements [82, 83].

Many practical challenges exist in translating microwave imaging algorithms to the clinical examinations as follows: living tissue with real blood flow, movement of patient, positioning of breast, constituent of breast, reflection at breast skin, attenuation in breast skin, etc.

To solve these issues, the following approaches are necessary with respect to hardware fast acquisition times (less than a minute), high signal-to-noise-ratio (greater than 30 dB), large bandwidth (greater than 10 GHz).

References

1. S. Chaudhary, R. Mishra, A. Swarup, and J. M. Thomas, Dielectric properties of normal & malignant human breast tissues at radiowave & microwave frequencies, *Indian J. Biochem. Biophys.*, vol. 21, no. 1, pp. 76–79, 1984.
2. A. J. Surowiec, S. S. Stuchly, J. R. Barr, and A. Swarup, Dielectric properties of breast carcinoma and the surrounding tissues, *IEEE Trans. Biomed. Eng.*, vol. 35, no. 4, pp. 257–263, 1988.
3. A. Campbell and D. Land, Dielectric properties of female human breast tissue measured in vitro at 3.2 GHz, *Phys. Med. Biol.*, vol. 37, no. 1, p. 193, 1992.
4. W. T. Joines, Y. Zhang, C. Li, and R. L. Jirtle, The measured electrical properties of normal and malignant human tissues from 50 to 900 MHz, *Med. Phys.*, vol. 21, no. 4, pp. 547–550, 1994b.
5. C. Gabriel, S. Gabriel, and E. Corthout, The dielectric properties of biological tissues: I. literature survey, *Phys. Med. Biol.*, vol. 41, no. 11, p. 2231, 1996a.
6. S. Gabriel, R. Lau, and C. Gabriel, The dielectric properties of biological tissues: II. measurements in the frequency range 10 Hz to 20 GHz, *Phys. Med. Biol.*, vol. 41, no. 11, p. 2251, 1996b.
7. S. Gabriel, R. Lau, and C. Gabriel, The dielectric properties of biological tissues: III. parametric models for the dielectric spectrum of tissues, *Phys. Med. Biol.*, vol. 41, no. 11, p. 2271, 1996c.
8. K. R. Foster, H. P. Schwan, Dielectric properties of tissues and biological materials: A critical review, *Crit. Rev. Biomed. Eng.*, vol. 17, pp. 25–104, 1989.
9. M. Lazebnik, L. McCartney, D. Popovic, C. B. Watkins, M. J. Lindstrom, J. Harter, S. Sewall, A. Magliocco, J. H. Booske, M. Okoniewski, and S. C. Hagness, A large-scale study of the ultrawideband microwave dielectric properties of normal breast tissue obtained from reduction surgeries, *Phys. Med. Biol.*, vol. 52, pp. 2637–2656, 2007.
10. M. Lazebnik, D. Popovic, L. McCartney, C. B. Watkins, M. J. Lindstrom, J. Harter, S. Sewall, T. Ogilvie, A. Magliocco, T. M. Breslin, W. Temple, D. Mew, J. H. Booske, M. Okoniewski, and S. C. Hagness, A large-scale study of the ultrawideband microwave dielectric properties of normal, benign and malignant breast tissues obtained from cancer surgeries, *Phys. Med. Biol.*, vol. 52, pp. 6093–6115, 2007.
11. T. Sugitani, S. Kubota, S. Kuroki, K. Sogo, K. Arihiro, M. Okada, T. Kadoya, M. Hide, M. Oda, and T. Kikkawa, Complex permittivities of

breast tumor tissues obtained from cancer surgeries, *Appl. Phys. Lett.*, vol. 104, no. 25, p. 253702, 2014; erratum: *Appl. Phys. Lett.*, vol. 107, p. 019902.

12. A. Martellosio, M., Pasian, M. Bozzi, L. Perregrini, A. Mazzanti, F. Svelto, P. Eugene Summers, G. Renne, L. Preda, and M. Bellomi, Dielectric properties characterization from 0.5 to 50 GHz of breast cancer tissues, *IEEE Trans. Microwave Theory Tech.*, vol. 65, no. 3, pp. 998–1011, 2017.
13. E. C. Fear, S. C. Hagness, P. M. Meaney, M. Okoniewski, and M. A. Stuchly, Enhancing breast tumor detection with nearfield imaging, *IEEE Microwave Magaz.*, vol. 3, no. 1, pp. 48–56, 2002.
14. E. C. Fear, P. M. Meaney, and M. A. Stuchly, Microwaves for breast cancer detection? *IEEE Potentials*, vol. 22, pp. 12–18, 2003.
15. N. K. Nikolova, *Introduction to Microwave Imaging*, Cambridge University Press, July 2017, ISBN: 9781107085565.
16. R. C. Conceição, J. J. Mohr, and M. O'Halloran, eds., *An Introduction to Microwave Imaging for Breast Cancer Detection*, Springer International Publishing AG Switzerland, 2016, ISBN 978-3-319-27865-0, ISBN 978-3-319-27866-7 (eBook).
17. N. K. Nikolova, Microwave imaging for breast cancer, *IEEE Microwave Magaz.*, vol. 12, no. 7, pp. 78–94, 2011.
18. A. Shahzad, Fast ultra wideband microwave imaging for early stage breast cancer detection, Doctoral thesis of Electrical and Electronic Engineering, National University of Ireland, Galway, Ireland, 2017.
19. M. A. Elahi, Confocal microwave imaging and artifact removal algorithms for the early detection of breast cancer, Doctoral thesis of Electrical & Electronic Engineering, College of Engineering & Informatics, National University of Ireland Galway, Ireland, 2018.
20. H. Song, Time-domain impulse radar imaging for breast cancer detection using CMOS integrated circuits, Doctoral thesis of Electrical and Electronic Engineering, Graduate School of Advanced Sciences of Matter, Hiroshima University, Higashi-Hiroshima, Japan, 2018.
21. D. D. O'Loughlin, Improving the sensitivity of radar-based breast imaging algorithms in diverse patient populations, Doctoral thesis of Electrical and Electronic Engineering, College of Engineering and Informatics, National University of Ireland Galway, Ireland, 2018.
22. S. L. Nass, I. C. Henderson, and J. C. Lashof, *Mammography and Beyond: Developing Technologies for the Early Detection of Breast Cancer*, National Academy Press, 2001.

23. R. E. Bird, T. Wallace, and B. Yankaskas, Analysis of cancers missed at screening mammograph, *Radiology*, vol. 184, pp. 613–617, 1992.
24. R. A. Hubbard, K. Kerlikowske, C. I. Flowers, B. C. Yankaskas, W. Zhu, and D. L. Miglioretti, Cumulativ after 10 years of screening mammography—a cohort study, *Annals of Internal Medicine*, vol. 155, no. 8, pp. 481–492, 2011.
25. R. D. Rosenberg, W. C. Hunt, M. R. Williamson, F. D. Gilliland, P. W. Wiest, C. A. Kelsey, C. R. Key, and M. N. Linver, Effects of age, breast density, ethnicity, and estrogen replacement therapy on screening mammographic sensitivity and cancer stage at diagnosis: Review of 183, 134 screening mammograms in Albuquerque, New Mexico, *Radiology*, vol. 209, no. 2, pp. 511–518, 1998.
26. C. M. Ronckers, C. A. Erdmann, C. E. Land, et al., Radiation and breast cancer: A review of current evidence, *Breast Cancer Res.*, vol. 7, no. 1, pp. 21–32, 2005.
27. WHO Classification of Tumours of the Breast. 4th ed., WHO Classification of Tumours, vol. 4, IARC WHO Classification of Tumours, no. 4. Lakhani, S. R., Ellis. I. O., Schnitt, S. J., Tan, P. H., van de Vijver, M. J., IARC, Switzerland, ISBN-13 9789283224334, ISBN-10 9283224337.
28. Japanese Breast Cancer Society, The general rules for clinical and pathological recording of breast cancer, *Japanese J. Surg.*, vol. 19, no. 5 pp. 612–632, 1989.
29. J. R. Harris, et al., eds., *Disease of the Breast*, 4th ed. Philadelphia, PA, USA, Wolters Kluwer/Lippincot Wiliams & Wilkins, pp. 321–407, 2010.
30. H. Song, S. Sasada, N. Masumoto, T. Kadoya, N. Shiroma, M. Orita, K. Arihiro, M. Okada, and T. Kikkawa, Detectability of breast tumors in excised breast tissues of total mastectomy by IR-UWB-radar-based breast cancer detector, *IEEE Trans. Biomed. Eng.*, vol. 66, no. 8, AUGUST 2019, pp. 2296–2305.
31. W. D. Hurt, Multiterm Debye dispersion relations for permittivity of muscle, *IEEE Trans. Biomed. Eng.*, vol. 32, pp. 60–64 1985.
32. M. Lazebnik, M. Okoniewski, J. H. Booske, and S. C. Hagness, Highly accurate Debye models for normal and malignant breast tissue dielectric properties at microwave frequencies, *IEEE Microw. Wireless Components Lett.*, vol. 17, no. 12, 2007.
33. D. Popovic, L. McCartney, C. Beasley, M. Lazebnik, M. Okoniewski, S. C. Hagness, and J. Booske, Precision open-ended coaxial probes

for in vivo and ex vivo dielectric spectroscopy of biological tissues at microwave frequencies, *IEEE Trans. Microw. Theory Tech.*, vol. 53, pp. 1713–1722, 2005.

34. D. A. G. Bruggeman, Berechnung verschiedener physikalischer Konstanten von heterogenen Substanzen. I. Dielektrizittskonstanten und Leitfhigkeiten der Mischkrper aus isotropen Substanzen, *Annalen der Physik*, vol. 416, no. 7, pp. 636–664, 1935.

35. S. C. Hagness, A. Taove, and J. E. Bridges, Two-dimensional FDTD analysis of a pulsed microwave confocal system for breast cancer detection: Fixed-focus and antenna-array sensors, *IEEE Trans. Biomed. Eng.*, vol. 45, no. 12, pp. 1470–1479, 1998.

36. E. Fear and M. Stuchley, Microwave system for breast tumor detection, *IEEE Microw. Guided Wave Lett.*, vol. 9, pp. 470–472, 1999.

37. J. Bourqui, J. Sill, and E. Fear, A prototype system for measuring microwave frequency reflections from the breast, *Int. J. Biomed. Imaging*, vol. 2012, Article ID 851234 https://doi.org/10.1155/2012/851234, 2012.

38. M. Klemm, I. Craddock, J. Leendertz, A. Preece, and R. Benjamin, Improved delay-and-sum beamforming algorithm for breast cancer detection, *Int. J. Antennas Propagation*, vol. 2008, p. 9, 2008.

39. M. Klemm, I. J. Craddock, J. A. Leendertz, A. Preece, and R. Benjamin, Radar-based breast cancer detection using a hemispherical antenna array experimental results, *IEEE Trans. Antennas Propagation*, vol. 57, pp. 1692–1704, 2009.

40. M. Klemm, J. Leendertz, D. Gibbins, I. Craddock, A. Preece, and R. Benjamin, Microwave radar-based breast cancer detection: Imaging in inhomogeneous breast phantoms, *IEEE Antennas Wireless Propagation Lett.*, vol. 8, pp. 1349–1352, 2009.

41. H. B. Lim, N. T. T. Nhung, E.-P. Li, and N. D. Thang, Confocal microwave imaging for breast cancer detection: Delay-multiply-and-sum image reconstruction algorithm, *IEEE Trans. Biomed. Eng.*, vol. 55, no. 6, pp. 1697–1704, 2008.

42. D. Byrne, M. O'Halloran, M. Glavin, and E. Jones, Data independent radar beamforming algorithms for breast cancer detection, *Prog. Electromagnetics Res.*, vol. 107, pp. 331–348, 2010.

43. D. Byrne and I. J. Craddock, Time-domain wideband adaptive beamforming for radar breast imaging, *IEEE Trans. Antennas Propagation*, vol. 63, no. 4, pp. 1725–1735, 2015.

44. A. Shahzad, M. O'halloran, E. Jones, and M. Glavin, Prefiltered beamforming for early-stage breast cancer detection, *IEEE Antennas Wireless Propagation Lett.*, vol. 12, pp. 500–503, 2013.

45. Y. Xie, B. Guo, L. Xu, J. Li, and P. Stoica, Multi-static adaptive microwave imaging for early breast cancer detection, *IEEE Trans. Biomed. Eng.*, vol. 53, pp. 1647–1657, 2006.

46. E. J. Bond, X. Li, S. C. Hagness, and B. D. Van Veen, Microwave imaging via space-time beamforming for early detection of breast cancer, *IEEE Trans. Antennas Propagation*, vol. 51, pp. 1690–1705, 2003.

47. M. O'Halloran, E. Jones, and M. Glavin, Quasi-multistatic mist beamforming for the early detection of breast cancer, *IEEE Trans. Biomed. Eng.*, vol. 57, pp. 830–840, 2010.

48. E. C. Fear, J. Bourqui, C. Curtis, D. Mew, B. Docktor, and C. Romano, Microwave breast imaging with a monostatic radar-based system: A study of application to patients, *IEEE Trans. Microw. Theory Tech.*, vol. 61, no. 5, pp. 2119–2128, 2013.

49. E. Porter, M. Coates, and M. Popovic, An early clinical study of time-domain microwave radar for breast health monitoring, *IEEE Trans. Biomed. Eng.*, vol. 63, no. 3, pp. 530–539, 2016.

50. A. W. Preece, I. Craddock, M. Shere, L. Jones, and H. L. Winton., MARIA M4: Clinical evaluation of a prototype ultrawideband radar scanner for breast cancer detection, *J. Med. Imag.*, vol. 3, no. 3, 2016, Art. no. 033502.

51. H. Song, S. Sasada, T. Kadoya, M. Okada, K. Arihiro, X. Xiao, and T. Kikkawa, Detectability of breast tumor by a hand-held impulse-radar detector: Performance evaluation and pilot clinical study, November 27, 2017, pp. 1–11. *Scientific Reports*, vol. 7, Article number: 16353, 2017.

52. H. Song, A. Azhari, X. Xiao, E. Suematsu, H. Watanabe, and T. Kikkawa, Microwave imaging using CMOS integrated circuits with rotating 4 × 4 antenna array on a breast phantom, *Int. J. Antennas Propagation*, vol. 2017, Article ID 6757048, p. 13, 2017.

53. H. Song, H. Kono, Y. Seo, A. Azhari, J. Somei, E. Suematsu, Y. Watarai, T. Ota, H. Watanabe, Y. Hiramatsu, A. Toya, X. Xiao, and T. Kikkawa, A radar-based breast cancer detection system using CMOS integrated circuits, *IEEE Access*, vol. 3, pp. 2111–2121, 29 Oct., 2015 Date of Current Version :12 Nov., 2015.

54. H. Song, S. Sasada, N. Masumoto, T. Kadoya, M. Okada, K. Arihiro, X. Xiao, and T. Kikkawa, A two-stage rotational surface clutter

suppression method for microwave breast imaging with multistatic impulse-radar detector, *IEEE Trans. Instrum. Meas.*, vol. 69, pp. 9586–9598, 2020.

55. D. O'Loughlin, M. O'Halloran, B. M. Moloney, M. Glavin, E. Jones, and M. A. Elahi, Microwave breast imaging: Clinical advances and remaining challenges, *IEEE Trans. Biomed. Eng.*, vol. 65, no. 11, pp. 2580–2590, 2018.

56. D. O'Loughlin, B. L. Oliveira, A. Santorelli, E. Porter, M. Glavin, E. Jones, M. Popovíc, and M. O'Halloran, Sensitivity and specificity estimation using patient-specific microwave imaging in diverse experimental breast phantoms, *IEEE Trans. Biomed. Eng.*, vol. 38, no 1, pp. 303–311, 2019.

57. P. M. Meaney, M. W. Fanning, D. Li, S. P. Poplack, and K. D. Paulsen, A clinical prototype for active microwave imaging of the breast, *IEEE Trans. Microwave Theory Tech.*, vol. 48, no. 11, pp. 1841–1853, 2000.

58. P. M. Meaney, K. D. Paulsen, B. W. Pogue, M. Miga, et al., Microwave image reconstruction utilizing log-magnitude and unwrapped phase to improve high contrast object recovery, *IEEE Trans. Med. Imaging*, vol. 20, no. 2, pp. 104–116, 2001.

59. P. Meaney, K. Paulsen, A. Hartov, and R. Crane, Microwave imaging for tissue assessment: Initial evaluation in multitarget tissue-equivalent phantoms, *IEEE Trans. Biomed. Eng.*, vol. 43, no. 9, pp. 878–890, 1996.

60. P. Meaney, K. Paulsen, M. Fanning, D. Li, and Q. Fang, Image accuracy improvements in microwave tomographic thermometry: Phantom experience, *Int. J. Hyperthermia*, vol. 19, no. 5, pp. 534–550, 2003.

61. P. M. Meaney, P. A. Kaufman, L. S. Muffly, M. Click, S. P. Poplack, W. A. Wells, G. N. Schwartz, R. M. di Florio-Alexander, T. D. Tosteson, Z. Li, et al., Microwave imaging for neoadjuvant chemotherapy monitoring: Initial clinical experience, *Breast Cancer Res.*, vol. 15, no. 2, pp. 1–16, 2013.

62. T. M. Grzegorczyk, P. M. Meaney, P. A. Kaufman, R. M. di Florio-Alexander, and K. D. Paulsen, Fast 3-d tomographic microwave imaging for breast cancer detection, *IEEE Trans. Med. Imaging*, vol. 31, no. 8, pp. 1584–1592, 2012.

63. P. M. Meaney, A. H. Golnabi, N. R. Epstein, S. D. Geimer, M. W. Fanning, J. B. Weaver, and K. D. Paulsen, Integration of microwave tomography with magnetic resonance for improved breast imaging, *Med. Phys.*, vol. 40, no. 10, p. 103101, 2013.

64. P. M. Meaney, M. W. Fanning, T. Raynolds, C. J. Fox, Q. Fang, C. A. Kogel, S. P. Poplack, and K. D. Paulsen, Initial clinical experience with microwave breast imaging in women with normal mammography, *Acad. Radiol.*, vol. 14, no. 2, pp. 207–218, 2007.

65. A. Fhager, M. Gustafsson, and S. Nordebo, Image reconstruction in microwave tomography using a dielectric Debye model, *IEEE Trans. Biomed. Eng.*, vol. 59, no. 1, pp. 156–166, 2012.

66. P. Mojabi and J. LoVetri, A prescaled multiplicative regularized Gauss-Newton inversion, *IEEE Trans. Antennas Propagation*, vol. 59, no. 8, pp. 2954–2963, 2011.

67. D. Kurrant and E. Fear, Regional estimation of the dielectric properties of inhomogeneous objects using nearfield reflection data, *Inverse Probl.*, vol. 28, no. 7, p. 075001, 2012.

68. G. Oliveri, L. Lizzi, M. Pastorino, and A. Massa, A nested multi-scaling inexact-Newton iterative approach for microwave imaging, *IEEE Trans. Antennas Propagation*, vol. 60, no. 2, pp. 971–983, 2012.

69. W. Chew and Y. Wang, Reconstruction of two-dimensional permittivity distribution using the distorted born iterative method, *IEEE Trans. Med. Imaging*, vol. 9, no. 2, pp. 218–225, 1990.

70. R. Scapaticci, I. Catapano, and L. Crocco, Wavelet-based adaptive multiresolution inversion for quantitative microwave imaging of breast tissues, *IEEE Trans. Antennas Propagation*, vol. 60, no. 8, pp. 3717–3726, 2012.

71. A. Zakaria and J. LoVetri, The finite-element method contrast source inversion algorithm for 2d transverse electric vectorial problems, *IEEE Trans. Antennas Propagation*, vol. 60, no. 10, pp. 4757–4765, 2012.

72. Z. Q. Zhang and Q. H. Liu, Three-dimensional nonlinear image reconstruction for microwave biomedical imaging, *IEEE Trans. Biomed. Eng.*, vol. 51, no. 3, pp. 544–548, 2004.

73. C. Gilmore, A. Abubakar, W. Hu, T. M. Habashy, and P. M. Van Den Berg, Microwave biomedical data inversion using the finite difference contrast source inversion method, *IEEE Trans. Antennas Propagation*, vol. 57, no. 5, pp. 1528–1538, 2009.

74. I. Catapano, L. Di Donato, L. Crocco, O. M. Bucci, A. F. Morabito, T. Isernia, and R. Massa, On quantitative microwave tomography of female breast, *Prog. Electromagnetics Res.*, vol. 97, pp. 75–93, 2009.

75. D. W. Winters, J. D. Shea, P. Kosmas, B. D. Van Veen, and S. C. Hagness, Three-dimensional microwave breast imaging: Dispersive dielectric

properties estimation using patient-specific basis functions, *IEEE Trans. Med. Imaging*, vol. 28, no. 7, pp. 969–981, 2009.

76. R. Scapaticci, P. Kosmas, and L. Crocco, Wavelet-based regularization for robust microwave imaging in medical applications, *IEEE Trans. Biomed. Eng.*, vol. 62, no. 4, pp. 1195–1202, 2015.
77. J. D. Shea, P. Kosmas, S. C. Hagness, and B. D. Van Veen, Three-dimensional microwave imaging of realistic numerical breast phantoms via a multiple-frequency inverse scattering technique, *Med. Phys.*, vol. 37, p. 4210, 2010.
78. J. Shea, P. Kosmas, B. Van Veen, and S. Hagness, Contrast-enhanced microwave imaging of breast tumors: A computational study using 3d realistic numerical phantoms, *Inverse Probl.*, vol. 26, no. 7, p. 074009, 2010.
79. L. Jofre, M. S. Hawley, A. Broquetas, E. de Los Reyes, M. Ferrando, and A. R. Elias-Fuste, Medical imaging with a microwave tomographic scanner, *IEEE Trans. Biomed. Eng.*, vol. 37, no. 3, pp. 303–312, 1990.
80. N. Irishina, M. Moscoso, and O. Dorn, Microwave imaging for early breast cancer detection using a shape-based strategy, *IEEE Trans. Biomed. Eng.*, vol. 56, no. 4, pp. 1143–1153, 2009.
81. M. El-Shenawee and E. L. Miller, Spherical harmonics microwave algorithm for shape and location reconstruction of breast cancer tumor, *IEEE Trans. Med. Imaging*, vol. 25, no. 10, pp. 1258–1271, 2006.
82. J. E. Johnson, T. Takenaka, K. Ping, S. Honda, and T. Tanaka, Advances in the 3-d forward-backward time-stepping inverse scattering technique 154 for breast cancer detection, *IEEE Trans. Biomed. Eng.*, vol. 56, no. 9, pp. 2232–2243, 2009.
83. T. Moriyama, Z. Meng, and T. Takenaka, Forward-backward time-stepping method combined with genetic algorithm applied to breast cancer detection, *Microw. Opt. Technol. Lett.*, vol. 53, no. 2, pp. 438–442, 2011.

Chapter 11

Ultrasonic Transducers and Non-Contact Measurement Technique for Medical and Agricultural Application/Flexible Acoustic Force Sensor

Marie Tabaru[a] and Kazuaki Nishimura[b]

[a]*Tokyo Institue of Technology, 4259 Nagatsuda-cho, Yokohama, Kanagawa 226-8503, Japan*
[b]*Tohoku University, 4-1 Seiryo-machi, Aoba-ku, Sendai 980-8575, Japan*

tabaru.m.ab@m.titech.ac.jp, knishimura@dent.tohoku.ac.jp

This chapter describes low-intensity ultrasonic transducer and airborne ultrasonic transducer. The chapter also introduces a novel technique by using the transducers for medical and agricultural application. Furthermore, a flexible force sensor by using acoustic characteristics of soft-tube is explained. The relating technical fields are so wide that each topic is described in an independent section.

Biomedical Engineering
Edited by Akihiro Miyauchi and Yuji Miyahara

ISBN 978-981-4877-63-3 (Hardcover), 978-1-003-14194-5 (eBook)
www.jennystanford.com

11.1 Impact of Ultrasound Therapy on Bisphosphonate-Related Osteonecrosis of the Jaw [1]

11.1.1 Introduction

Bisphosphonates (BPs) are drugs of osteoclastic resorption used to treat impairment of bone remodeling and, therefore, to prevent bone loss and be conserved in the integrity of the bone structure. They are indicated in osteoporosis, bone metastases, multiple myeloma, and malignant hypercalcemia. However, with increasing use of a new generation of BPs which have higher potency than earlier generation of BPs, evidence from the side effects of BPs implied that patients taking BPs are at risk of developing BP-related osteonecrosis of the jaw (BRONJ). BRONJ is a serious oral complication associated with antiresorptive and antiangiogenic therapies; it results in progressive bone and soft tissue destruction in the maxillofacial region. It has been more than 15 years since it was first reported in 2003; the pathogenesis of BRONJ remains unclear. Moreover, preventive treatment and definitive treatment strategies for BRONJ have not been developed due to its uncertain mechanisms. We have previously demonstrated that the presence of oral bacteria is required for the onset of BRONJ and that diminished production of keratinocyte growth factor (KGF) in the lesion may be associated with the pathogenically retarded epithelial wound healing processes [2]. Moreover, we revealed a critical pathogenic engagement of Semaphorin 4D (Sema4D), which potently inhibits bone formation, produced by γδT cells in the development of BRONJ [3]. We focused on the development of a novel prevention and treatment method that uses low-intensity pulsed ultrasound (LIPUS), which accelerates bone healing and decreases the amount of biofilm. The purpose of this study is to investigate the effects of ultrasound using the BRONJ mouse model, collect basic data for future clinical application to human, and prepare and adjust ultrasonic generators.

11.1.2 Materials and Methods

Animals and experiment design: C57BL/6J wild-type (WT mice) 6–8-week-old females were obtained from the Charles River Laboratory. BRONJ was induced following a method reported previously [2, 3]. Briefly, after 4 weeks of pretreatment with Zoledronate (Zol) or control saline, the mice received extraction of upper first molar, followed by oral inoculation with *Fusobacterium nucleatum* (Fn; 10^9 CFU) or PBS every other day for 14 days.

Low-intensity pulsed ultrasound device: A function generator (SG-4105 IWATSU), an oscilloscope (DS-5105 B IWATSU), a power amplifier (HSA 4101 NF corporation), and a port driven vibrator (KAIJO) (Fig. 11.1) were connected and used as an ultrasound stimulator. Around the extraction socket area received ultrasound treatment as follows; ultrasound intensity 451 mW/cm^2, frequency 3 MHz, pulse width 200 μs, the 1 kHz pulse wave was repeated and treatment lasted for 14 days, once daily, 20 min for each radiation [4].

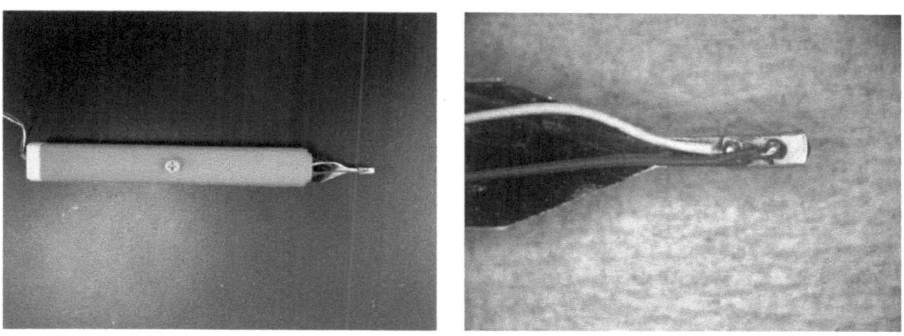

Figure 11.1 Developed ultrasonic transducer for oral treatment of mouse.

11.1.3 Results and Discussion

Evaluation of the efficacy of LIPUS in the prevention of BRONJ development: LIPUS-group (Zol + Fn + LIPUS) showed almost complete healing of the extraction socket. However, in the BRONJ-group, unhealed epithelial wounds and persistently exposed extraction sockets were observed at Day 15 (Fig. 11.2).

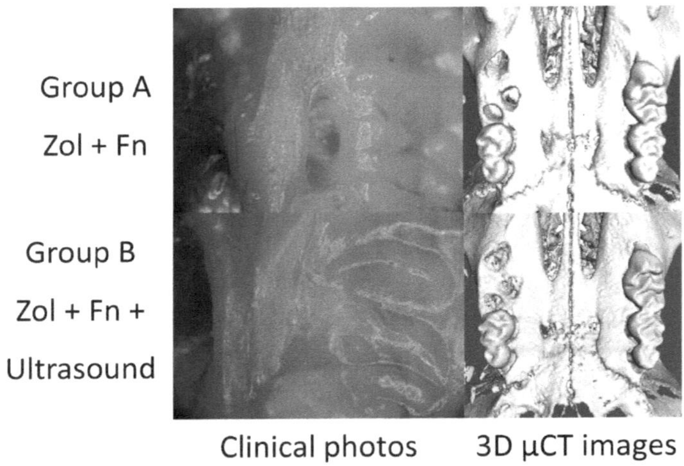

Figure 11.2 Clinical and μCT evaluation of ultrasound on BRONJ-like lesions. Group B (Zol+Fn+ultrasound) showed complete healing of the epithelial wounds. However, in Group A (Zol+Fn) showed unhealed epithelial wounds and persistently exposed extraction sockets were observed at Day 15.

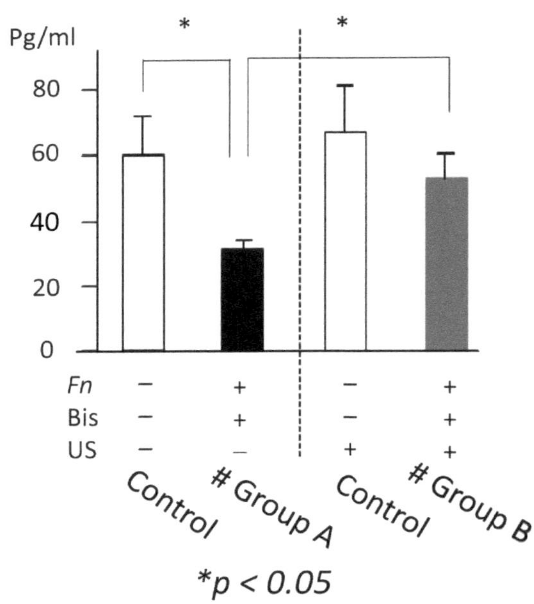

Figure 11.3 KGF production in gingival tissue on day 15 measured by ELISA.

To evaluate the levels of cytokines in the mouse BRONJ model, murine gingival tissues were homogenized and the concentrations of KGF* and Sema4D** were measured by ELISA (enzyme-linked immuno sorbent assay).

The production level of KGF was significantly decreased in Group A (Zol + Fn) than the control. However, in Group B (Zol + Fn + Ultra sound), the production level of KGF recovered to the control level (Fig. 11.3). Sema4D concentration were significantly higher in Group A (Zol + Fn) than the control, whereas in Group B (Zol + Fn + Ultra sound), Sema4D concentration were at the same level as the control (Fig. 11.4).

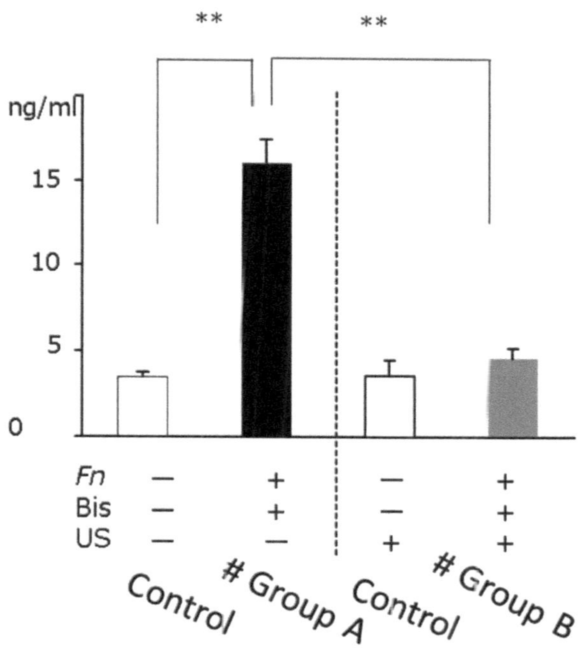

Figure 11.4 Sema4D production in gingival tissue on day 15 measured by ELISA.

11.1.4 Conclusions

These findings suggest that LIPUS stimulation may prevent the development of BRONJ and affect the production level of KGF and Sema4D.

*KGF: Keratinocyte growth factor (KGF), a member of the fibroblast growth factor (FGF) family, is a growth factor produced by stromal cells in epithelial tissues. It plays an important role in the growth control of epithelial cells.

**Sema4D: Semaphorin-4D is a coupling factor expressed on osteoclasts and plays an important role as a suppressor of bone formation.

11.2 Non-Contact Hardness Measurement of Fruits Using Airborne Ultrasound [5]

11.2.1 Introduction

The demand for high-quality fruits has increased, and various sensors are integrated in sorting factories [6]. Although hardness is one of the criteria for fruits' quality [7], it is still measured by hands. There is a conventional hardness meter for fruits. However, since the conventional one is a contact type, fruits may be damaged. Therefore, it is necessary to develop a non-contact method to measure the hardness of fruits. We have studies about the non-contact method using airborne ultrasound, where the surfaces of fruits were excited by focusing airborne ultrasound and produced vibrations were measured with a laser Doppler velocimeter (LDV) [8]. In this study, we observed the time-dependent changes in the hardness parameters of 12 kinds of fruits using the proposed technique.

11.2.2 Methods

In this study, the viscoelastic properties of fruits are based on the Kelvin–Voigt model [9, 10]. We assume that the spring constants and center frequencies decrease as fruits ripen, and the maximum displacements and damping coefficients increase. Twelve kinds of fruits were chosen as samples: strawberries, grapes, cherry, American cherry, mandarin orange, banana, oranges, kiwifruit, Japanese pear, peach, apple, melons (small floral pattern, middle, and bottom). The numbers of samples were 10 for strawberries and grapes, 3 for melons and oranges, and 1 for the others. Measurement periods were 4 weeks (measured once a week) for apples and oranges, 40 days for kiwifruit (measured every 4 days). Other samples were measured for 5 days (measured once a day). The samples were placed on trays in laboratory without covering during the measurement period.

Figure 11.5 shows the measurement system [8]. A high-power planar ultrasonic transducer (NGC100-D50, Ultran) was driven with burst sine waves (100 kHz, 5 waves, 160 Vp-p). The planar ultrasonic wave was focused on the fruits' surfaces by using an offset-type parabolic reflector. Then, vibration was produced on the fruits surfaces due to acoustic radiation pressure. The vibrations of the fruit surface were measured using a LDV and data were stored into a personal computer (PC). The maximum displacements, center frequencies, and damping coefficients were calculated by performing integral calculation and frequency analysis. Figures 11.6a–c show the examples of input wave, velocity waveform, and displacement waveform. The frequency spectrum of velocity waveform was also calculated. In order to investigate the trends of change of hardness properties over time, linear approximations were performed and gradients were estimated. In addition, the hardness of the sample was measured using a fruit hardness tester. The samples were categorized into group 1 with larger sizes and larger elastic moduli such as apples, pears and oranges, and group 2 with smaller sizes and smaller elastic moduli such as cherries and strawberries.

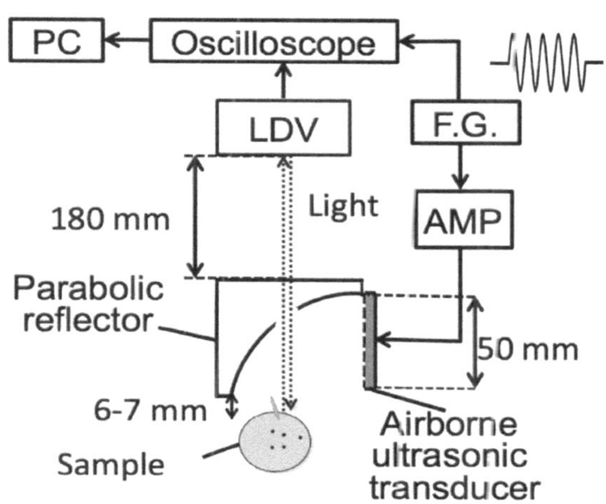

Figure 11.5 Schematic of the experimental system.

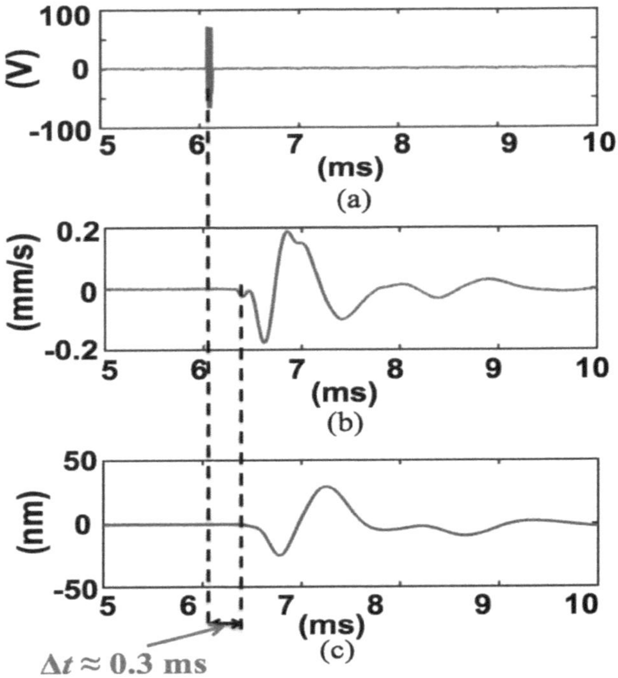

Figure 11.6 Procedure of signal processing. (a) Input wave (burst sine wave), (b) measured velocity, and (c) calculated displacement.

11.2.3 Results and Discussion

Figures 11.7a–c show the gradient l_1 for the maximum displacements, l_2 for the center frequencies, and l_3 for the damping coefficients, respectively. As assumed with the Kelvin–Voigt model, the damping coefficients and maximum displacements increased (l_1 and l_3 were positive), and the center frequencies decreased (l_2 was negative) as the fruits ripened. The results also show that the absolute values of all the gradients are smaller in the group 1. On the contrary, the samples in the group 2 had the larger gradients for all the parameters. The fruits such as peaches and kiwifruits tended to have the large standard deviations. One of the reasons is that these samples have a rough surface and the laser waves were scattered on the fruits' surfaces. The differences of positions of melon samples were not large except l_2.

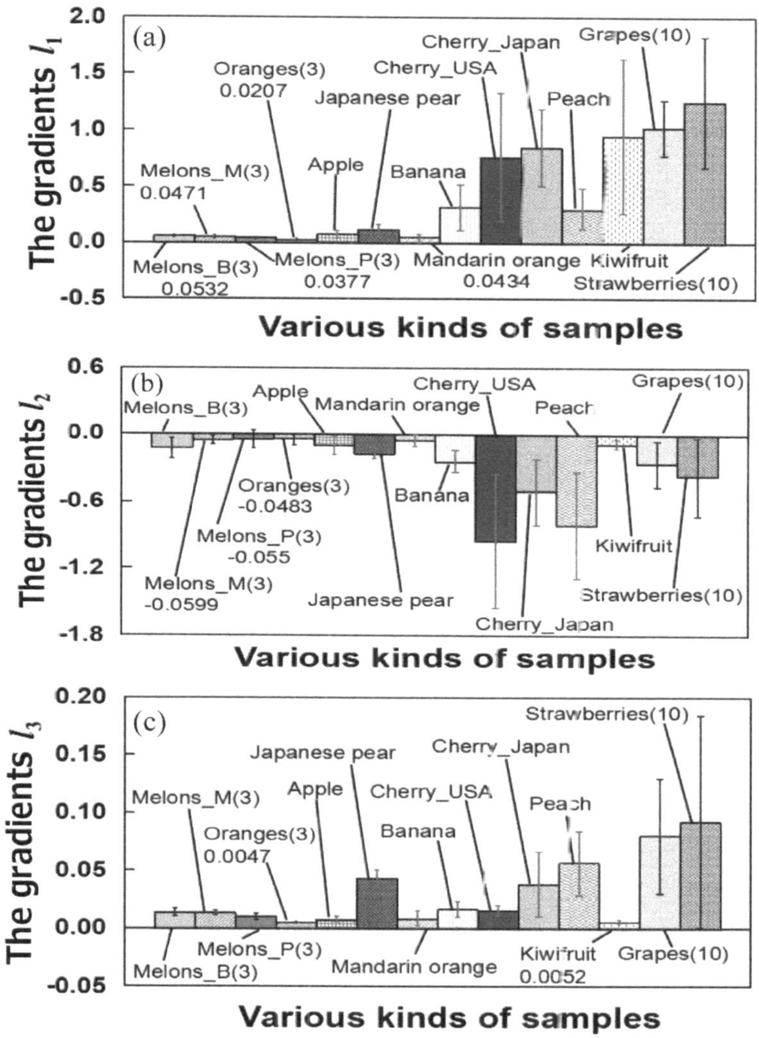

Figure 11.7 The gradients (a) l_1, (b) l_2, and (c) l_3 of various kinds of samples.

11.2.4 Conclusion

The changes with time of 12 kinds of fruits were successfully measured with the proposed non-contact method. The results showed that the changes of the elastic properties were the same as expected. In addition, it was possible to classify the differences of the gradients with time in the two groups. Therefore, we confirm that the proposed non-contact measurement system could be effective for judging the maturity of fruits. It is necessary to improve the measurement method for the fruits which have rough surfaces, such as peach and kiwifruit.

11.3 The Soft and Sensitive Door-Pinching Sensor Utilizing Acoustic Characteristics of an Elastic Tube [11]

11.3.1 Introduction

Door-pinching accidents in trains have become a serious problem. A force sensor utilizing acoustic characteristics of an elastic tube can be potentially used as a soft and sensitive door-pinching sensor to detect the pinching of small objects such as a string, a stick, and the wheel of a baby car. Nakamura et al. proposed a distributed-force sensor by utilizing acoustic characteristics of tube [12]. In the previous system, it was difficult to detect which position is closer to the sound source because of the proximity of the DC component. In this section, we introduce the improvement in the performance of the proposed sensor by removing the DC component, utilizing polynomial approximation, and detection of 1 mm deformation in the range of 100–2100 mm became possible by applying dual sound sources.

11.3.2 Methods

Figure 11.8 shows an experimental setup. A rubber tube of a door head (inside diameter: 15 mm, length: 2200 mm), which is generally used in a train door, was examined. Static deformations from 1 to 10 mm were applied at 1 mm intervals. Each deformation, sweep wave (2–9 kHz, 0.2 V_{pp}) was outputted from an earphone and propagated inside the tube. Part of the wave reflected at the deformation position and the other parts of the wave transmitted. Simultaneously, interference wave was inputted into the microphone. The data was stored with a sampling period of 6.4 × 10^{-5} s into a PC via an oscilloscope for following signal processing. Firstly, Fourier spectrum was calculated by fast Fourier transform (FFT). Signals were 95% overlapped so that resulted spectrum has a resolution of 3.9 Hz. Next, position response was calculated by second FFT. Here, position response can be written as

$$p(x) = p_0^2 \left\{ (1 + r^2)\,\delta(x) + r\delta\left(x \pm 2\pi \frac{2x_L}{c} \right) \right\}, \tag{11.1}$$

where p_0 is the incident acoustic pressure, c is The sound speed in air (= 340 m/s), x_L is the deformation position, and r is the reflection coefficient of sound pressure at the deformation position. Before the second FFT, the signal without deformation was subtracted from the signal after deformation. The DC component was also removed by polynomial approximation to detect the deformation at the positions less than x_L = 300 mm.

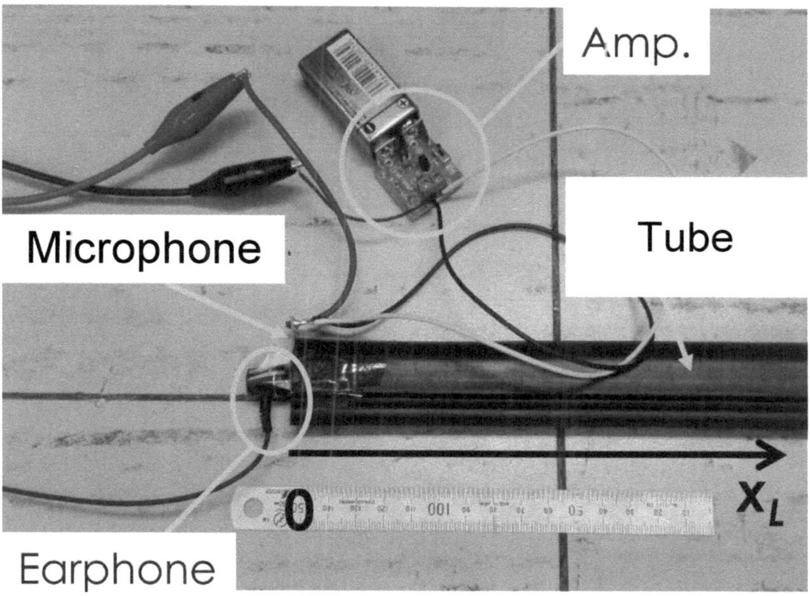

Figure 11.8 Experimental setup.

11.3.3 Results and Conclusion

Figure 11.9 shows the position response for the deformation of 3 mm at x_L = 100 mm. The figure shows it is possible to detect the peak at x_L = 100 mm after removal of DC component.

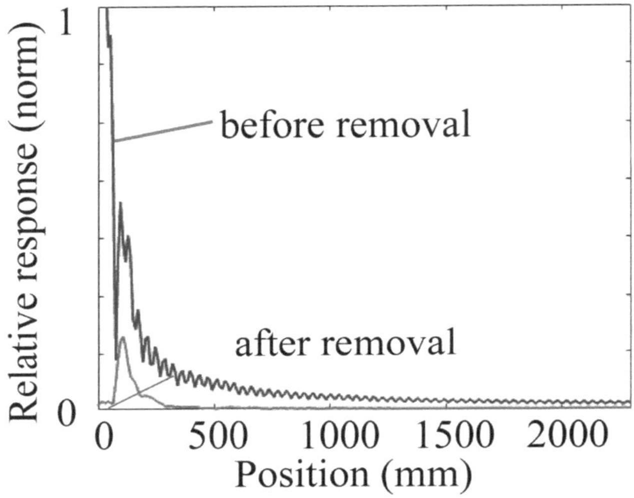

Figure 11.9 The position response before and after the removal of DC component.

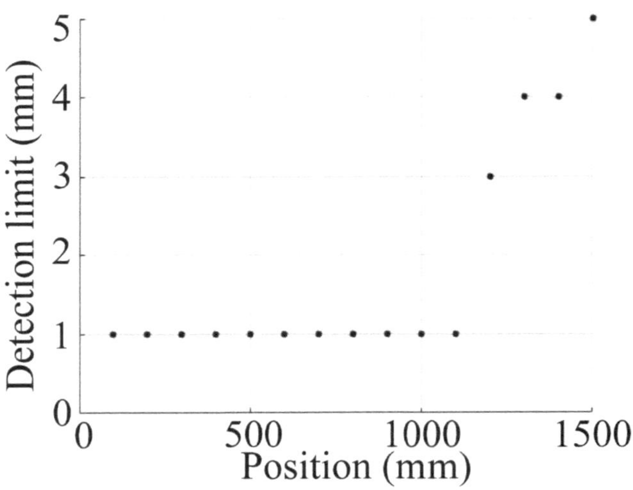

Figure 11.10 Detection limit vs. position.

Figure 11.10 shows that the minimum detectable deformation as a function of detective positions. Deformations of 1 mm were detected at x_L = 100–1100 mm. By applying dual sound sources at the both ends of the tube, deformations of 1 mm were successfully detected at the range of x_L = 100–2100 mm. The results confirm that the proposed sensor can be used to as a soft and sensitive door-pinching sensor.

11.4 Viscoelasticity Measurement for Living Tissue Using Airborne Ultrasonic Doppler Method [13]

11.4.1 Introduction

Non-contact viscoelasticity measurements have been required in various fields, such as management of fruits and vegetables, development of medical materials, and diagnosis of inflammatory skin [14, 15]. Conventional non-contact viscoelasticity measurement techniques often use light wave such as laser Doppler velocimeter for vibration measurement. Measurements using light wave are highly accurate; however, they are affected by the surface condition (unevenness or transparent material) of the target materials. The purpose of this study is to establish a measurement technique that enables non-contact viscoelasticity measurement even in such a situation by using MHz airborne ultrasonic for vibration measurement. In this section, we introduce non-contact vibration measurement system using airborne ultrasonic transducer. The viscoelastic properties of an elastic phantom and a chicken sample were examined for confirmation.

11.4.2 Experimental Method

(i) Measurement system

We applied a contact measurement technique of viscoelastic properties [16] to non-contact method by using airborne ultrasound. Figure 11.11 shows the experimental setup.

A vibrator was set on a sample surface for vibration excitation. In this study, a piezoelectric actuator (MTKK16S400F170R, Mechano Transformer) was used as a vibrator. The surface wave is detected by an airborne ultrasonic transducer (HAR1907225, Japan Probe) with center frequency of 1 MHz, aperture diameter of 24 mm, focal length of 18.5 mm, focal width of 0.7 mm, and focal depth of 5.7 mm. Figure 11.12 shows the two-dimensional distribution of energy of the airborne ultrasonic transducer calculated using Huygens' principle [17].

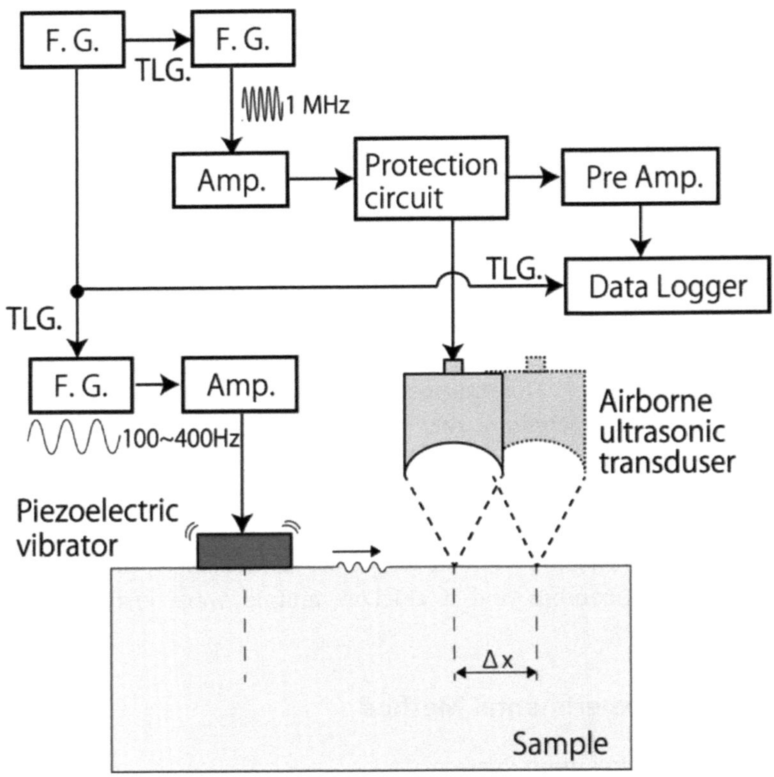

Figure 11.11 Experimental setup.

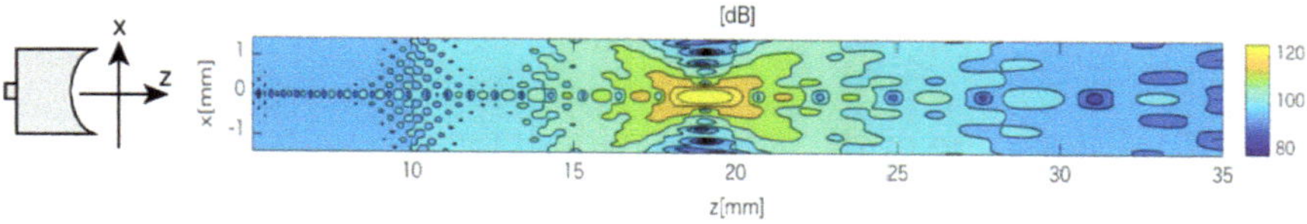

Figure 11.12 Pressure distribution of an airborne ultrasonic transducer.

(ii) Estimation principle of viscoelasticity

The phase velocity of a surface wave is expressed by the following equation:

$$c_s(\omega_s) = \omega_s \Delta x / \Delta\phi \tag{11.2}$$

where Δx is the distance between two points, $\Delta\phi$ is the phase difference, and ω_s is the center frequency of the surface wave [16]. It is known that Rayleigh waves propagate on a solid surface such as a living tissue. The propagation speed of the Rayleigh wave is approximated by the following equation:

$$c_s = \frac{1}{1.06}\sqrt{\frac{\mu_1}{\rho}} \tag{11.3}$$

where μ_1 is the shear modulus and ρ is the density. When the Voigt model is applied to Eq. (11.2), the equation containing the viscosity coefficient is obtained as shown in Eq. (11.3).

$$c_s(\omega_s) = \frac{1}{1.06}\sqrt{\frac{2(\mu_1^2 + \omega_s^2\mu_2^2)}{\rho(\mu_1 + \sqrt{\mu_1^2 + \omega_s^2\mu_2^2})}} \tag{11.4}$$

Here, μ_1 is a shear modulus and μ_2 is a viscosity coefficient. In this experiment, phase velocity of surface wave was obtained from Eq. (11.1), and the shear moduli and the viscosity coefficients were obtained from Eq. (11.3). If a viscoelastic material is assumed to have Poisson's ratio close to 0.5, the shear modulus, μ_1, can be related to Young's modulus E by $E \fallingdotseq 3\mu_1$.

(iii) Estimation of viscoelastic parameters

An elastic phantom (100 × 100 × 50 mm^3, Young's modulus: 30 kPa, OST) and a chicken wing were used as samples. Sine waves (100, 200, 300, 400 Hz; 3 waves; 104 V_{pp}) were inputted to the piezoelectric actuator for excitation. For the detection of surface waves, sine waves (1 MHz, 5 waves, PRF = 8 kHz, 124 V_{pp}) were inputted to the airborne ultrasonic transducer. The reflected ultrasonic waves from the sample surface were received by the airborne ultrasonic transducer. The received signals were acquired using a data logger (MR6000, Hioki) at a sampling frequency of 50 MHz. The distances from the piezoelectric actuator to the ultrasonic transducer were set to 30, 31, 32, 33, and 34 mm. Displacements were calculated by conventional correlation calculation method.

11.4.3 Experimental Results

Figure 11.13 shows the calculated displacements at 30 and 34 mm when the excitation frequency was 200 Hz. Figure 11.13 shows that surface waves are observed in 10 ms < t < 30 ms, and the phases of the waves at the positions of x = 30 and 40 mm are different. Figure 11.14 shows the calculated phase for each position. Figure 11.15 shows the phase velocity of the surface wave obtained by substituting the inverse of the slope of Fig. 11.14 into Eq. (11.1). When fitting was performed using Fig. 11.15 and Eq. (11.3), viscoelasticity was estimated as μ_1 = 10.7 kPa and μ_2 = 0.7 Pa·s. Young's modulus was estimated to 32.1 kPa. From the estimated results, the error was 7% for the phantom Young's modulus of 30 kPa. The result shows that viscosity was small value, which agreed with the reference [16]. Figure 11.16 shows the phase velocity of the surface wave of the chicken sample. Viscoelasticity was estimated as μ_1 = 3.1 kPa and μ_2 = 3.1 Pa·s. Young's modulus μ was estimated to 9.3 kPa. The estimated viscosity coefficient of the chicken was higher than that of phantom.

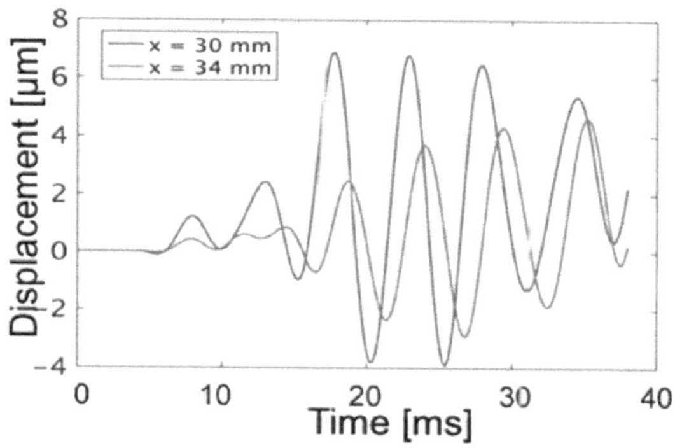

Figure 11.13 Calculated displacements of surface wave.

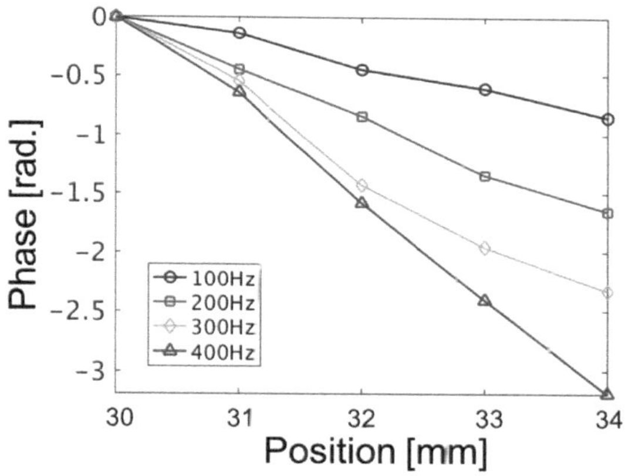

Figure 11.14 Phase vs. position (phantom).

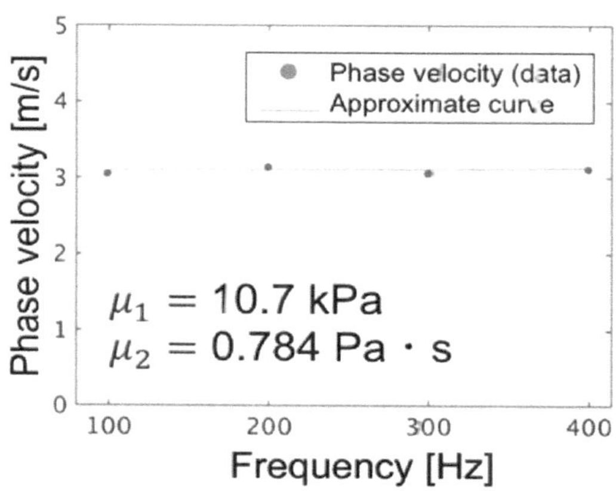

Figure 11.15 Estimated phase velocity (phantom).

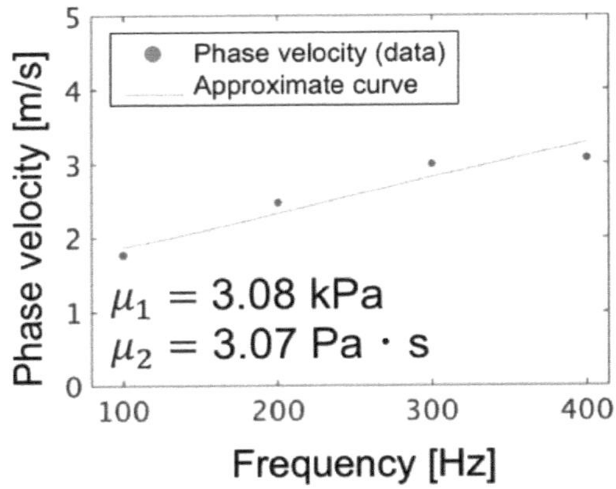

Figure 11.16 Estimated phase velocity (chicken).

11.4.4 Summary and Future Study

The viscoelasticity of the elastic phantom and chicken was successfully measured by the developed airborne ultrasonic Doppler system. For a future study, we will consider non-contact vibration.

Acknowledgments

Section 11.1: The part of this work was supported by Murata Science Foundation.

Section 11.2: The part of this work was supported by Ono Acoustics Research Fund.

Section 11.3: This work was supported by JSPS KAKENHI Grant Number 15K20991 and 18K04009. The part of this work was supported by Takano Science Foundation and Eno Science Foundation.

Section 11.4: The authors are grateful to Japan Probe for airborne ultrasonic transducers. The part of this work was supported by Ono Acoustics Research Fund.

References

1. K. Satomi, K. Nishimura, M. Tabaru, and K. Nakamura, *Proc. 4th International Symposium on Biomedical Engineering (ISBE2019)*, 2019, p. 130.

2. H. Mawardi, et al., *J. Dental Res.*, 2011, 90, 1339–1345.
3. A. Movila, et al., *Biochem. Biophys. Res. Commun*, 2016, 480, 42–47.
4. K. Nishimura, et al., Annual report of the Cooperative Research Project of Research Center for Biomedical Engineering, 2019, 106.
5. H. Hashimoto, C. Wu, and M. Tabaru, *The 4th International Symposium on Biomedical Engineering (ISBE2019)*, 2019, p. 120.
6. http://www.shibuya-sss.co.jp/case/case03.html.
7. P. Chen and Z. Sun, *J. Agric. Eng. Res.*, 1991, 49, 85.
8. M. Tabaru et al., *Proc. Spring Meeting Acoust. Soc. Japan*, 2015, 1-9-5, 1121.
9. H. Hosaka, *Introduction to Mechanical Vibrations*, 2005, 41–67.
10. S. Terasaki et al., *J. Japan. Soc. Hort. Sci.*, 2001, 70(5), 572–580.
11. S. Shimomura, K. Fujii, M. Tabaru, *International Workshop on Piezoelectric Materials and Applications in Actuators (IWPMA2018)*, 2018, p. 133.
12. K. Nakamura, S. Odajima, and M. Tabaru, *Acoust. Sci. Tech.*, 2017, 38, 80–86.
13. R. Sando, S. Hirata, M. Tabaru, *Viscoelasticity measurement for living tissue using airborne ultrasonic Doppler method, USE2019*, 2019, 1P2-13.
14. M. Tabaru and K. Nakamura, *Proc. of ASJ spring meeting*, 2015, p. 2. [in Japanese].
15. Ł. Ambroziński, et al., *Sci. Rep.*, 2016, 6, p. 11.
16. S. Chen, et al., *J. Acoustic. Soc. Am.*, 2004, 115, 2781.
17. T. L. Szabo, *Diagnostic Sound Imaging: Inside Out* (Elsevier, MA, USA), 2014.

Chapter 12

Time-Resolved CMOS Image Sensors for Biomedical Applications

Shoji Kawahito, Yuya Shirakawa, Keiichiro Kagawa, Keita Yasutomi, and De Xing Lioe

Research Institute of Electronics, Shizuoka University, 3-5-1 Johoku, Naka-ku, Hamamatsu, Shizuoka 432-8011, Japan

skawahito@gmail.com

This chapter presents semiconductor imaging devices using time-resolved pixel architectures that have been designed for use in biomedical applications. A complementary metal–oxide–semiconductor (CMOS) technology provides an opportunity to implement two types of time-resolved semiconductor-based imaging systems. These are a time-correlated single-photon counting (TCSPC) system, which consists of a single-photon avalanche diode (SPAD) detector, and a time-gating-based time-resolved imaging system, which uses lock-in pixels based on a CMOS image sensor technology. In general, TCSPC-based systems exhibit high accuracies and high time resolution at the cost of complicated logic circuits that are required for almost every pixel to measure the photon-arrival times directly and simultaneously.

Biomedical Engineering
Edited by Akihiro Miyauchi and Yuji Miyahara

ISBN 978-981-4877-63-3 (Hardcover), 978-1-003-14194-5 (eBook)
www.jennystanford.com

In contrast, time-gating-based systems are characterized by high spatial resolution with relatively simple lock-in pixels. The obtained time-resolution can be very high upon utilization of multiple time-gating windows with multi-tap lock-in pixels and usage of demodulators designed for fast carrier-response. This chapter focuses on time-resolved lock-in-pixel CMOS image sensors for time-gating-based imaging systems and discusses the principle and design of multi-tap lock-in pixels and biomedical applications using time-resolved CMOS image sensors for fluorescence-lifetime imaging microscopy (FLIM), time-resolved near-infrared spectroscopy (NIRS), time-of-flight (TOF)-based spectroscopy, and stimulated Raman spectroscopy (SRS).

12.1 Basic Pixel Structures

A conceptual schematic of the time-resolved lock-in pixel image sensors with multi-tap outputs is shown in Fig. 12.1. The photocurrent i_{ph} generated in a photo detector, typically a photo diode, flows into a capacitor or a charge integrator at the i-th tap output, y_i (i = 1, 2,..., n) if the switch controlled by w_i (i = 1, 2, ..., n) is turned on, and then the output is expressed as

$$y_i = G_c \int_{o}^{MT_c} i_{ph}(t) w_i(t) dt, \tag{12.1}$$

where G_c is the charge-to-voltage conversion gain, M is the number of cycles, T_c is the cycle time of lock-in operation, and w_i is the charge sampling window function of the i-th tap, where w_i assumes 1 for the switch being turned on and 0 for the switch being turned off, respectively. An example of the timing for multiple-phase sampling is shown in Fig. 12.1 (b). Using multiple-phase sampling with multiple short time-windows, multiple time-correlated components are obtained at one time.

This pixel-level multiple time-correlated sampling is an effective method for highly time-resolved imaging. A time window for charge draining w_D, as shown in Fig. 12.2, is necessary for reducing noise and offset via draining of unwanted charges due to ambient light and dark current.

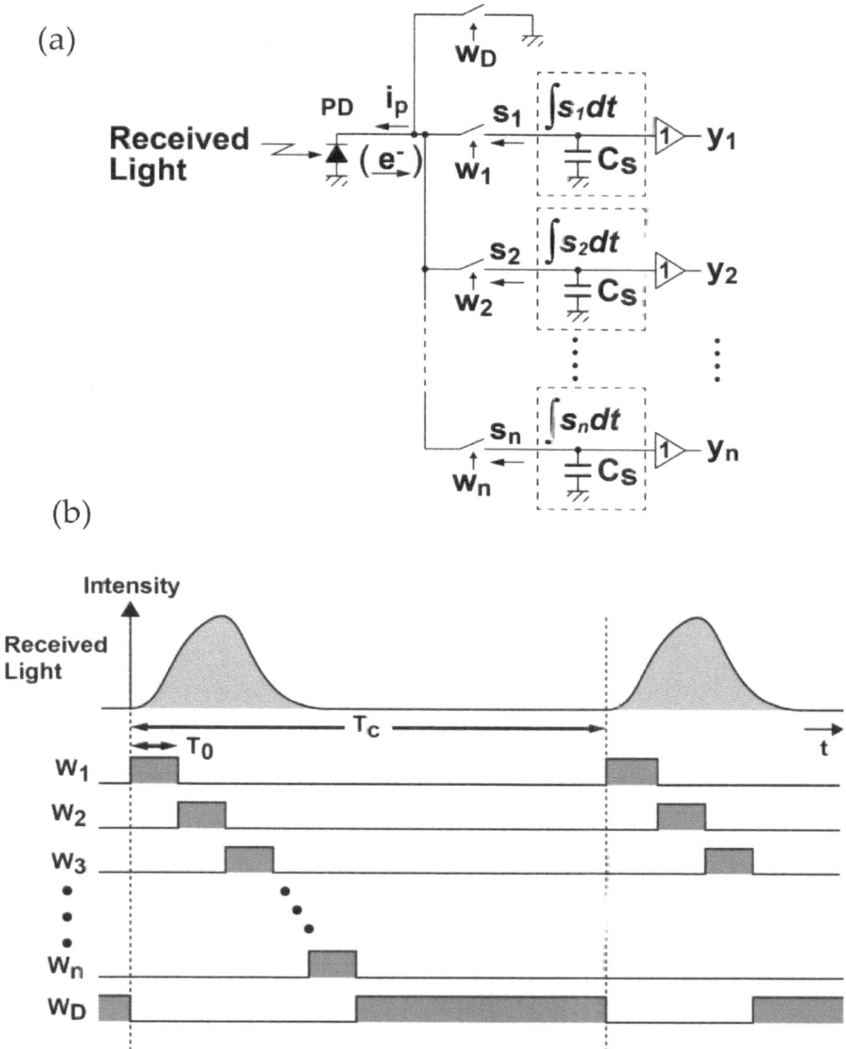

Figure 12.1 Multi-tap lock-in pixel and short multiple-phase sampling for time-resolved imaging. Multi-tap demodulation pixel. Gating in one cycle.

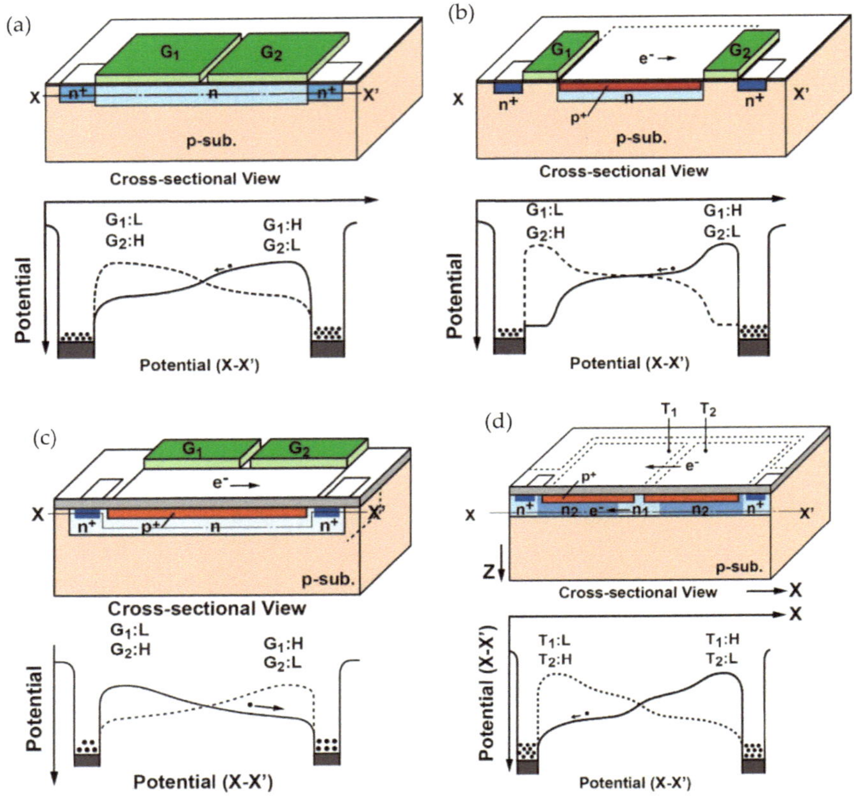

Figure 12.2 Various demodulator designs. (a) Photogate. (b) PPD with transfer gates. (c) PPD with LEFM gates. (d) Tapped PPD.

Time-resolved imaging for biomedical applications requires a time resolution of sub-100 picoseconds. A high-speed demodulator design is one of the key points for highly time-resolved image sensors. Figure 12.2 shows various demodulator designs. The photogate shown in Fig. 12.2a is a traditional demodulator introduced in the 1990s and is mainly used for TOF range imagers [1, 2]. CMOS-based buried-channel photogate demodulators using an additional n-type doping layer [3] and a p-/n-stacked layer [4] are useful for high-speed photocarrier transfer. The operation of the demodulator is described as follows. On application of a high (H) level to gate G_1 and a low (L) level to gate G_2, the depleted channel potential (solid line) for attracting the photocarriers (electrons) to be transferred to the left charge sensing node (n+) is created; On application of L to G_1 and H to G_2, the potential profile (dashed line) for transferring the photocarrier to the right is created. The photogate demodulators present an issue of reflection and absorption of light by the above-silicon structure if front-side illumination is employed. Recently, back-side illumination (BSI)-based photogate demodulators with high quantum efficiency for indirect TOF imagers have been reported [5, 6]. A pinned photodiode (PPD) has been a key technology for attaining high image quality in image sensors since its introduction in interline-transfer CCD image sensors in the 1980s [7]. Figures 12.2b,c, and d show PPD-based demodulators compatible with PPD CMOS image sensor technology. The demodulator with the PPD and transfer gates (Fig. 12.2b) [8] has relatively high potential barriers to prevent un-demodulated leakage when the transfer gates are turned off. A possible problem of this structure is slower photocarrier response at the central region of the PPD if the length of the light aperture size is large, and some electrons fall back to the PPD when a large gate voltage is applied. The demodulator with the PPD and the lateral electric field charge modulator (LEFM) gates (shown in Fig. 12.2c) is relatively effective for high-speed photocarrier transfer if the width of the channel is small and there are fewer fallback electrons to the PPD [9–11]. These PPD-based modulators are not always fast if the light aperture size becomes large because the modulation of the potential profiles is performed at the PPD edge. The tapped PPD demodulator shown in Fig. 12.2 can directly modulate the potential profiles at the central region of the PPD, and very-high-speed carrier transfer is expected [12].

Low-noise time-resolved imaging owing to the limited number of available signal photons is often required for biomedical applications. A demodulator with intermediate storage is useful for a low-noise signal readout based on true-correlated double sampling (true-CDS). A circuit schematic of the lock-in pixel using a 2-tap demodulator with intermediate storage and a drain is shown in Fig. 12.3. Figure 12.4 shows the pixel device structure of a 2-tap demodulator with intermediate storage and potential diagrams for showing the operation of this demodulator [13]. The demodulator type is a PPD with LEFM gates. The charge storage, expressed as C_{i1} and C_{i2} in Fig. 12.3, is implemented by an additional doping layer n_2, as shown in Fig. 12.4, to create a sufficient potential well capacity. In the demodulation phase, by switching the gates G_1 and G_2 between the H and L levels, the photogenerated carriers are transferred to the right or left storage depending on the applied gate voltage levels of G_1 and G_2 as a result of the demodulation. After sufficient lock-in measurement cycles, the accumulated signal is read using the true-CDS process. To accomplish this, the charge sensing node, or floating diffusion node (n+), is reset and then the transfer gates TX_1 and TX_2 are turned on by applying H level to TX_1 and TX_2, and the signal charges are transferred to the charge sensing node and stored in capacitors C_{s1} and C_{s2}. kTC noise is cancelled by the true-CDS via the difference between the reset level (before charge transfer) and the photosignal level (after charge transfer) of the pixel output. In the 4-tap lock-in pixel with intermediate storage, a readout noise level of 1.2e- has been obtained [14].

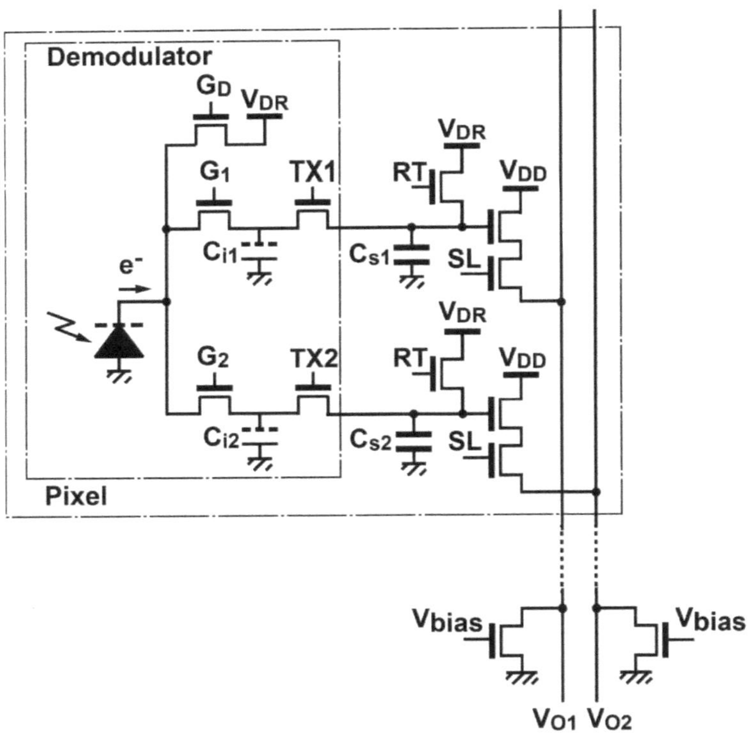

Figure 12.3 Two-tap lock-in pixel with charge storage and drain.

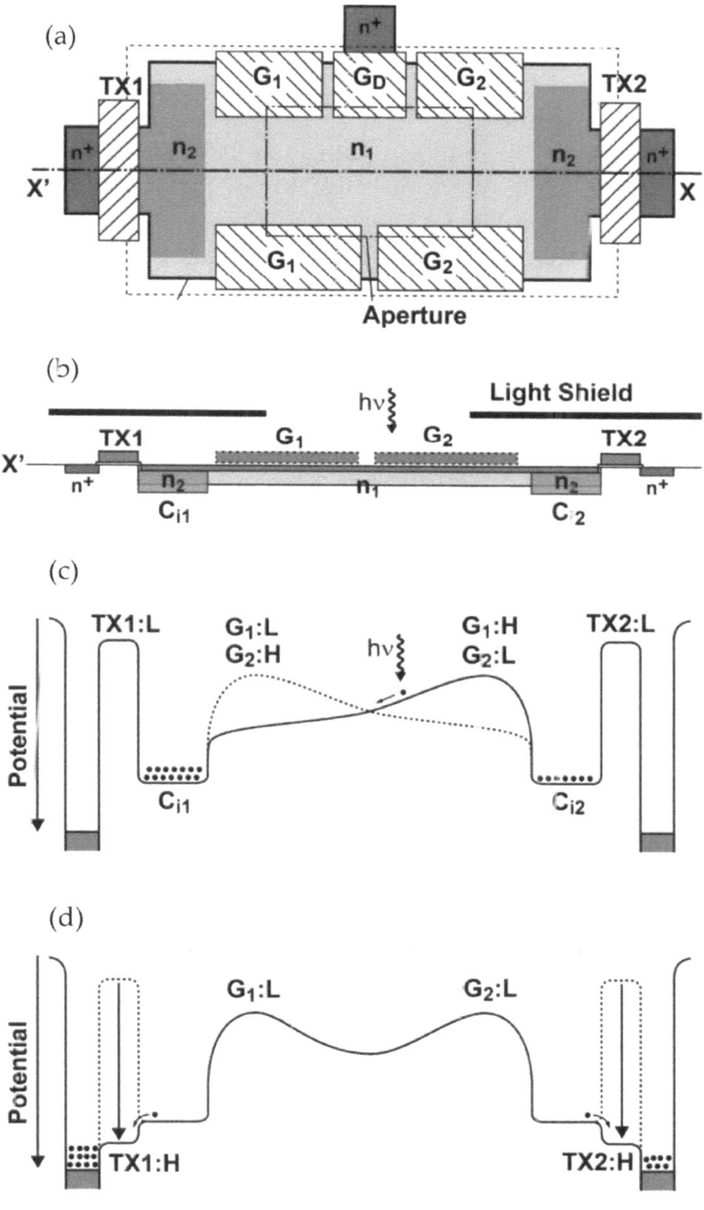

Figure 12.4 Demodulator with intermediate charge storage and operation. (a) Top view. (b) Cross-sectional view. (c) Potential profile (demodulation). (d) Potential profile (signal readout).

Using the basic 2-tap demodulator structures shown in Figs. 12.2 and 12.3, various designs of n-tap (n>2) demodulators are achievable. Figure 12.5 shows a 4-tap time-resolved lock-in pixel using a demodulator with 4 signal-taps and a drain [15]. The demodulator is designed using the PPD and LEFM gates shown in Fig. 12.2b. With this pixel, a 4-phase sampling lock-in operation shown in Fig. 12.1 for $n = 4$ is realized. The operation is similar to that of the 2-tap pixel, except that it has five modulation gates. For the case of sampling by G_1, for example, the H level is applied to the G_1 gate, and the L level is applied to G_2, G_3, G_4 and G_D, following which photo carriers generated in the PPD are transferred to a signal-tap S_1. For draining the unwanted photo carriers, the H level is applied to G_D and L level is applied to G_1, G_2, G_3 and G_4.

Figure 12.6a shows the demodulator of the 8-tap lock-in pixel. A pinned-photodiode (PPD) is located at the center of the structure as a photo detector. The flow of photo carriers to eight directions is controlled by eight LEFM gates [16, 17]. This pixel uses eight intermediate charge storages to perform true-CDS for canceling the reset noise. The intermediate charge storages are implemented with pinned storage diodes (SDs) together with a charge-transfer assisting (CA) gate. During the demodulation phase, for transferring photocarriers from the PPD to SD, the potential well of the SD is deepened by the CA gate voltage to be biased to the H level. When the accumulated signal charges stored in the SDs are read, the potential well depth of the SD is lowered by the CA gate to be biased to the L level.

Figures 12.6b,c show the 3D device simulation results obtained via SPECTRA (Link Research Corporation) when the generated photocarriers are to be transferred to SD_7. The LEFM gate G_7 and CA gates are biased to the H level, and the other LEFM gates are biased to the L level. A potential gradient is generated to transfer photocarriers to SD_7, as shown in Fig. 12.6c. In Fig. 12.6b, red points denote the initial positions of electrons generated by a photon, and black dotted lines indicate the movement trace of an electron. As shown in this simulation, a pixel can generate eight time-windows by consecutively driving the LEFM gates.

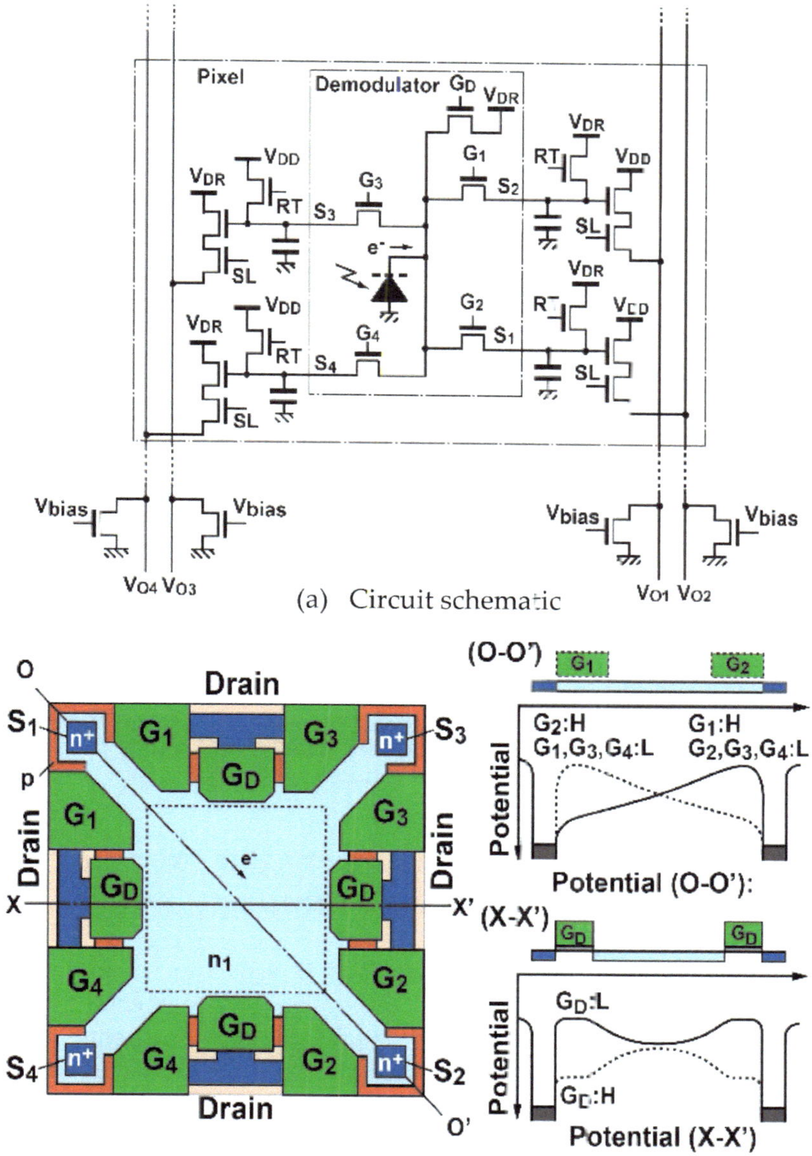

(a) Circuit schematic

(b) 4-Tap demodulator with a drain

Figure 12.5 Four-tap lock-in pixel with 4 signal-taps and a drain. (a) Circuit schematic. (b) 4-tap demodulator with a drain.

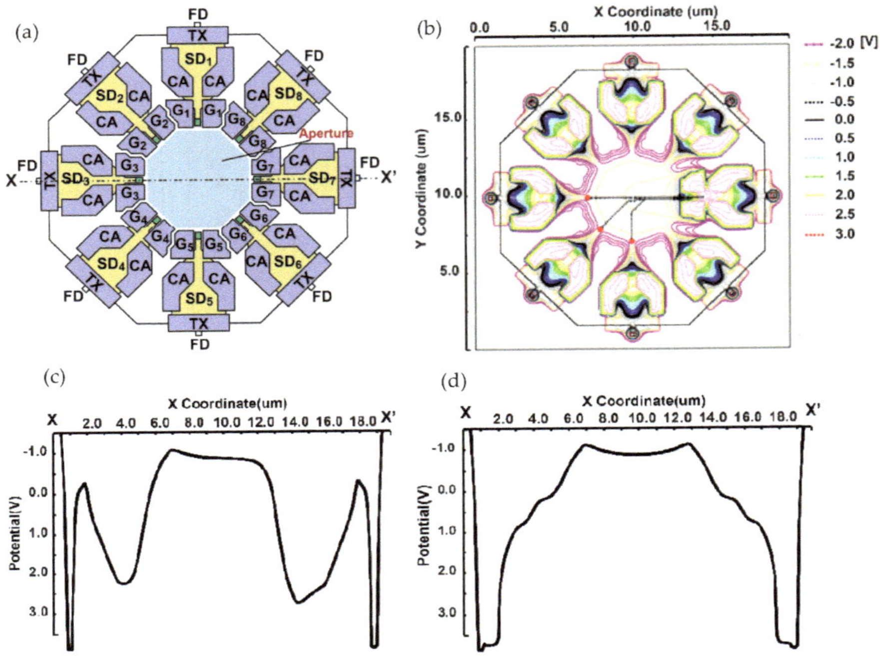

Figure 12.6 Eight-tap lock-in pixel and its 3D device simulation results. (a) Structure of the 8-tap lock-in pixel, (b) charge transportation result, (c) potential diagram of SD accumulation mode (X-X′), and (d) potential diagram for charge transfer mode from the SD to FD (X-X′).

12.2 Fluorescence Lifetime Imaging for Macro-Imaging and Microscopy

Fluorescence lifetime is a value that is useful for quantifying micro-chemical and physical molecular environments [18]. Because fluorescence intensity is absorbed by pigments and dependent on fluorophore concentration, it cannot be very quantitative. Ratiometry based on fluorescence intensities for multiple emission wavelengths is widely used to alleviate the error caused by fluorophore concentrations and light absorption. In contrast, fluorescence lifetime imaging (FLI) is much less susceptible to disturbances in nature. The fluorescence lifetime reveals information on the temperature, pH, quencher concentration, and fluorescence resonance energy transfer (FRET), among other factors. For example, cellular metabolism is quantitatively measured as the lifetimes of autofluorescence from endogenous coenzymes such as flavin adenine dinucleotide and nicotinamide adenine dinucleotide [19–22]. FLI is a powerful tool for both macro- and micro-imaging.

The measured temporal fluorescence response, $g(t)$, is calculated as follows:

$$g(t) = f(t) * h(t) \tag{12.2}$$

$$f(t) = \sum a_i \exp\left(-\frac{t}{\tau_i}\right) \tag{12.3}$$

Here, $h(t)$ is a system impulse response function that includes an excitation light waveform and the impulse response of the photodetector. The function $f(t)$ is a multi-component decay function of fluorescence. Typically, FLI is categorized into a time-domain and frequency domain. The digital frequency domain (DFD) method [23] is a very effective approach for combining the time-domain and frequency domain methods. In this method, measurement is performed in the time domain; thus, the function $g(t)$ is measured by a time-resolving photodetector. Next, the measured value is Fourier-transformed on a computer. A complex frequency component for frequency ν normalized by total intensity is given by

$$F^*(\upsilon) = \frac{1}{\sum a_i \tau_i}\left[\sum \frac{a_i/\tau_i}{1/\tau_i^2 + (2\pi\upsilon)^2} + i\sum \frac{2\pi a_i \upsilon}{1/\tau_i^2 + (2\pi\upsilon)^2}\right] \tag{12.4}$$

$F^*(\nu)$ is the complex conjugate of $F(\nu)$. Figure 12.7 shows the phasor plot of Eq. 12.4 on the complex number plane. The plot is on or inside the hemi-circle with a radius of 0.5 and center of $0.5+0i$. For the lifetimes of 0 and ∞, the plotted positions become $1.0+0i$ and $0+0i$, respectively. If a fluorophore has a single component, the plot is on the hemi-circle. For multiple-component fluorophores, the plot is inside the hemi-circle and given by a weighted linear combination of the complex components, which is completely a linear system.

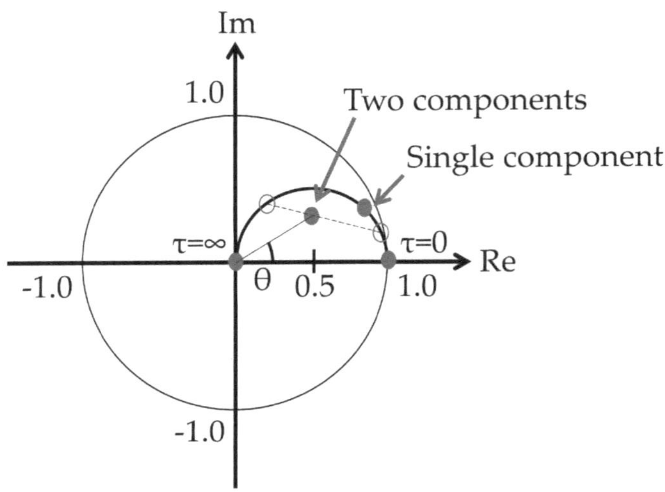

Figure 12.7 Phasor plot.

The DFD method is very useful because multi-component fluorophores can be compared on a single two-dimensional plane without any fitting. An example of the footprint of popular fluorophores is shown in Fig. 12.2 in Ref. 21. The synthesized fluorescence lifetime is calculated as the angle based on the origin of the coordinate, θ, as follows:

$$\tau_{\text{syn}} = \frac{\tan\theta}{2\pi v} \tag{12.5}$$

$$\tan\theta = \frac{\sum \dfrac{2\pi a_i v}{1/\tau_i^2 + (2\pi v)^2}}{\sum \dfrac{a_i/\tau_i}{1/\tau_i^2 + (2\pi v)^2}} \tag{12.6}$$

To obtain the original signal $F^*(v)$ from the measured signal $G^*(v)$, a single-component fluorophore with a known lifetime is typically measured as a reference. If the calculated normalized frequency component with Eq. 12.4 for a certain lifetime τ is given by $F'^*(\nu)$ and the measured value is $G'^*(\nu)$, the calibrated frequency component where the system response is excluded is obtained by multiplying a factor of $F'^*(\nu)/G'^*(\nu)$ by the measured $G^*(\nu)$.

Multi-tap charge modulators are suitable for use with the DFD method because they can be used for wide-field imaging without any scanning, have a high charge transfer efficiency, exert no pile-up effect, and have a high-charge capacity unlike time-correlated single photon counting which is a popular method in the time-domain FLI. The feasibility of the 2-tap time-resolving CMOS image sensor is described in Ref. [24]. However, because the number of taps on the multi-tap charge modulator is low, additional delay scanning is required, as shown in Fig. 12.8. In this example, a two-tap modulator is assumed, and eight images are captured for different delays. Because all charges are accumulated and read out for multi-tap modulators, the images for complementary time window functions are also read out (not shown in the figure). This scanning slows the image acquisition rate because multiple images must be acquired to analyze the data, whereas using multiple images can improve the signal to noise ratio, which can be solved by increasing the frame rate of the image sensor.

There are some limitations to DFD FLI. The synthesized lifetime given by Eq. 12.5 depends on the analysis frequency, ν. Therefore, to compare data measured with different configurations, the analysis frequency should be identical. If the sampling frequencies are different, resampling is required. The second issue occurs when the fluorescence lifetime components are not explicit. If there are unknown fluorophores, it is difficult to understand what is happening from the phasor plot. In such a case, decomposition of the lifetime elements is necessary. However, decomposition of the fluorophore elements based on a statistical method such as principal component analysis (PCA) and independent component analysis (ICA) is possible only when a variety of mixing ratios of the components are obtained from samples. To overcome this issue, fitting in the temporal frequency domain is performed, although comparison of multiple-lifetime-component fluorophores without fitting is an crucial advantage of DFD-FLI. In our method, a set of multiple amplitudes and lifetimes, $\{a_i, \tau_i\}$, are estimated for every pixel. Then, the lifetime histogram for all the $\{a_i, \tau_i\}$ sets is combined with the phasor plot. Fitting is performed using the following equation. j is the order of analysis frequency.

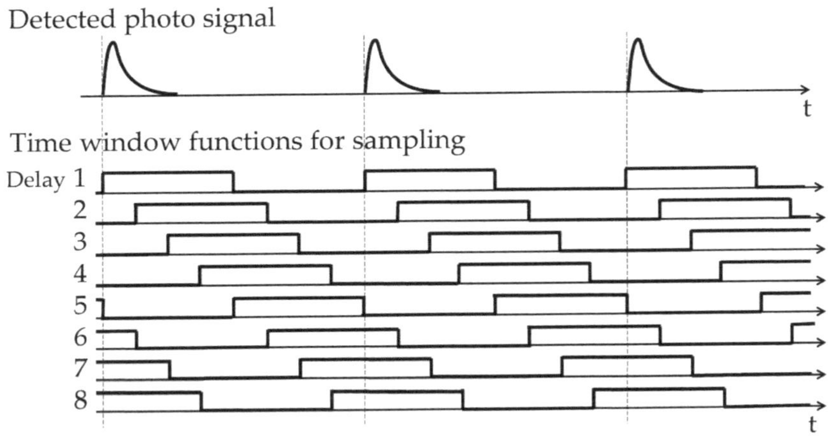

Figure 12.8 Delay scanning for DFD FLI for two-tap CMOS image sensors.

$$\underset{\{a_i,\tau_i\}}{\operatorname{argmin}} \sum_j \left\| \frac{1}{\sum_i a_i\tau_i} \left[\sum_i \frac{a_i/\tau_i}{1/\tau_i^2 + (2\pi v)^2} + i \sum_j \frac{2\pi a_i v}{1/\tau_i^2 (2\pi v)^2} \right] - F_j \right\|^2 \quad (12.7)$$

Figure 12.9 shows an example of the extended phasor plot. Fluorescent acrylic plates were stacked, and the mixing condition was not uniform. Therefore, on the phasor plot, the distribution becomes linear because there are two different types of fluorescence. In this experiment, two components were assumed during fitting. The peak positions were approximately 1.25 and 10 ns for violet and orange acrylic plates, respectively. The field of view was approximately 10 mm sq. A pulsed semiconductor laser (Tama Electric, Inc., Model OPG-1000PL, wavelength of 405 nm) was used for excitation. The number of delay steps was 32. The fundamental frequency used for analysis was 20 MHz.

The image acquisition efficiency or signal-to-noise ratio of the fluorescence lifetime can be improved by increasing the number of taps and decreasing the time window durations. Multi-tap time-resolving CMOS image sensors are very promising for wide-field imaging for both microscopy and macro-imaging in biology. For example, they enable endoscopes to be used for wide-field cancer imaging based on their autofluorescence-based metabolic-state imaging capability.

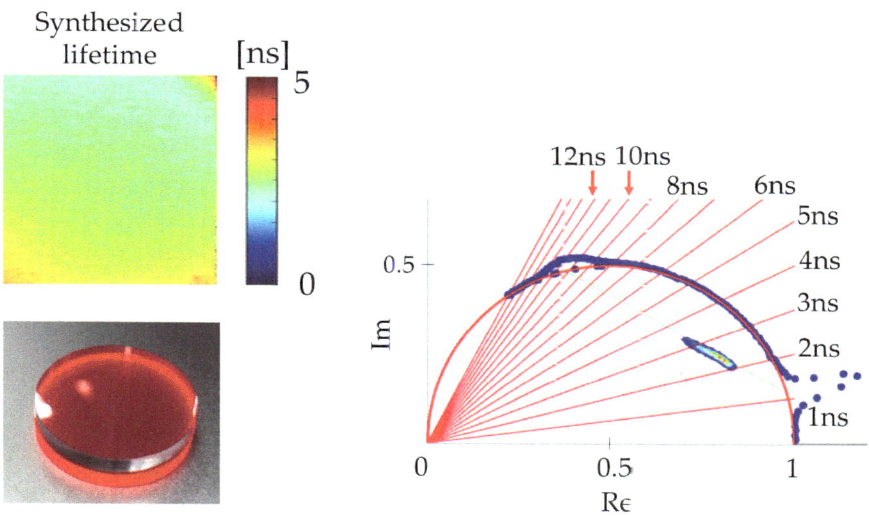

Figure 12.9 Example of extended phasor plot.

12.3 Time of Flight Imaging for Biomedical Applications

Time-of-flight (TOF) imaging is a type of active optical range imaging that is used to obtain depth images and intensity images by sensing round-trip TOF from a light source (Fig. 12.10). The distance, L, is calculated as follows:

$$L = \frac{c}{2} t_{\text{TOF}}, \tag{12.8}$$

where c is the speed of light. Because of the simple calculation, a real-time, low-latency acquisition system can be built. Unlike active triangulation methods such as structured light, a long baseline between the light source and the sensor is not required in TOF cameras; the camera module can be compact. Thus, TOF range cameras are used for a variety of applications, such as AR/VR/MR, security systems, drones, robots, and vehicles. They also offer new possibilities in biomedical applications, such as a 3D imaging guide device for endoscopic surgery.

There are two methods that can be used to measure the TOF: direct TOF (D-TOF) measurement [25, 26], and indirect TOF (I-TOF) measurement [1, 3–6, 8, 10, 27, 28]. In the D-TOF method, the photon arrival time is directly sensed by a single-photon avalanche diode (SPAD) and a time-measurement circuit, such as a time-to-digital converter. In the I-TOF measurement, the TOF is estimated by the mechanism of time-dependent photo charge modulation using a lock-in pixel. The pixel size of lock-in pixels is simple and compact compared to SPAD-based pixels, and I-TOF range imagers are suitable for applications requiring high spatial resolution.

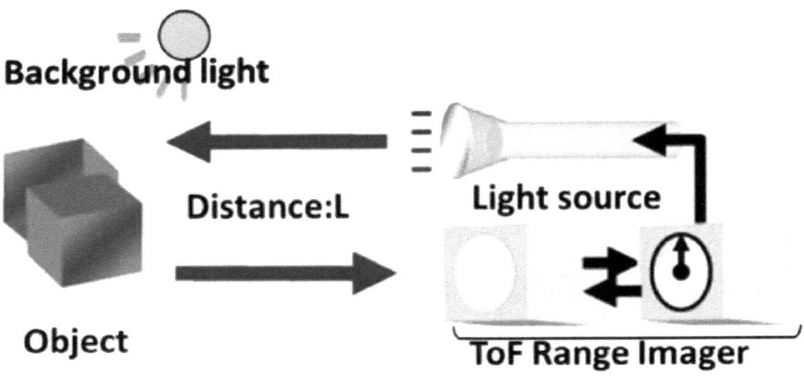

Figure 12.10 Time-of-flight range imaging.

In general, TOF range cameras have a range resolution (1) of several millimeters, which is relatively poor compared to active triangulation methods. To obtain better range resolution in the I-TOF measurement, the authors have proposed a new I-TOF measurement technique, employing an impulse photocurrent response [29, 30]. Instead of using the squared or sinusoidal modulated light source adopted by general I-TOF range imagers, a short-pulse laser with a pulse width of <100 ps is used for the light source, as shown in Fig. 12.11a. Due to the short light pulse, the photocurrent response at the lock-in pixel can be regarded as an impulse response. As a result, the range resolution is determined only by the photocurrent response. To facilitate this capability, the lateral electric field charge modulator (LEFM) concept is used in the lock-in pixel. Figure 12.12b shows an example of the high-speed lock-in pixel design with a 3-tap output. By using the proposed I-TOF measurement with an LEFM-based lock-in pixel, a high range resolution of 64 μm_{rms} is achieved in the prototype, which corresponds to a 430 fs time resolution [31].

In the I-TOF measurement technique, assuming a Gaussian function for the photocurrent response, the distance calculated by the TOF is given by

$$L = \frac{c}{2}(\sqrt{2\pi\tau}X + T_{ofs}), \tag{12.9}$$

where τ is the intrinsic response time of the photocurrent, T_{ofs} is the time offset that determines the minimum distance of the measurable range, and X is the signal charge ratio, which is defined as

$$X = \frac{N_2 + N_3}{N_1 + N_2 - 2N_3}, \tag{12.10}$$

where N_1, N_2, and N_3 are accumulated electrons by the time window of TW1-TW3 or by the gating clocks of G1–G3. In an example of design [30], the measurable range is approximately 30 mm, corresponding to $\sqrt{2\pi\tau}$ = 200 ps. Although the measurable range is typically smaller than that of general TOF range imagers, the limited measurable range can be expanded by using a range-shift technique in pulse-based TOF measurements [15, 32], in which the measurable range is shifted by controlling a trigger delay of the light source (i.e., T_{ofs}). Another important technique is on-chip skew calibration [30, 31] in order to apply the modulation technique to the 2D pixel array.

Figure 12.12 shows an example of the 3D measurement results using our prototype high-range resolution TOF range imager.

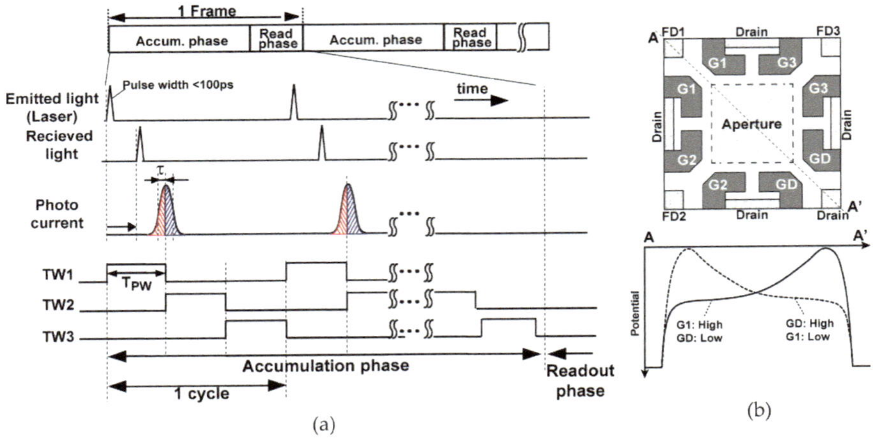

Figure 12.11 I-TOF measurement method with impulse photocurrent response. (a) Timing diagram, and (b) a design example of 3-tap LEFM.

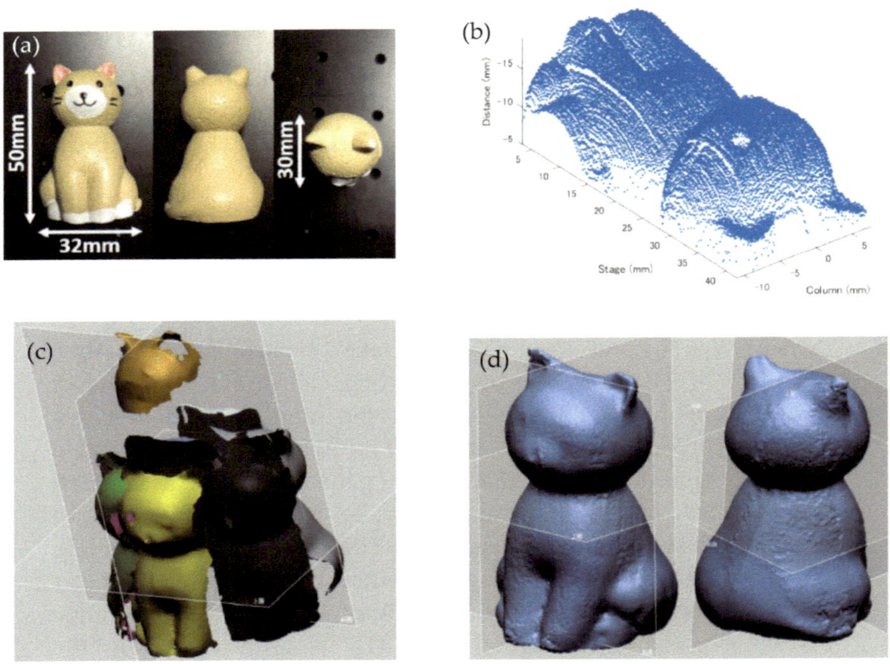

Figure 12.12 Example of 3D measurement results for cat miniature. (a) Object: cat miniature, (b) point cloud data of single scanning, (c) seven mesh data and alignment, and (d) complete 3D CAD model generated by synthesized mesh data.

The captured target is a cat miniature having dimensions of 32×30×50 mm^3, as shown in Fig. 12.12a. Since the prototype is a line sensor, a 1D mechanical stage is used to capture the 3D image. After taking the distance data, point cloud data are created, as shown in Fig. 12.12b. After post-processing of the point cloud, where potential error points are corrected or removed, mesh data are created using standard 3D modeling software. To obtain a complete CAD model, the point cloud data are taken and processed from seven different angles, as shown in Fig. 12.12c. Figure 12.12d shows synthesized CAD data using 3D modeling software. Accurate and complete 3D models of small objects are successfully acquired by the prototype TOF range imager.

12.4 Sensors for Near Infrared Spectroscopy and Stimulated Raman Spectroscopy

12.4.1 Near-Infrared Spectroscopy

Near-infrared spectroscopy (NIRS) has long been studied as a technique of non-invasive applications in monitoring blood oxygenation. There are several methods in realizing a NIRS system, with the most common being the continuous-wave (CW) approach. CW observes the light attenuation at a distance from the light source [33]. The observed attenuation is due to the different optical properties in the absorption and scattering of the tissue. The CW method can only determine the change in the absorption coefficient, μ_a, but not in the scattering coefficient. In contrast to CW, the time-resolved (TR) approach enables the determination of absolute values of the optical properties, including the absorption coefficient (μ_a) and reduced scattering coefficient ($\mu_{s'}$) [34]. CW is commonly used in NIRS applications owing to its simplicity and relatively inexpensive implementation, despite the advantages shown by TR-NIRS. A widely employed detector in TR-NIRS is a photo-multiplier tube, with recent works demonstrating the use of single-photon avalanche diodes (SPADs) and silicon photo-multipliers [35, 36].

The requirement to perform the TR technique is the necessity of having a fast intrinsic response time. The lateral electric field charge modulator (LEFM) concept is used to realize a TR-NIRS detector using CMOS image sensor technology [11]. The image sensor has a pixel array of 128 × 128 pixels with a pixel pitch of 22.4 μm × 22.4 μm. A pixel consists of a pinned photodiode (PPD) at the center, four pairs of transfer gates, four pinned-storage diodes (PSD), a pair of draining gates, four floating diffusions (FDs), and a pulse generator. The two-stage charge transfer mechanism of transferring the charge from PPD to PSD before finally transferring to FD enables the operation of true-correlated double sampling (true-CDS), which minimizes the noise signal. The pulse generator (PG) with local capacitors allows high-speed charge modulation and generates a narrow time-window of approximately 900 ps.

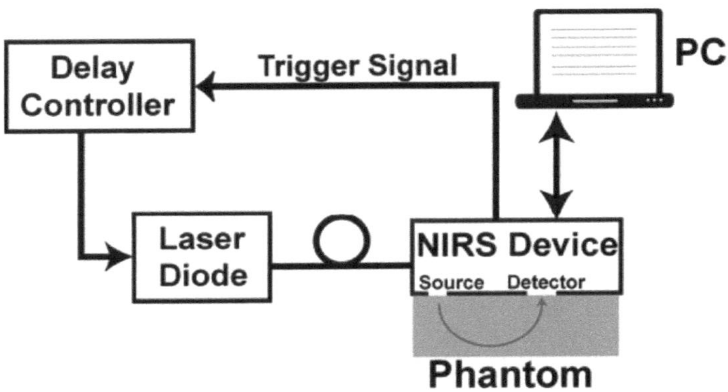

Figure 12.13 Schematic diagram of the NIRS experimental setup. The light source-detector distance is 30 mm, with a laser wavelength of 780 nm.

The experimental setup for the proof-of-concept is shown in Fig. 12.13. The NIRS device consists of a time-resolved CMOS image sensor and a field-programmable gate array (FPGA). The source-detector separation is 30 mm. A trigger signal is generated from the FPGA to the delay controller (DG645, Stanford Research Systems, US). The trigger signal is programmed to sweep across a certain delay range for the time window to scan through the entire reflected signal range, as shown in Fig. 12.14, where the reflectance signal is a function of μ_a and $\mu_{s'}$. The pulse laser diode (LDB-100B-780F, Tamadenshi, Japan) has a pulse width of 100 ps at a wavelength of 780 nm. The phantom used is a solidified liquid solution.

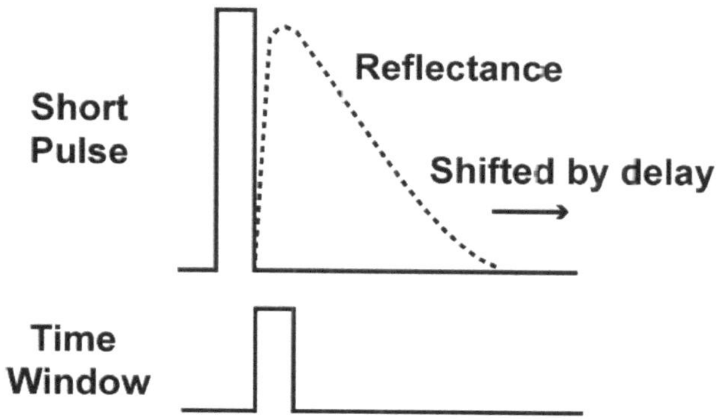

Figure 12.14 The trigger signal to the laser diode is time-shifted to obtain the full reflectance.

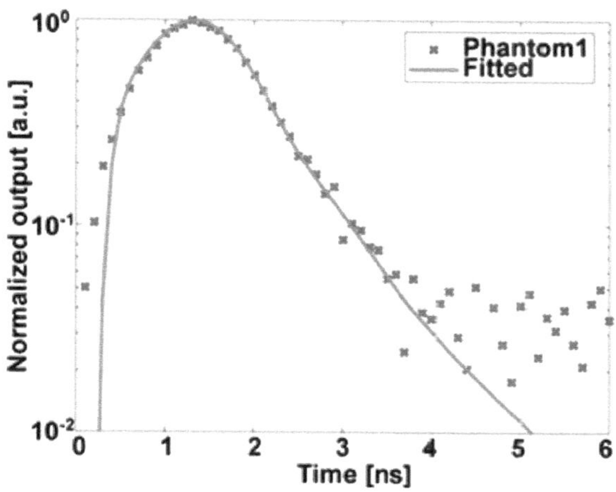

Figure 12.15 The TR-NIRS reflectance from a solidified phantom and the resulting fitting curve. Absorption coefficient and reduced scattering coefficient can be obtained from the curve.

Figure 12.15 shows the TR-NIRS measured result of the reflectance mode. The measured data is fitted to

$$R(\rho,t) = (4\pi Dc)^{-\frac{3}{2}} z_0 t^{-\frac{5}{2}} \exp(-\mu_a ct)\exp\left(-\frac{r^2 + z_0^2}{4Dct}\right), \qquad (12.11)$$

where R is the reflectance, D is the diffusion coefficient, z_0 is initially scattered depth, c is the speed of light in the tissue, and ρ is the source-detector separation. This allows μ_a and $\mu_{s'}$ to be obtained, which can be further used to attain the hemoglobin concentration and oxygen saturation through the measurement of two different wavelengths.

12.4.2 Stimulated Raman Scattering

Another application is detection of the Raman scattering, which has been explored extensively as label-free and noninvasive imaging to investigate biological samples [37]. The widely used spontaneous Raman scattering is not suitable for dynamic biological samples due to the long acquisition time. Stimulated Raman scattering (SRS), being a type of coherent Raman scattering (CRS) that enhances the Raman signal, does not exhibit a non-resonant background. Another CRS, coherent anti-Stokes Raman scattering (CARS), does exhibit a non-resonant background. SRS requires two laser sources, the pump (ω_p) and the Stokes (ω_s), to stimulate a sample. When the frequency difference between the two lasers, $\Omega = \omega_p - \omega_s$, matches a particular molecular vibration frequency, the SRS signal is stimulated. Figure 12.16 shows the principle of the SRS signal generation. The generated SRS signal, ΔIp is very small relative to the background signal, on the order of 10^{-5}. The conventional method uses a single photodiode and a lock-in amplifier, but such a technique is not suitable for multi-point parallel measurement.

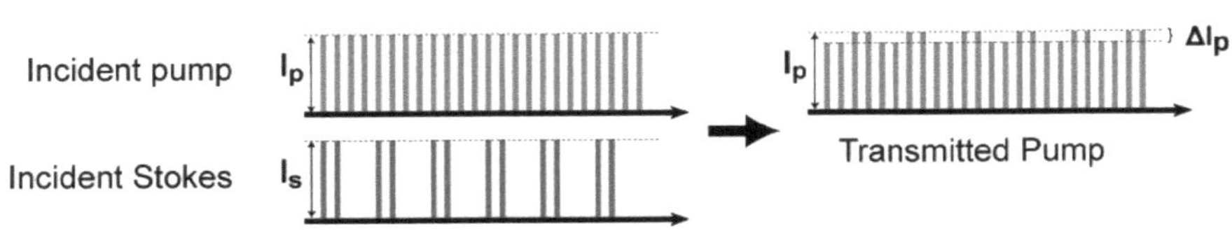

Figure 12.16 SRS signal detection scheme. The pump laser and Stokes laser overlap spatially and temporally, and the resulting pump signal is observed.

The CMOS image sensor approach embeds the functions of both a photodiode and a lock-in amplifier in a pixel [38]. Figure 12.17 shows a schematic of the lock-in pixel with a 2-tap demodulator, a low-pass filter, a sample-and-hold circuit, and an integrator. The 2-tap pixel configuration is locked with the modulation frequency to measure the Stokes-on and Stokes-off instant in a pixel. This configuration enables the parallel detection in an array of lock-in pixels before reading out from the sensor. Considering the signal-to-noise ratio of the SRS signal, a large area demodulator, instead of an array of small sub-pixels, is employed [39]. The aperture of the PPD is 32 μm × 32 μm. To achieve high-speed charge transfer, two-step ion implantation incorporating LEFM technology is used for the demodulator. Such a technique ensures a high electric field in the PPD to transfer the charge to the transfer gates. The simulated transfer time is less than 4 ns, which is well below the laser repetition frequency of 80 MHz. The signal from the demodulator then goes through the low-pass filter. The outputs of the low-pass filter contain the demodulated signal and the offset signal. These signals are sampled in the sample-and-hold circuit, and the difference of the two outputs, which consists only of the demodulated signal, is integrated multiple times to achieve a certain gain.

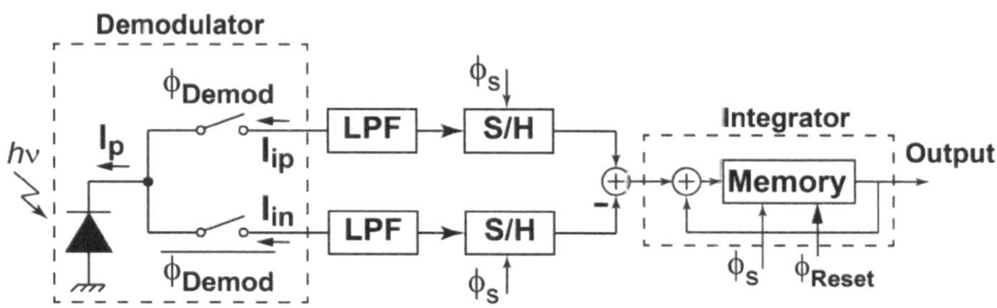

Figure 12.17 Schematic diagram of the lock-in pixel with 2-tap demodulator, low-pass filter, sample-and-hold circuit, and integrator.

The ability to detect a very small signal from a large background is confirmed with the experiment using stearic acid. Figure 12.18 shows the results of the stearic acid measured simultaneously using the CMOS lock-in pixel and a CARS system. The difference is due to the non-resonant background exhibited by the CARS system.

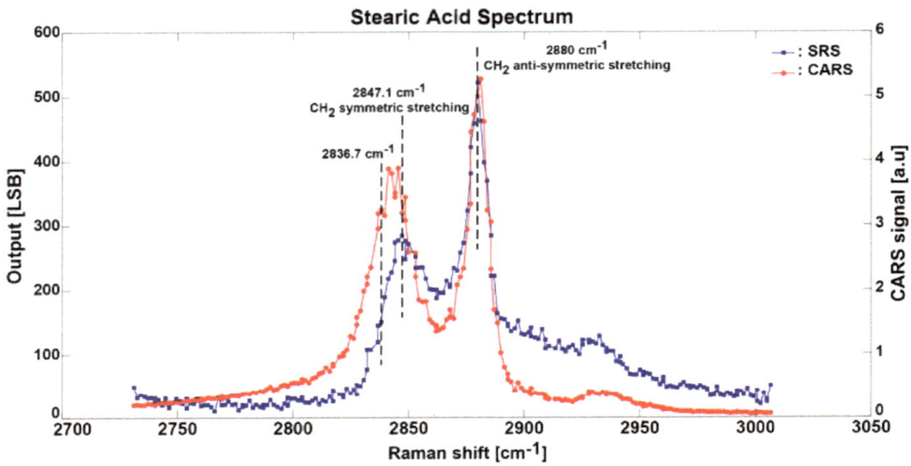

Figure 12.18 Stearic acid measurement results performed simultaneously using the CMOS lock-in pixel and a CARS system.

References

1. T. Spirig, P. Seitz, O. Vietze, and F. Heitger, The lock-in CCD-two-dimensional synchronous detection of light, *IEEE J. Quantum Electron.*, vol. 31, no. 9, pp. 1705–1708 (1995).
2. R. Lange and P. Seitz, Solid-state time-of-flight range camera, *IEEE J. Quantum Electron.*, vol. 37, no. 3, pp. 390–397 (2001).
3. S. Kawahito, I. A. Halin, T. Ushinaga, T. Sawada, et al., A CMOS time-of-flight range image sensor with gates-onfield-oxide structure, *IEEE Sens. J.*, vol. 7, no. 12, pp. 1578–1586 (2007).
4. D. Stoppa, N. Massari, L. Pancheri, M. Malfatti, M. Perenzoni, and L. Gonzo, A range image sensor based on 10 μm lock-in pixels in 0.18 μm CMOS imaging technology, *IEEE J. Solid-State Circuits*, vol. 46, no. 1, pp. 248–258 (2011).
5. C. S. Bamji, S. Mehta, B. Thompson, et al., 1 Mpixel 65 nm BSI 320 MHz demodulated TOF sensor with 3.5 um global shutter pixels and analog binning, *Dig. Tech. Papers, ISSCC*, pp. 94–95 (2018).
6. M. S. Keel, Y. G. Jin, Y. Kim, et al., A 640 × 480 indirect time-of-flight CMOS image sensor with 4-tap 7 um global shutter pixel and fixed-pattern phase noise self-compensation scheme, *Dig. Tech. Papers, Symp. VLSI Circuits*, no. C21-3, pp. 258–259 (2019).

7. N. Teranishi, A. Kohno, Y. Ishihara, and K. Arai, No image lag photodiode structure in the interline CCD image sensor, *Tech. Dig., Int. Electron Device Meeting*, pp. 324–327 (1982).

8. S.-J. Kim, D. K. Kim, B. Kang, and K. Lee, A CMOS image sensor based on unified pixel architecture with time-division multiplexing scheme for color and depth image acquisition, *IEEE J. Solid-State Circuits*, vol. 47, no. 11, pp. 2834–2845 (2012).

9. S. Kawahito, G. Baek, Z. Li, S. M. Han, M. W. Seo, K. Yasutomi and K. Kagawa. CMOS lock-in pixel image sensors with lateral electric field control for time-resolved imaging, *In Proc. Int. Image Sensor Workshop (IISW)*, Snowbird, UT, USA, pp. 361–364 (2013).

10. S. M. Han, et al., A time-of-flight range image sensor with background canceling lock-in pixels based on lateral electric field charge modulation, *IEEE J. EDS*, pp. 1–9 (2014).

11. M.-W. Seo, Y. Shirakawa, Y. Kawata, K. Kagawa, K. Yasutomi, and S. Kawahito, A time-resolved four-tap lock-in pixel CMOS image sensor for real-time fluorescence lifetime imaging microscopy, *IEEE J. Solid-State Circuits*, vol. 58, no. 8, pp. 2319–2330 (2018).

12. S. Kawahito, K. Kondo, K. Yasutomi, and K. Kagawa, A time-resolved lock-in pixel image sensor using multiple-tapped diode and hybrid cascade charge transfer structure, *Proc. Int. Image Sensor Workshop*, no. R28 (2019).

13. M. W. Seo, K. Kagawa, K. Yasutomi, Y. Kawata, N. Teranishi, Z. Li, I. A. Halin, and S. Kawahito, A 10 ps time-resolution CMOS image sensor with two-tap true-CDS lock-in pixels for fluorescence lifetime imaging, *IEEE J. Solid-State Circuits*, vol. 51, no. 1, pp. 141–154 (2016).

14. M.-W. Seo, and S. Kawahito, A 7ke- SD-FWC 1.2e-rms temporal random noise 128×256 time-resolved CMOS image sensor with two in-pixel SDs for biomedical applications, *IEEE Trans. Biomed. Circuits Syst.*, vol. 11, no. 6 (2017).

15. T. Kasugai, S.-M. Han, H. Trang, T. Takasawa, S. Aoyama, K. Yasutomi, K. Kagawa, and S. Kawahito, A time-of-flight CMOS range image sensor using 4-tap output pixels with lateral-electric-field control, *in Proc. of IS&T International Symposium on Electronic Imaging 2016*, pp. IMSE-048.1-6 (2016).

16. Y. Shirakawa, M. W. Seo, K. Yasutomi, K. Kagawa, N. Teranishi, and S. Kawahito. Design of an 8-tap CMOS lock-in pixel with lateral electric field charge modulator for highly time-resolved imaging, *In Silicon Photonics XII*; Publisher: San Francisco, United States (2017).

17. Y. Shirakawa, K. Yasutomi, K. Kagawa, S. Aoyama, and S. Kawahito. An 8-tap CMOS lock-in pixel image sensor for short-pulse time-of-flight measurements, *Sensors 2020*, 20, 1040.
18. A. Periasamy and R. M. Clegg, *Flim Microscopy in Biology And Medicine*, CRC Press, Boca Raton (2010).
19. M. C. Skala, K. M. Riching, A. Gendron-Fitzpartick, J. Eickhoff, K. W. Eliceiri, J. G. White, and N. Ramanujam, In vivo multiphoton microscopy of NADH and FAD redox states, fluorescence lifetimes, and cellular morphology in precancerous epithelia, *PNAS*, vol. 104, no. 49, pp. 19494–19499 (2007).
20. V. I. Shcheslavskiy, M. V. Shirmanova, V. V. Dudenkova, K. A. Lukyanov, A. I. Gavrina, A. V. Shumilova, E. Zagaynova, and W. Becker, Fluorescence time-resolved microimaging, *Opt. Lett.*, vol. 43, no. 13, pp. 3152–3155 (2018).
21. C. Stringari, A. Cinquin, O. Cinquin, M. A. Digman, P. J. Donovan, and E. Gratton, Phasor approach to fluorescence lifetime microscopy distinguishes different metabolic states of germ cells in a live tissue, *PNAS*, vol. 108, no. 33, pp. 13582–13587 (2011).
22. C. Stringari, J. L. Nourse, L. A. Flanagan, and E. Gratton, Phasor fluorescence lifetime microscopy of free and protein-bound NADH reveals neural stem cell differentiation potential, *Plos One*, vol. 7, Issue 11, e48014 (2012).
23. R. A. Colyer, C. Lee, and E. Gratton, A novel fluorescence lifetime imaging system that optimized photon efficiency, *Microsc. Res. Tech.*, vol. 71, pp. 201–213 (2008).
24. H. Chen, N. Ma, K. Kagawa, S. Kawahito, M. Digman, and E. Gratton, Widefield multi-frequency fluorescence lifetime imaging using a two-tap CMOS camera with lateral electric field charge modulators, *J. Biophonics*, vol. 12, no. 5, e201800223 (2019).
25. C. L. Niclass, et al., Design and characterization of a CMOS 3-D image sensor based on single photon avalanche diodes, *IEEE JSSC*, vol. 40, no. 9, pp. 1847–1854 (2005).
26. C. Niclass, et al., A 0.18 μm CMOS SoC for a 100-m-Range 10-Frame/s 200×96 pixel time-of-flight depth sensor, *IEEE JS*, vol. 49, no. 1, pp. 315–330 (2014).
27. C. S. Bamji, et al., A 0.13 um CMOS system-on-chip for a 512 × 424 time-of-flight image sensor with multi-frequency photo-demodulation up to 130 MHz and 2 GS/s ADC, *IEEE J. Solid-State Circuits*, vol. 46, no. 1, pp. 248–258 (2015).

28. Y. Kato, et al., 320×240 back-illuminated 10 μm CAPD pixels for high-speed modulation time-of-flight CMOS image sensor, *IEEE J. Solid-State Circuits*, vol. 53, no. 4, pp. 1071–1078 (2018).

29. K. Yasutomi, T. Usui, S. Han, T. Takasawa, K. Kagawa, and S. Kawahito, An indirect time-of-flight measurement technique with impulse photocurrent response for sub-millimeter range resolved imaging, *Opt. Express*, vol. 22, no. 16, pp. 18904–18913 (2014).

30. K. Yasutomi, T. Usui, S.-M. Han, T. Takasawa, K. Kagawa, and S. Kawahito, A submillimeter range resolution time-of-flight range imager with column-wise skew calibration, *IEEE Trans. Electron Devices*, vol. 63, no. 1, pp. 182–188 (2016).

31. K. Yasutomi, Y. Okura, K. Kagawa and S. Kawahito, A Sub-100 μm-range-resolution time-of-flight range image sensor with 3-tap lock-in pixels, Non-overlapping gate clock, and reference plane sampling, *IEEE J. Solid-State Circuits*, vol. 54, no. 8, pp. 2291–2303 (2019).

32. T. Sawada, K. Ito, M. Nakayama, and S. Kawahito, TOF range image sensor using a range-shift technique, *in Proc. IEEE Sensors 2008*, pp. 1390–1393 (2008).

33. M. Ferrari, Progress of near-infrared spectroscopy and topography for brain and muscle clinical applications, *J. Biomed. Opt.*, vol. 12, no. 6, p. 062104 (2007).

34. J. Steinbrink, H. Wabnitz, H. Obrig, A. Villringer, and H. Rinneberg, Determining changes in NIR absorption using a layered model of the human head, *Phys. Med. Biol.*, vol. 46, no. 3, pp. 879–896 (2001).

35. Y. Yamada, H. Suzuki, and Y. Yamashita, Time-domain near-infrared spectroscopy and imaging: A review, *Appl. Sci.*, vol. 9, no. 6, p. 1127 (2019).

36. R. Re, E. Martinenghi, A. D. Mora, D. Contini, A. Pifferi, and A. Torricelli, Probe-hosted silicon photomultipliers for time-domain functional near-infrared spectroscopy: phantom and in vivo tests, *Neurophotonics*, vol. 3, no. 4, p. 045004 (2016).

37. G. J. Thomas, Raman spectroscopy of protein and nucleic acid assemblies, *Annu. Rev. Biophys. Biomol. Struct.*, vol. 28, no. 1, pp. 1–27 (1999).

38. D. Lioe, et al., A stimulated Raman scattering CMOS pixel using a high-speed charge modulator and lock-in amplifier, *Sensors*, vol. 16, no. 4, p. 532 (2016).

39. K. Mars, et al., Label-free biomedical imaging using high-speed lock-in pixel sensor for stimulated Raman scattering, *Sensors*, vol. 17, no. 11, p. 2581 (2017).

Chapter 13

High-Resolution Optical Microscopy for Bio-Imaging

Wataru Inami and Yoshimasa Kawata

Shizuoka University, 3-5-1 johoku, Naka-ku, Hamamatsu 432-8561, Japan

inami.wataru@shizuoka.ac.jp

This chapter introduced the principle of the super-resolution optical microscope (EXA microscope) by electron beam excitation and the experimental results of bio-imaging. In this microscope, a focused electron beam is irradiated onto a fluorescent film to excite a nanometric light source below the diffraction limit. A nanometric light source is scanned by scanning an electron beam to form the image of a specimen on the phosphor film. By separating the vacuum and atmospheric pressure with a fluorescent membrane, it is possible to observe the dynamics of living biological specimen under atmospheric pressure. The absorption distribution and refractive index distribution of the specimen can be dynamically observed with the EXA microscope. The results of evaluating the resolution of the microscope by numerical analysis combining Monte-Carlo simulation [1] and the

Biomedical Engineering
Edited by Akihiro Miyauchi and Yuji Miyahara

ISBN 978-981-4877-63-3 (Hardcover), 978-1-003-14194-5 (eBook)
www.jennystanford.com

finite-difference time-domain method [2, 3] and observing the dynamics of biological cells are shown.

13.1 Introduction

The optical microscope is considered to have been invented around the 16th century, and its history is old. However, it is still used as a major method for observing biological specimen with high resolution. This is because there is little restriction on the usage environment, such as atmospheric pressure or liquid, without giving damage to the sample. In combination with spectroscopic measurement, qualitative analysis can be performed. Observing the dynamics of a living specimen is indispensable for elucidating biological functions, and an optical microscope is most suitable for this purpose. It is well known that the spatial resolution of an optical microscope is determined by the diffraction limit [4] and is on the order of a wavelength (several hundred nanometers). Therefore, it is necessary to develop an optical microscope with higher spatial resolution in order to elucidate the interaction between multiple molecules or micro-organs and the mechanism of information transmission. One of the most recent developments in optical microscopes is the development of super-resolution fluorescence microscopes capable of observing specimens with a spatial resolution of several tens of nanometers. Super-resolution fluorescence microscopes such as STED microscope [5], PALM [6], STORM [7], SIM [8] SAX microscope [9], etc. are capable of achieving a spatial resolution below the diffraction limit. These super-resolution microscopes have been reported to achieve a spatial resolution of about 20 nm, which has been difficult to observe with conventional optical microscopes. The structure and dynamics of proteins in several tens of nanometers are introduced in this chapter.

13.2 Principle and Features of Super-Resolution Microscope with Electron Beam Excitation

Figure 13.1 shows the configuration of the developed super-resolution optical microscope using electron beam excitation [10].

In the developed system, an inverted compact scanning electron microscope is used to irradiate an electron beam on a fluorescent film on the area of several nanometers. The excited fluorescence is absorbed and scattered by the specimen on the fluorescent film, the transmitted light is collected by the objective lens, and the light is detected by the upper optical microscope. The electron beam is scanned to obtain a two-dimensional image of the specimen.

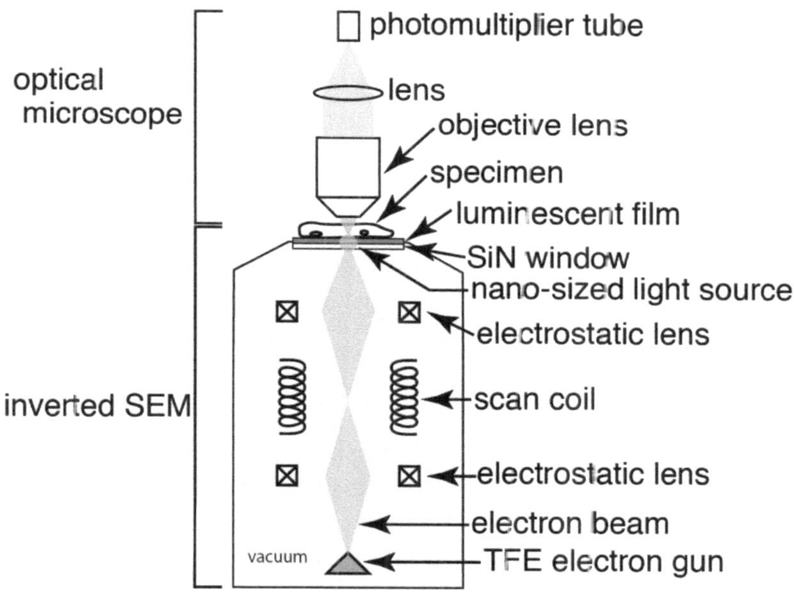

Figure 13.1 Schematic diagram of super-resolution optical microscope using electron beam excitation.

In this microscope, a nano-sized point light source is excited on the fluorescent film by a focused electron beam, the specimen is directly placed on the fluorescent thin film, and the sample is illuminated by the nano-sized point light source on the fluorescent film. When the distance between the specimen and the fluorescent thin film is as small as the wavelength, the sample can be observed with an evanescent wave of a nano-sized point light source generated by electron beam excitation, and resolution exceeding the diffraction limit can be realized.

By scanning the electron beam, the light emission region is scanned, and an image is acquired.

In this system, the optical microscope part and the electron microscope part are separated at the fluorescent thin film part where the specimen is placed. Therefore, the specimen does not need to be placed in a vacuum or deposited with a metal film and can be used in the same environment as a normal optical microscope.

In general, this method has the following advantages [11–15].

1. Nanometer order resolution

Since the fluorescent thin film is excited by the convergent electron beam, a nanometric point light source that does not depend on the diffraction limit of light can be generated. Therefore, it is possible to achieve a resolution that greatly exceeds the resolution of conventional optical microscopes.

2. Observation of optical constants such as absorption and refractive index distribution

The light transmitted through a specimen from the micro light source or the fluorescence excited by the nanometric point light source is detected in this system. Therefore, this system can measure the optical constant distribution such as absorption distribution and refractive index distribution of the specimen. This is a significant feature compared to other super-resolution microscopy such as PALM (photoactivated localization microscopy), SAX (Saturated excitation), and STED (Stimulated emission depletion) microscopy that can only be applied to fluorescent labeled specimen. Moreover, the information obtained is completely different from the transmission X-ray images, electron microscope images, and topographic images by atomic force microscope.

3. High-speed observation by scanning electron beam

By scanning an electron beam, a nanometric point light source can be easily scanned. Therefore, high-speed observation is possible. In a normal near-field optical microscope [16, 17], the observation speed is often limited because the nanoaperture is scanned with high accuracy in the vicinity of the sample surface.

4. High functionality by selecting fluorescent thin film materials

By using fluorescent thin films with various functions (emission wavelength characteristics, polarization characteristics, nonlinear optical response, etc.), it is possible to realize optical nanoimaging techniques with various functions.

A thin fluorescent thin film with high quantum efficiency is required for EXA microscope in order to obtain an image with high spatial resolution and high signal-to-noise ratio. It is desired that the fluorescent film emits light with high brightness in a low acceleration voltage range, particularly 5 kV or less. This voltage limitation is due to preventing the damage for specimen by transmitted electron beam through the fluorescent film. In conventional electron microscopes, it has been reported that the specimen is damaged by electron beam irradiation [18, 19]. When an electron beam with a high acceleration voltage irradiates a fluorescent film with a thickness of several tens of nanometers, most of the electron beam passes through the film. Therefore, when an electron beam is irradiated at a high acceleration voltage, the sample is considered to be damaged by the electron beam passed through the fluorescent film. By irradiating an electron beam with a low acceleration voltage, it is necessary to reduce the transmittance of the electron beam and suppress damage to the sample. Therefore, it is desired to emit light with high brightness in a low acceleration voltage range of 5 kV or less.

In order to observe a specimen at high spatial resolution and high signal-to-noise ratio, in addition to high quantum efficiency, the spatial emission uniformity of the flucrescent film is important. If the spatial uniformity of the emission intensity is low, the background intensity of the image fluctuates greatly. It is necessary to optimize the deposition method to form a single crystal film or a thin film with small grains. In general, when annealing is performed to increase quantum efficiency, the grain size of the fluorescent film increases.

A thin fluorescent film can reduce the electron beam scattering in the fluorescent film compared to a thick fluorescent film. Therefore, since the CL (cathodoluminescence) emission volume can be reduced, and a smaller optical spot can be generated, the spatial resolution of the EXA microscope is improved.

13.3 Observation Results of Unstained Biological Cell with EXA Microscope

Figure 13.2 shows a comparison of (a) EXA microscope image and (b) phase contrast microscopic image of unstained MARCO (Macrophage Receptor with Collagenous Structure)-expressing CHO (Chinese Hamster Ovary) cells [20]. The MARCO-expressing CHO cells were fixed with 1% glutaraldehyde. Comparing Figs. 13.2a,b, it is found that the EXA microscope can be clearly imaged the outline and nanostructures of the cell. The fluorescent thin film that emits high-intensity light with spatially uniform intensity contribute to high signal-to-noise ratio. In addition, the spatial resolution of the EXA microscope is higher than that of the phase contrast microscope, which is the factor that enables the EXA microscope to clearly observe the cell outline.

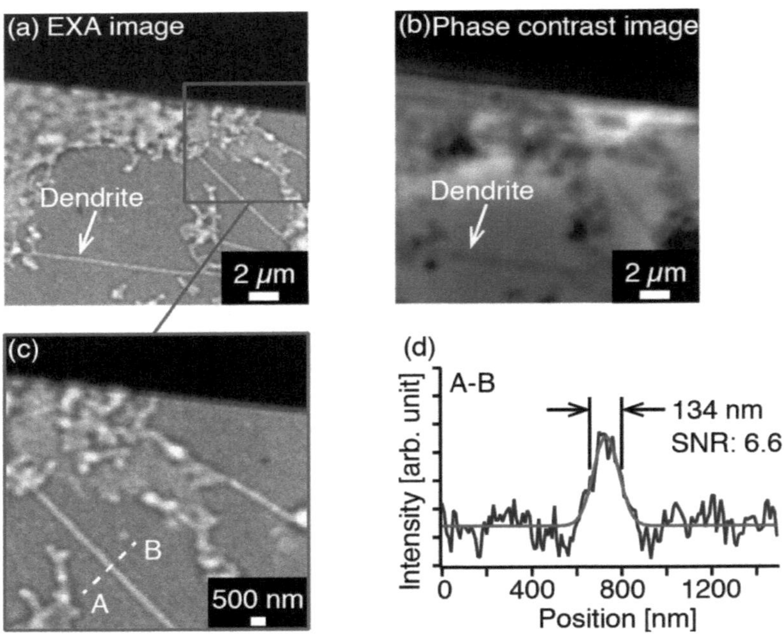

Figure 13.2 (a) EXA microscope image of unstained MARCO-expressing CHO cells, (b) phase contrast microscope image of unstained MARCO-expressing CHO cells, (c) Enlarged image of the box in (a), (d) Intensity profile between A and B in (c).

Further, in Fig. 13.2a,b, the dendritic cell membrane structure (dendrites) of MARCO-expressing CHO cells is shown by arrows. By introducing the MARCO receptor gene into MARCO-expressing CHO cells, dendritic structures appear from the cell membrane. A dendritic cell membrane structure that is difficult to observe with a phase contrast microscope can be clearly seen with an EXA microscope. Figure 13.2c shows an enlarged view of the region surrounded by the square in Fig. 13.2a. The fine structures were difficult to observe in phase contrast microscope due to the blur caused by the resolution limit. However, they were observed clearly in the EXA microscope image. Figure 13.2d shows the intensity profile between A and B in Fig. 13.2c. From Fig. 13.2d, the full width at half maximum of the dendrite image was 134 nm. Therefore, it is found that the specific structure of unstained MARCO-expressing CHO cells can be observed with a spatial resolution below the diffraction limit.

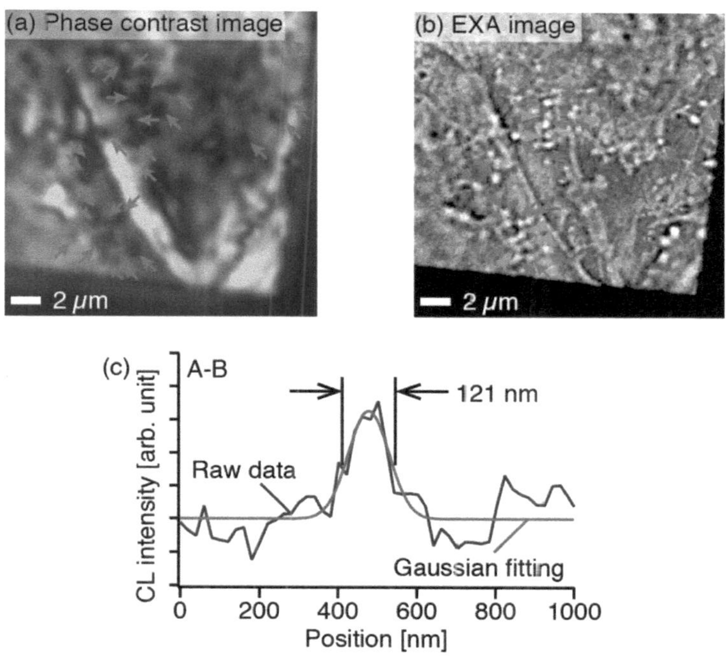

Figure 13.3 (a) Phase-contrast microscope image of granules of an unstained MARCO-expressing CHO cell, (b) EXA microscopy image of unstained MARCO-expressing CHO cell in the same place as (a), (c) Intensity profile between A and B in (b).

Figure 13.3 shows the observation results of intracellular granules of an unstained MARCO-expressing CHO cell using ZnO luminescent film deposited by the ALD (Atomic Layer Deposition) method [20]. Figure 13.3a shows the phase contrast microscope image, and Fig. 13.3b shows the EXA microscope image of the intracellular granules. Comparing Figs. 13.3a,b, the intracellular granules common to both images are shown by red arrows. In Fig. 13.3b, the granules shown as green arrows are only observed in the EXA image. In the phase contrast microscope, several particles are indistinctly observed like one agglomeration because of insufficient spatial resolution. Since the EXA microscope has high spatial resolution, they were clearly resolved as some granules. Figure 13.3c shows the intensity profile of the fiber structure between A and B in Fig. 13.3b. From this intensity profile, the full width at half maximum was 121 nm. Therefore, in addition to the extracellular structure shown in Fig. 13.3, we succeeded in observing the intracellular microstructure of unstained cell with high spatial resolution.

Next, observation of living cell with EXA microscope is described. Figure 13.4 shows the results of time-lapse imaging of living MARCO-expressing CHO cells with the EXA microscope [21]. The acceleration voltage is 5 kV, the irradiation current is 1 nA, and the frame rate is 1 fps. The image size is 512 × 512 pixels. From Fig. 13.4, we were able to observe the dynamics of living cells, especially the movement of nucleolus and the collection of intracellular granules as follows. The intracellular granules indicated in the circle region at 150 sec are concentrated in the circle area at 250 sec. There was a nucleolus near the circled area, and intracellular granules aggregated near the nucleolus. The nucleolus indicated by the arrow head disappears once in 300 sec and reappears at 450 sec. This is considered to be because the cell nucleus has come out of the depth of field. The EXA microscope can observe a range of several hundred nanometers from the fluorescent thin film surface with high resolution, because the evanescent wave of the nanometric light source decays as the distance from the fluorescent thin film increases.

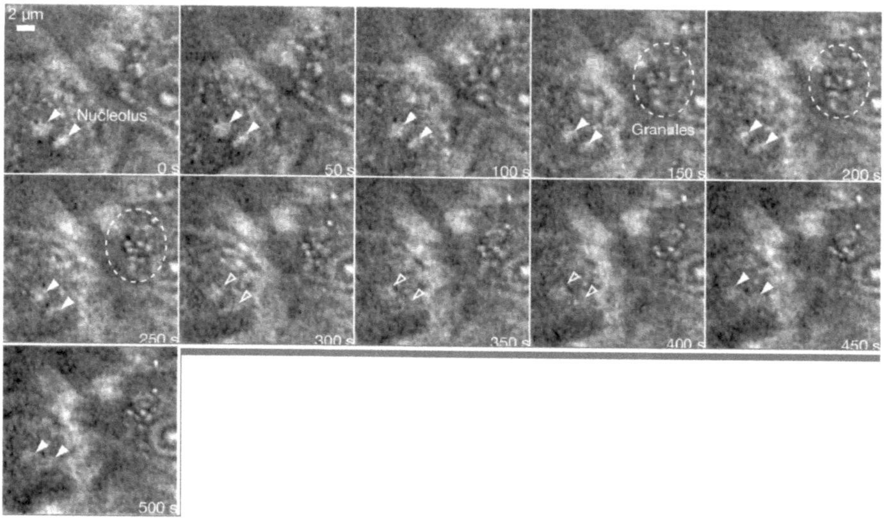

Figure 13.4 Results of time-lapse imaging of living MARCO-expressing CHO cells with the EXA microscope.

13.4 Evaluation of Spatial Resolution of EXA Microscope by Numerical Simulation

We combined the electron beam scattering analysis by Monte Carlo simulation [1] with the light propagation analysis by the finite difference time domain method [2] to analyze the emission distribution of the CL by electron beam excitation [22]. This analysis technique enabled evaluation of spatial resolution by light propagation, emission intensity distribution outside the fluorescent film, and analysis of reflection and absorption in the multilayer structure, which could not be realized by Monte Carlo simulation.

Figure 13.5 shows a schematic diagram of the analysis method of the emission distribution of CL by combining Monte Carlo simulation and FDTD (Finite-difference time-domain) method [22]. First, electron beam trajectory is calculated using Monte Carlo simulation, and the emission position and intensity of CL are calculated from the energy loss of the electron due to the scattering. At each light emission position, light emission by a dipole was assumed. The light propagation from all dipoles was calculated by the FDTD method, and the light intensity distribution inside and outside the fluorescent film was obtained by superimposing these distributions.

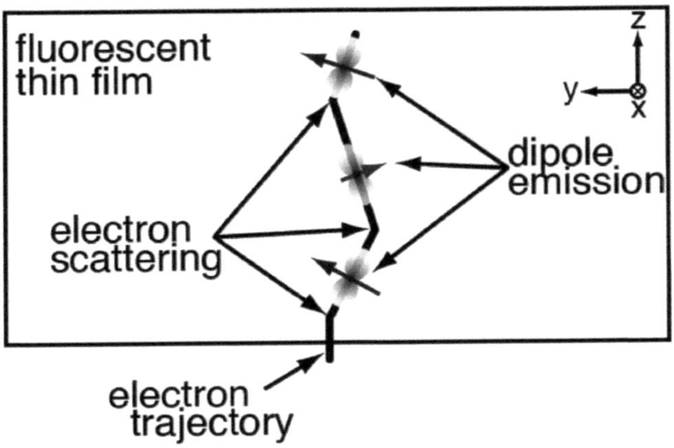

Figure 13.5 Schematic diagram of the analysis method of the emission distribution of CL generated by electron beam by combining Monte Carlo simulation and FDTD method

Figure 13.6 shows the spot size and peak intensity of the spot generated by the electron beam as a function of Si_3N_4 thin film thickness [22]. The acceleration voltage of the incident electron beam was 5 kV. When the electron beam distribution spreads laterally on the surface opposite to the electron beam incident surface, the size of the light spot increases. Since the electrons are almost completely scattered during propagation through the thicker film, the spread of the lateral electron distribution is increased. Therefore, the spot size increased with the film thickness.

The light intensity decreases as the thickness of Si_3N_4 increases. As the thickness of the thin film increased, the number of electrons reaching the surface opposite to the incident surface of the electron beam decreased. The light emission near the opposite surface was a major factor in the central peak light intensity of the spot. As a result, the light intensity of the light spot decreases with increasing film thickness.

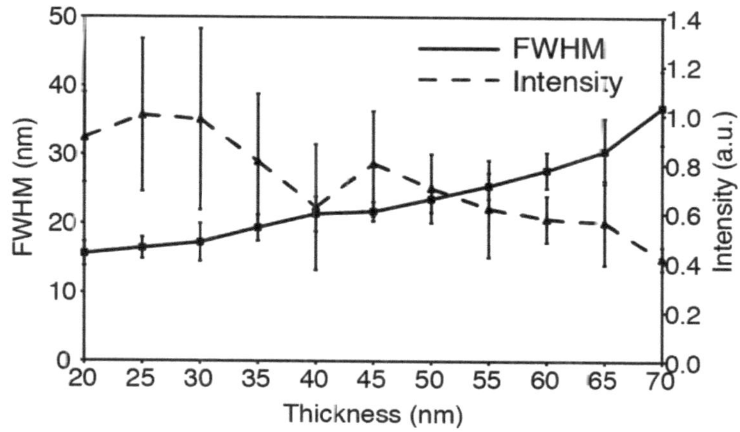

Figure 13.6 The size and peak intensity of the spot generated by the electron beam as a function of Si3N4 thin film thickness.

Figure 13.7 shows the acceleration voltage of the incident electron beam dependence of the spot size and peak intensity [22]. The thickness of the Si_3N_4 thin film was 50 nm. The full width at half maximum of the spot gradually decreases in the range of 2 to 10 keV. Since the nanometric optical spot size is determined by the spread of the electron beam, the spot size is reduced by the higher accelerating voltage of the electrons because electron scattering in the thin film is reduced. The peak light intensity decreases when the voltage is between 3.5 and 10 keV, and has the peak between 2.5 and 3.5 keV. When the acceleration voltage falls below 2.5 keV, the intensity begins to decline rapidly, because the incident electron beam does not reach the surface opposite to the incident surface.

It is also important to prevent damage of specimen from electron beam irradiation. The reduction of the electron beam transmittance due to the addition of the gold thin film is described. Gold is a material that has high density and is difficult to transmit electron beams [23–25]. It has also been reported that coating a thin gold film reduces the electron beam transmittance to 10% and suppresses damage to biological samples [26]. Here, by inserting a thin gold film between ZnO and the cell, the damage to the cell is suppressed by reducing the electron beam transmittance.

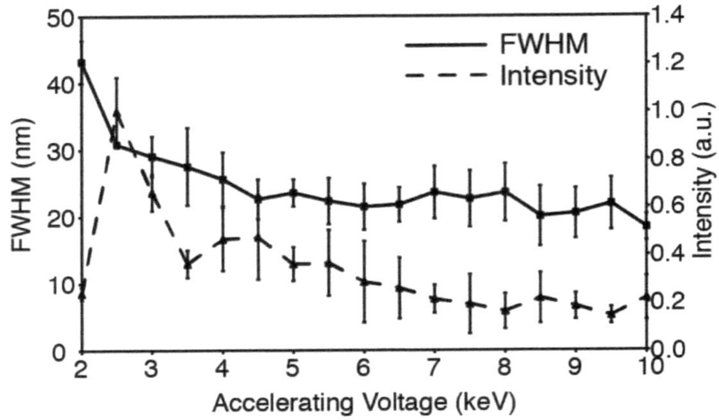

Figure 13.7 The acceleration voltage of the incident electron beam dependence of the spot size and peak intensity.

Figure 13.8 shows the dependence of electron beam transmission on the gold film thickness calculated by Monte Carlo simulation [27]. The acceleration voltage is 3 kV. The electron beam transmission decreases as the gold film thickness increases. When the gold film thickness is 15 nm, the electron beam transmittance is 0%. The minimum gold film thickness required to prevent transmission of electron beams is 15 nm. The optical spot size generated by electron beam irradiation under this condition was calculated. It was evaluated whether the gold thin film would reduce the spatial resolution. Figure 13.9 shows the result of analyzing the electric field intensity distribution of CL generated in the Si_3N_4 film with a gold film [27]. The Si_3N_4 and gold film thicknesses were 50 and 15 nm, respectively. We estimated the CL spot size on the surface of the gold thin film by the numerical analysis method combining Monte Carlo simulation and the finite difference time domain method. According to Fig. 13.9, CL generated in the Si_3N_4 layer penetrates the gold thin film. The peak CL intensity was reduced by 36% compared to the case without the gold film because the gold film hindered the permeation of CL. The full width at half maximum (FWHM) of the electric field intensity was 45 nm at a distance of 10 nm from the surface of the gold thin film. With the addition of the thin gold film, the EXA microscope can observe with better spatial resolution than

200 nm without irradiating the specimen with an electron beam. From Figs. 13.8 and 13.9, the optimal thickness of the gold film is 15 nm. As described above, coating the substrate with gold can reduce radiation damage of a specimen without reducing the spatial resolution beyond the diffraction limit of the light.

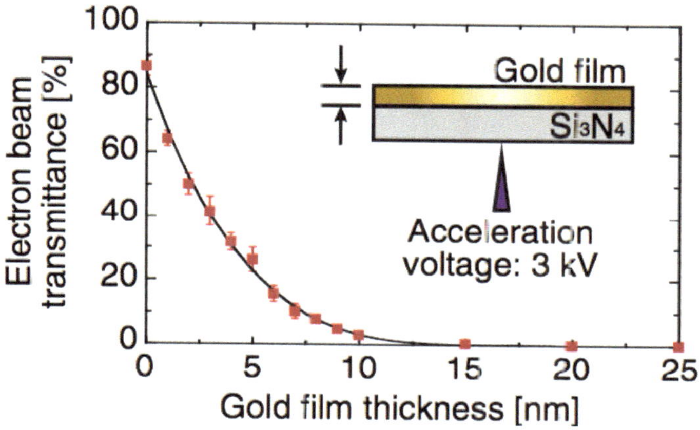

Figure 13.8 The dependence of electron beam transmission on the gold film thickness calculated by Monte Carlo simulation.

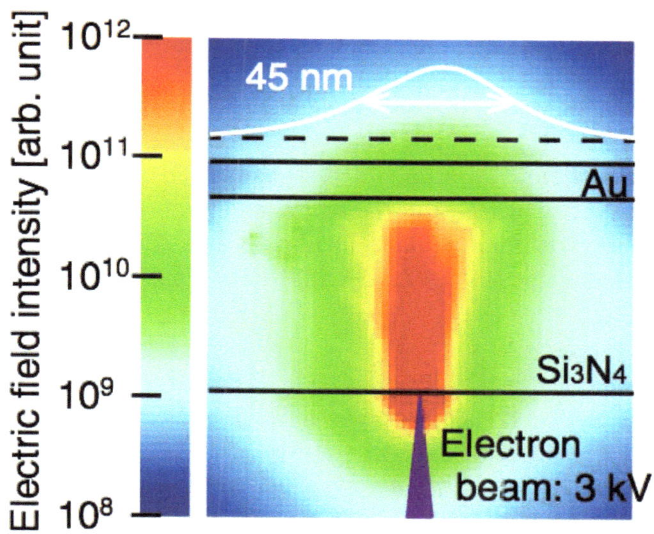

Figure 13.9 The simulated electric field intensity distribution of CL generated in the Si_3N_4 film with a gold film.

13.5 Summary

This chapter described the super-resolution microscope using electron beam. A focused electron beam is irradiated to the fluorescent thin film to generate a nanometric light spot below the diffraction limit. Since the electron beam can realize a spot diameter of several nanometers, the light emitting area of the luminescent film can be reduced. The generated spot size depends on the acceleration voltage and the thickness of the luminescent thin film. In this microscope, since light is used, information on the refractive index, absorption coefficient, and polarization characteristics of a specimen can be obtained, which has not been described in this chapter owing to space limitation. Further, by making the luminescent thin film highly functional, it becomes possible to acquire various optical information of the sample. When the fluorescent thin film emits white light, the spectral characteristics can be measured. This super-resolution EXA optical microscope will make it possible to elucidate biological phenomena in small areas that could not be observed ever and will greatly contribute to the progress of nanobiotechnology.

Acknowledgments

The authors would like to thank Prof. Terakawa, Dr. Miyakawa, Dr. Lin, Dr. Nawa, Dr. Furukawa, Dr. Fukuta and Dr. Masuda for simulations, experiments and useful discussions. We also would like to thank Prof. Nakanishi and Prof. Kominami for the preparation of fluorescent thin film. A part of this chapter was supported by the (CREST) and KAKENHI of Japan.

References

1. Joy, D. C. (1999). *Monte Carlo Modeling for Electron Microscopy and Microanalysis*, Oxford University Press.
2. Yee, K. (1966). Numerical solution of initial boundary value problems involving Maxwell's equations in isotropic media, *IEEE Trans. Antennas Propagation,* **14**(3), pp. 302–307.

3. Reuter, C. E., Joseph, R. M., Thiele, E. T., Katz, D. S., and Taflove, A. (1994). Ultrawideband absorbing boundary condition for termination of waveguiding structures in FDTD simulations, *IEEE Microw. Guided Wave Lett.*, **4**(10), pp. 344–346.

4. Abbe, E. (1873). Beitrage zur Theorie des Mikroskops und der mikroskopischen. Wahrnehmung, *Arch. Mikrosk. Anat.*, **9**, pp. 413–468.

5. Hell S. W., and Wichmann, J. (1994). Breaking the diffraction resolution limit by stimulated emission: Stimulated-emission-depletion fluorescence microscopy, *Opt. Lett.*, **19**(11), pp. 780–782.

6. Betzig, E., Patterson, G. H., Sougrat, R., Lindwasser, O. W., Olenych, S., Bonifacino, J. S., Davidson, M. W., Lippincott-Schwartz, J., and Hess H. F. (2006). Imaging intracellular fluorescent proteins at nanometer resolution, *Science*, **313**(5793), pp. 1642–1645.

7. Huang, B., Wang, W., Bates, M., and Zhuang, X. (2008). Three-dimensional super-resolution imaging by stochastic optical reconstruction microscopy, *Science*, **319**(5864), pp. 810–813.

8. Gustafsson, M. G. (2000). Surpassing the lateral resolution limit by a factor of two using structured illumination microscopy, *J Microsc.*, **198**(2), pp. 82–87.

9. Fujita, K., Kobayashi, M., Kawano, S., Yamanaka, M., and Kawata S. (2007). High-resolution confocal microscopy by saturated excitation of fluorescence, *Phys. Rev. Lett.*, **99**(22), pp. 228105

10. Inami, W., Nakajima, K., Miyakawa, A., and Kawata, Y. (2010). Electron beam excitation assisted optical microscope with ultra-high resolution, *Opt Express*, **18**(12), pp. 12897–12902.

11. Furukawa, T., Kanamori, S., Fukuta, M., Nawa, Y., Kominami, H., Nakanishi, Y., Sugita, A., Inami, W., and Kawata, Y. (2015). Fabrication of bright and thin Zn_2SiO_4 luminescent film for electron beam excitation-assisted optical microscope, *Opt. Express*, **23**(14), pp. 18630–18637.

12. Miyake, A., Kanamori, S., Nawa, Y., Inami, W., Kominami, H., Kawata, Y., and Nakanishi, Y. (2014). Formation of ZnO luminescent films on SiN films for light source of high-resolution optical microscope, *J. J. Appl. Phys.*, **53**(4S), 04EH11.

13. Sugita, A., Kamiya, M., Morita, C., Miyake, A., Nawa, Y., Masuda, Y., Inami, W., Kominami, H., and Nakanishi, Y. (2014). Nanometric light spots of cathode luminescence in Y_2O_3:Eu^{3+} phosphor thin films excited by

focused electron beams as ultra-small illumination source for high-resolution optical microscope, *Opt. Mater. Exp.*, **4**(1), pp. 155–161.

14. Masuda, Y., Nawa, Y., Inami, W., and Kawata, Y. (2015). Carboxylic monolayer formation for observation of intracellular structures in HeLa cells with direct electron beam excitation-assisted fluorescence microscopy, *Biomed. Opt. Exp.*, **6**(8), pp. 3128–3133.
15. Inami, W., Fukuta, M., Kawata, Y., and Terakawa S., (2019). Visualization of absorption distribution beyond the diffraction limit of light with by electron-beam excitation assisted optical microscope, *J. Microsc.*, **276**(1), pp. 46–50.
16. Ash, E. A., and Nicholls, G. (1972). Super-resolution aperture scanning microscope, *Nature,* **237**(5357), pp. 510–512.
17. Pohl, D. W., Denk, W., and Lanz, M. (1984). Optical stethoscopy: Image recording with resolution $\lambda/20$, *Appl. Phys. Lett.*, **44**(7), pp. 651–653.
18. Thach, R. E., and Thach, S. S. (1971). Damage to biological samples caused by the electron beam during electron microscopy, *Biophys. J.*, **11**(2), pp. 204–210.
19. Royall, C. P., Thiel, B. L., and Donald, A. M. (2001). Radiation damage of water in environmental scanning electron microscopy, *J., Microsc.*, **204**(3), pp. 185–195.
20. Fukuta, M., Ono, A., Nawa, Y., Inami, W., Shen, L., Kawata, Y., and Terekawa, S. (2017). Cell structure imaging with bright and homogeneous nanometric light source, *J. Biophotonics,* **10**(4), pp. 503–510.
21. Fukuta, M., Kanamori, S., Furukawa, T., Nawa, Y., Inami, W., Lin, S., Kawata, Y., and Terakawa, S. (2015). Dynamic nano-imaging of label-free living cells using electron beam excitation-assisted optical microscope, *Sci. Rep.,* **5**, Article number: 16068.
22. Inami, W., Fujiwara, J., Fukuta, M., Ono, A., and Kawata, Y. (2012). Analysis of electron and light scattering in a fluorescent thin film by combination of Monte Carlo simulation and finite-difference time-domain method, *Appl. Phys. Lett.*, **101**(15), p. 151104.
23. Bohr, N. (1913). I. On the constitution of atoms and molecules, *Phil. Mag.*, **26**(151), pp. 1–25.
24. Bethe, H. (1930). Zur Theorie des Durchgangs schneller Korpuskularstrahlen durch Materie, *Ann. Physik.*, **5**(3), pp. 325–400.
25. Joy, D. C., and Luo, S. (1989). An empirical stopping power relationship for low-energy electrons, *Scanning*, **11**(4), pp. 176–180.

26. Ogura, T. (2012). High-contrast observation of unstained proteins and viruses by scanning electron microscopy, *Plos One*, **7**(10), e46904.

27. Fukuta, M., Nawa, Y., Inami, W., and Kawata, Y. (2017). Prevention of electron beam transmittance for biological cell imaging using electron beam excitation-assisted optical microscope, *Opt. Rev.*, **24**(2), pp. 237–241.

Chapter 14

X-Ray Semiconductor Imaging Device Technology and Medical-Imaging Application

Toru Aoki, Katsuyuki Takagi, Hiroki Kase, and Akifumi Koike

Research Institute of Electronics, Shizuoka University, 3-5-1 Johoku, Nakaku, Hamamatsu 432-8011, Japan

aoki.toru@shizuoka.ac.jp

X-ray and γ-ray imaging devices using the semiconductors such as CdTe, CdZnTe, and TlBr are suitable for photon-counting detection and imaging because photons of X-rays and γ-rays can be directly converted into the electric charges. Since the energy of photons can be detected by counting the charge for each photon, there is a possibility that new X-ray imaging using energy information will be achieved in this region. This chapter describes the photon-counting and charge-counting by semiconductor radiation detectors, and describes the development of new X-ray imaging using these X-ray imaging devices.

Note that X-rays and γ-rays are the same in the detector of the imaging device. Therefore, both of them are referred as an X-ray device in this chapter.

Biomedical Engineering
Edited by Akihiro Miyauchi and Yuji Miyahara

ISBN 978-981-4877-63-3 (Hardcover), 978-1-003-14194-5 (eBook)
www.jennystanford.com

14.1 Introduction: Nanovision-Science in X-Ray Imaging

Nanovision-science [1] is an ambitious effort to pioneer a new imaging technology by incorporating optical and electronic nanotechnology into existing image engineering. Pursuit of unlimited immersive image technology has led to precise control of electrons and photons by incorporating nano-sized processing technology into pixels. Now, in addition to these, the imaging technology beyond human eyes by Nanovision-science has come to have great significance as an input device of accurate data such as deep-learning and artificial intelligence (AI). In addition, Nanovision-science is changing a treatment of photons and electrons, which have been treated as a statistically and collectively in image technology, into individual photons and electrons, and opens up entirely new image technologies.

The X-ray imaging devices introduced in this chapter play two major significant roles in Nanovision-science: (1) visualization of X-ray imaging, which is an invisible light for human eye, and (2) individual handling of photons and electrons. The former has been widely used in society since the discovery of X-rays by Röntgen in 1895. The latter is that photon energy is detected and utilized by counting an identical charge which is generated in a semiconductor-radiation-detector [2]. In this chapter, the latter photon-counting and charge-counting techniques in X-ray detection are explained, and applications to a new X-ray imaging are described.

14.2 X-Ray Imaging Device

An X-ray imaging device is a device that receives X-rays and captures images. X-ray films have been used for a long time since the discovery of X-rays. X-ray film needs such as a development process and, in some cases, a printing for imaging. Both processes require chemical treatments and equipment. In addition, there is a problem that these processes take time, and a sensitivity of X-ray films is low because the films are too thin to absorb enough X-ray. In order to solve these problems, an imaging plate using a stimulable luminescent material has been developed. In this method, radiation is received with high sensitivity and recorded as trapping of electrons or holes in trap levels in the imaging plate. The trapped charges are excited by infrared laser scanning, and an image is read out as the recombination map of charges on the plate. Therefore, a digitalized image becomes possible without the processes of development and/or printing. The imaging plate captures the image as data. Therefore, it has been widely used as a digital device because of its good sensitivity and easy handling. Furthermore, there is an advantage that the data can be erased, and it is economical to use repeatedly.

However, comparing a general digital camera which can handle a captured digital image on the spot where the image is taken, the imaging plates need to be moved to a place where the captured image can be readout. In recent years, since the processing of X-ray images into a computer such as Computed Radiography (CR) has become widespread, the imaging plates have become widely used instead of films. Further, as Digital Radiography (DR) represented by X-ray Computed Tomography (X-ray CT) has advanced, an X-ray camera has become equivalent to a general digital camera and popular. In the early days, an X-ray image tube was developed and used for a visible light video camera, and a high-sensitive X-ray image intensifier (X-ray I.I.) with a photomultiplier function. However, flat panel detectors (FPDs) using semiconductor detectors have been developed because the X-ray image tube was too large for handling and the image distortion due to the strong magnetic field often seen in medical fields. Many FPDs are as thin as IPs and can be connected to computers using only thin cables or wireless, so they can be replaced where IPs were used. Of course, since data is directly taken into a computer as digital data, various processes and large-scale data accumulation and distributed processing using a cloud server or the like are possible.

There are various types of FPDs, but an indirect conversion type and a direct conversion type are classified according to a conversion method from X-rays to electric signals, namely a charge-integration type (current processing) and a photon-counting type (pulse processing). The type is grouped by the processing of the converted signal.

An indirect conversion method uses a scintillator which emits visible light when receiving X-rays, and the visible light is converted by imaging devices such as CMOS (complementary metal oxide semiconductor), CCD (charge coupled device), etc. This method is widely used in FPDs because various types of scintillator can be selected and various kinds of radiation can be handled. A very high performance of CMOS image sensor can be used by the latest semiconductor technology. However, there is a problem that blur occurs due to light scattering in the scintillator. Also, most indirect conversion type FPDs use a charge integration method therefore energy information of X-ray photons cannot be obtained due to the problem of collection efficiency of generated photons.

On the other hand, a direct conversion type is a method in which X-rays are directly converted into electric charges by semiconductor or the like. In order to receive X-rays, materials having a large atomic number and a high density are desired. However, these materials tend to have a small band gap. Therefore, the generation of thermal noise increases, and this makes difficult to use at room temperature. (Please note that a number of X-ray photons is orders of magnitude smaller than that of visible light.) For this reason, there are very few choices for semiconductor-materials for X-ray receiving. There are also no recipes for manufacturing these special semiconductors. Therefore, it is necessary to research and develop the manufacturing method of these semiconductor materials. However, it is possible to take out the charge generated by the reception of X-ray photons without spreading by an applied electric field from the outside. There is little blur like a scintillator, and there is a possibility that noise can be suppressed by high X-ray absorption. In addition, since the charge collection efficiency of the charges generated by the X-ray photons is high, and it is suitable for photon-counting signal processing that processes each photon, research and development of photon-counting cameras as well as charge-integration cameras are active.

This chapter focuses on photon-counting X-ray imaging devices using CdTe [3] or TlBr [4] which have high X-ray absorption efficiency, large band gap, and excellent electric field mobility in semiconductors.

14.3 Photon-Counting

Photon-counting by CdTe is explained in this section. Photon-counting is a method counting of photons in one pixel. In a visible-light range, one photon generates one electron-hole pair in a semiconductor detection-element because the energy of semiconductor band-gap and the photon are similar. Therefore, the number of photons can be obtained by counting the number of generated electron-hole pairs. However, X-ray photons have very high energies that are orders of magnitude higher than the band gap of semiconductors. For example, it is 10 keV to 1 MeV, in which case the photon energies are 10,000 to 1 million times higher than the band gap energy of the semiconductor. Therefore, the principle of charge generation differs between visible-light range and X-ray, and the generated charge is proportional to the energy of the X-ray photon. This means that the number of generated charges depends on the energy of one X-ray photon, and the number of photons and the number of charges are proportional only when receiving a single energy photon such as a specific gamma ray source. In a white ray source such as X-rays, the number of photons cannot be estimated even if the number of charges is counted.

However, the energy of the X-ray photon can be known by counting the number of generated charges each time when one photon is incident because the number of generated charges is proportional to the energy of an X-ray photon. Although it is an enormous amount of processing, the energy spectrum of the incident X-ray can be known if the generated charge is counted for each incident photon and a histogram is created at a unit time such as the frame rate. This is used as a one-pixel detector for the energy analysis function of a scanning electron microscope (SEM). A charge-sensitive preamplifier is placed near a semiconductor detector which is connected to a main amplifier with a waveform-shaping function. A peak value is digitized by an analog-to-digital converter (ADC) with sampling and holding circuits and each peak value is stored in memory. Then, after a certain period of time, it is read out as a histogram. If a large number of photons enter in a certain time during the signal processing, a state called pile-up occurs in which the energy and number of the photons become unknown. Therefore, high-speed processing including the semiconductor detector and the signal processing circuit is required.

In general, the processing circuit has a maximum speed of about 20 k count per second (cps) when a continuous uniform pulse is applied. In actual X-rays with fluctuations, the upper limit is about one tenth of the maximum speed that is estimated under sufficiently small pileup [5].

In order to use the photon-counting in the X-ray image detector, it is necessary to integrate the above high-speed circuits for each small pixel. The required process speed is at least 10^6 photons/mm^2/s. However, it is extremely difficult at present to fabricate highly integrated signal circuits on CdTe or TlBr, and signal processing circuits must rely on silicon LSIs. Therefore, it is necessary to connect a pixel of CdTe or TlBr, which is a pixelated semiconductor X-ray detection element to a signal readout processing LSI for each pixel.

For the photon counting operation in X-ray region, signal reading by general scanning technique as in the visible light cannot be used. Therefore, a new processing circuit is required for every pixel, and this makes the signal processing LSI very complicated. Further, a large size X-ray imaging device is required because a lens cannot be used in X-ray region. Large-size manufacturing of a compound semiconductor such as CdTe or TlBr is difficult because these materials are brittle and difficult to handle, and cause a lower yield in mass-production. Considering the yield of large-scale signal processing LSIs, it is necessary to arrange small modules of about 1 to 2 cm^2 side by side and tile them to increase the device area.

In this way, the development of post-processes, such as the conversion of compound semiconductor X-ray detectors to pixel devices, high-precision cutting for tiling, bumping of signal processing LSIs and detectors, and the connection of external devices to multilayer devices, are also underway. It is an important process for realization. However, X-ray imaging using the energy information of X-ray photons opens up a whole new world of X-ray imaging by adding a new physical axis, and photon-counting is one of the inevitable methods.

14.4 Charge Counting

Accurate charge counting is very important for ensuring the accuracy of X-ray photon energy detection by photon-counting as in the previous section. X-ray photons generate the charges in the semiconductor detector. In many cases, it is not easy to perform a signal processing as it is on amount of electric charges. Therefore, the signal is converted into a voltage and then processed (in the case of simple processing, a charge output may be treated as a voltage output, but this is not characteristic). For example, in the case of photoelectric conversion by absorption in a CdTe detector, one charge is generated at about 4.4 eV at room temperature, so that about 2,300 electrons are generated by one photon of 10 keV. However, in photon-counting signal processing, since signals are processed for each X-ray photon, the signal processing must be performed using only this number of electrons, so ultra-low noise signal processing is required. In addition, in compound semiconductors such as CdTe, the mobility of electrons and holes differs by orders of magnitude, so it is necessary to devise signal processing. In addition, the device usually needs a millimeter-level thickness to absorb X-rays which has extremely high penetrating power. And in the case of high electric field, high bias voltage is required and the leakage current of the element itself becomes a problem. For these reasons, various devices have been reported, such as forming a diode structure with the element itself, providing a guard ring structure, using AC coupling for connection and so on.

The output from the semiconductor radiation detector is several thousand to ten-thousands of charges per pulse, and the pulse width is 1 ns to 1 μs. Generally, a charge-sensitive preamplifier is used to amplify and convert the voltage with low noise. Although the circuit is an integrating circuit, the signal is reset using the decay time-constant. The output is subjected to waveform-shaping by a main amplifier which have an analog waveform-shaping circuit. The waveform-shaping amplifier performs a waveform-shaping and an amplification by combining differentiation and integration having a shaping time-constant, and outputs a waveform as a pulse having a pseudo Gaussian distribution. The pulse-height value of the shaped pulse is digitized by an analog-to-digital converter (ADC) of about 10 to

14 bits, and a count number is stored in memories for each pulse-height value to know the energy spectrum of the X-ray photons. In the case of integration as a LSI for signal processing, the circuits of X-ray imaging device should be designed for reducing the circuit area, but this method is generally adopted as a basic rule.

On the other hand, in recent years, integrated circuit technology and digital circuit technology have rapidly advanced. The authors make the most of these, transfer the generated charge in CdTe or TlBr to the capacitor of the charge-sensitive preamplifier, and use the charge-to-digital conversion (QDC) to count the transferred charge directly [6]. We are developing a signal processing LSI. Due to the problems of device, noise, and limitations of read time, the performance on the counting per electron has not been achieved, but at present time, a 4-bit 1Mcps/pixel read circuit has been obtained within a size of 80 μm^2. The signal processing LSI integrated into 96 × 96 pixels has been developed. Unfortunately, it is not possible to make a capacitor that can accumulate the charge generated in the semiconductor detector, so the generated charge is temporarily transferred to the capacitor of the charge-sensitive preamplifier (integrator), and the charge in this capacitor is transferred to the switched capacitor. The charge is directly converted into a digital signal by counting the number of charge-transfer time until the all storage-charge becomes 0 by repeating a charge injection. This operation itself is similar to the delta-sigma ADC, but it is unique that the charge itself generated in the detector is directly manipulated and digitized [7].

The conventional analog circuit technology exhibits excellent noise characteristics, which is attractive to achieve a high energy resolution for the radiation signal-processing systems. However, in the case of pile-up in which multiple X-ray photons are incident within one pulse signal processing time, removal is limited and separation is not possible, and circuit constants such as an optimal time constant are set for each detector. Because of the necessity of the adjustment, it is difficult to make the LSI versatile in an LSI that is difficult to adjust and requires a large amount of manufacturing cost. However, in the QDC type, the pile-up separation can be performed under certain conditions by devising an algorithm, and it is possible to cope with high incident dose rates, and highly versatile signal processing is realized by adjusting the switched-capacitor and clock-frequency. It has been reported that the signal-processing LSI for QDC-type imaging sensor using CdTe detectors are designed to be used as an imaging device by directly connecting it to TlBr with different numbers of generated charges and carrier transfer characteristics. In addition, by realizing a Modified Digital Energy Integration algorithm and circuit that mixes charge-integration mode and photon-counting mode, it achieves 5 x 10^8 cps/mm^2. However, a higher counting rate is required and for X-ray CT as an imaging device [8]. In addition, a Schottky diode type CdTe detector that realizes a low leakage current for high energy resolution is commercially available. In the authors' laboratory, by further reducing of leakage current and arranging the junction inside the bulk CdTe, it is easy to perform post-processes such as a bumping, and the need for a guard ring structure eliminates the need for a tiling with no gap as an imaging device. We are developing a possible pn-junction type CdTe diode device using our unique laser diode technology.

Thus, X-ray imaging devices of a new generation have begun to be developed utilizing the latest digital technology, semiconductor technology, and LSI manufacturing technology while referring to the conventional radiation measurement device technology and signal processing technology. Photon-counting signal processing that can make full use of the high sensitivity (= low exposure) and energy resolution potential of semiconductor detectors such as CdTe and TlBr due to the high X-ray absorptance. The upper limit of dynamic range has been greatly expanded, and a highly versatile charge-counting signal processing LSI that can handle a variety of semiconductor detectors has been realized. Furthermore, a photon/charge counting type X-ray imaging sensor utilizing the most advanced 3D LSI technology has been realized. With the use of low-noise, high-contrast energy-resolved imaging, we are opening up a new world of X-ray imaging, including low exposure, high image quality, and high-performance imaging.

14.5 Low Exposure and High-Performance X-Ray Imaging

Photon/charge counting type X-ray semiconductor imaging devices incorporating the latest semiconductor and electronic circuit technologies have interesting features that can be applied to a medical imaging. The first is the realization of high-contrast images with high sensitivity and low noise, enabling imaging at low exposures. The second is to use energy information to emphasize the bands that require contrast and to use multi-energy [8]. This is a high-performance X-ray imaging such as material analysis type CT imaging by CT.

Noise that must be considered in X-ray imaging devices includes so-called fixed noise due to variations in the sensitivity and energy resolution of the sensor and circuit itself for each pixel, electrical noise for each pixel and for the entire sensor and circuit, and shot noise due to fluctuation of incident X-ray photons are main noise sources. Among these, at present, the fixed noise tends to be larger than the indirect conversion type FPD because the variation in the manufacturing process and the need for an amplification circuit for each pixel require a large variation in the semiconductor FPD. In the charge-integration type semiconductor FPD, this fixed noise has been considerably reduced, but still needs to be improved. In a photon-counting type semiconductor FPD, the circuit is complicated for each pixel, and noise due to energy resolution appears as fixed noise, which is relatively large. Since much of the fixed noise due to the circuit is due to variations in the analog processing circuit LSI in the first stage, it can be significantly reduced by direct charge digital conversion (QDC) by charge counting described in the previous section. On the other hand, noise due to energy resolution can be suppressed considerably by setting the energy threshold off the peak of the energy spectrum of X-ray photons, but this limits the free use based on the theory of energy information. Therefore, it is important to improve the energy resolution and reduce this variation as much as possible. For this purpose, it is indispensable to improve the detector materials, such as CdTe and TlBr, and the signal processing circuits by using algorithms that understand the principles well.

Electrical noise can be reduced by improving circuits and mounting techniques, and in the photon-counting type, noise can be eliminated by cutting low-pulse signals at a fixed threshold. Actually, this electrical noise degrades the energy resolution, so when performing an energy calculation, even if it is a photon-counting type, this noise cannot be ignored and sufficient noise reduction measures are indispensable.

Shot noise is more noticeable in the photon-counting type because other noise is less noticeable. In particular, it is difficult for the conventional photon-counting processing circuit to cope with a high incidence rate, that is, a high X-ray intensity. At present, the photon/charge counting type CdTe-FPD described in the previous section also supports high incident rates, so imaging is performed by increasing the dose to the minimum dose that provides good image quality by balancing shot noise and exposure dose.

In the application of X-ray imaging devices, especially high-quality imaging with a low dose is important for reducing exposure of imaging. Figure 14.1 shows an example of CT imaging of an acrylic phantom using the same CdTe material and preparing two types of detectors with only the difference between a charge-integration type and a photon-counting type signal processing system for comparison.

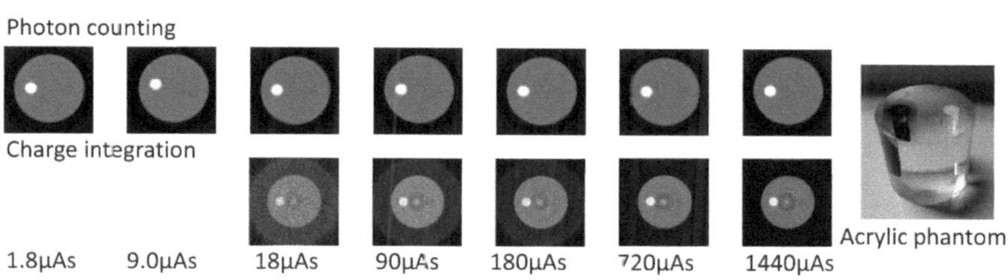

Figure 14.1 Comparison of X-ray CT images between the photon-counting and charge-integration devices using CdTe with various X-ray intensities. The inserted figure is a picture of the acrylic phantom.

As shown in the Fig. 14.1, the product of the X-ray tube current of the X-ray source and time is proportional to the dose (A-s). The acrylic phantom contains a strong white iodine contrast agent in the tomographic image, and the Root Mean Square (RMS) of granularity of acrylic, iodine contrast, and air were measured as shown in Fig. 14.2.

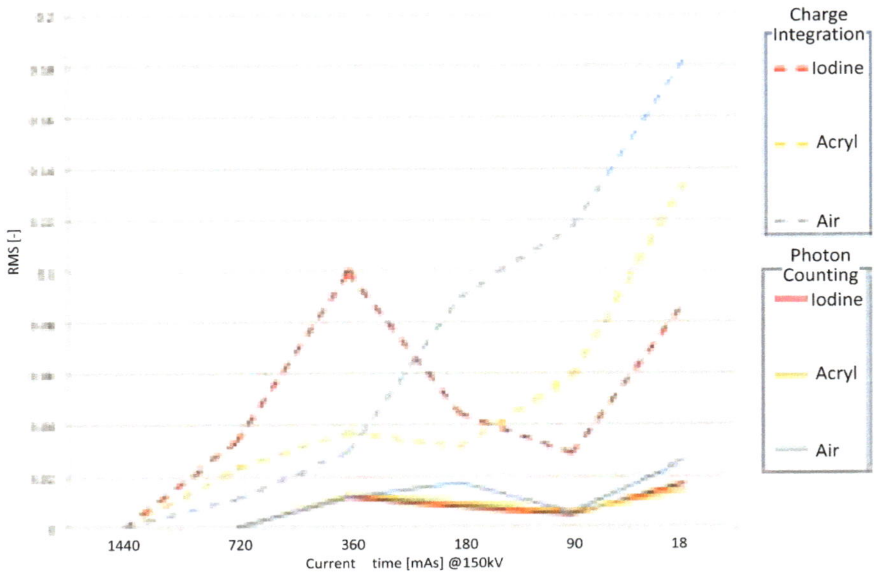

Figure 14.2 RMS of granularity in X-ray CT images of acrylic, iodine contrast and air. The charge-integration and photon-counting imaging devices with CdTe were used.

In the part where the X-ray dose is large at the right end, both images are reconstructed sufficiently well (artifact noise on the ring is noticeable in the charge-integration type, but it is due to fixed noise and should be ignored in this discussion). When the current value is reduced and the dose is reduced, almost no change in image quality is observed in the photon-counting type, whereas the radial artifact noise due to electrical noise increases in the charge-integration type, resulting in 9.0 μAs, the reconstructed image can no longer be constructed as a tomographic image. This is also evident in the graph summarized in Fig. 14.2, where the RMS of granularity increases linearly with decreasing dose in the charge-integration type, while it increases only slightly in the photon-counting type. This shows the same tendency even when observed at the output of the detector. Figure 14.3 shows a comparison between the charge accumulation type and the photon-counting type as NPS (Noise Power Spectrum). Since the measurement conditions are not the same as those in Figs. 14.1 and 14.2, simple comparisons cannot be made, in the photon-counting type is smaller than a substantially constant threshold value, the noise increases drastically. From the analysis of noise frequency characteristics, it is estimated that the electrical noise is dominant in the charge-integration type, and the shot noise is the photon-counting type noise that is noticeable below a certain tube voltage. As described above, the photon-counting type is capable of X-ray imaging with good image quality at a low dose, and has a possibility of low-exposure imaging in the future medical field.

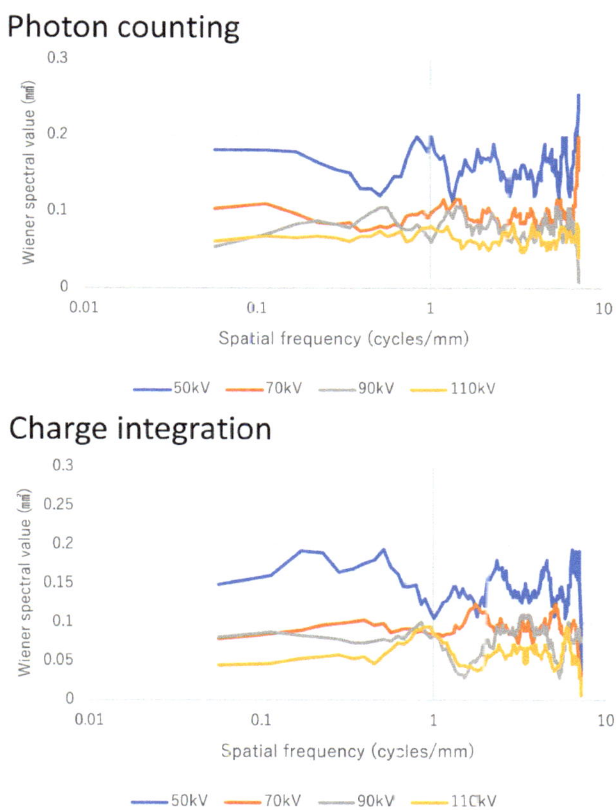

Figure 14.3 Observed NPS (Noise Power Spectrum) of the charge-integration and the photon-counting imaging device using CdTe.

Figure 14.4 shows an X-ray CT tomogram of the teeth (provided by Tohoku University Graduate School of Dentistry). A tooth is dense and difficult to image by a conventional X-ray CT. We used the CdTe photon-counting detector in this experiment. Although the artifacts due to the fixed noise were still noticeable, the internal structures of the teeth were clearly observed in these photographs. In the future, this low-noise and high-contrast X-ray imaging device is expected to be applied to such conventionally difficult imaging regions.

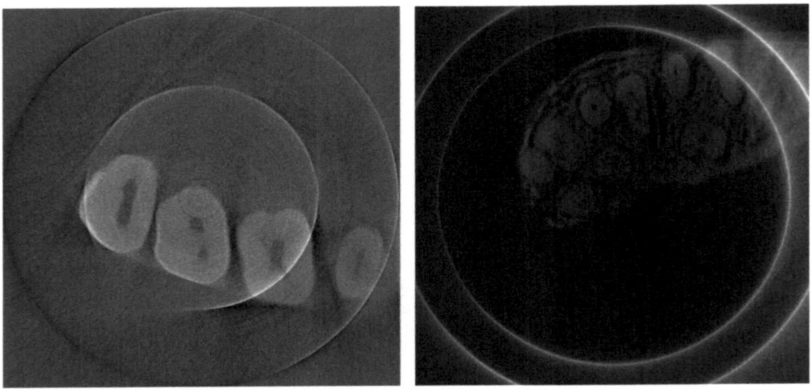

Figure 14.4 X-ray CT tomogram of teeth (provided by Tohoku University) by CdTe photon-counting imaging device.

On the other hand, functional imaging enables enhancement imaging of contrast agents and discrimination imaging of multiple contrast agents as currently performed by dual energy X-ray CT, and can reduce artifacts in principle by removing beam-hardening effect. Figure 14.5 shows an example of discrimination imaging of a plurality of contrast agents. Iodine-, gadolinium-, and barium-based X-ray and MRI contrast agents provide contrast when taken simultaneously, but are difficult to distinguish clearly. Since these contrast agents can be extracted and imaged by calculation of different energy bands, it is easy to create a colored tomogram for each contrast agent by performing only one image and repeating the calculation of different energy bands on a computer only once.

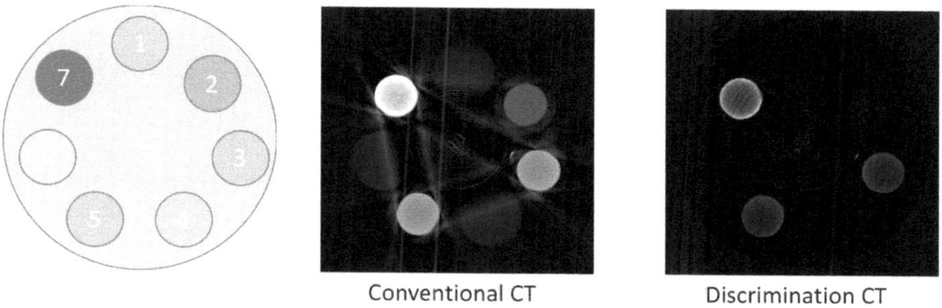

Figure 14.5 X-ray CT images of acrylic cylinders filled with contract medium: (1) Ferucarbotran; (2) Gadopentetate Meglumine; (3) Iopamidol; (4) NSS; (5) Iohexol; (6) Bothdel Oral Sloution; and (7) Baricon meal.

Figure 14.6 shows a photograph of an attempt to discriminate healthy teeth from carious teeth using energy information acquired by a photon-counting X-ray imaging sensor. In the dual energy X-ray CT shows the CT value distribution. Images can be separated into tomographic images of two physical values, "electron density" and "effective atomic number." Dental dentin and enamel have different densities even after atomic number and can be easily separated. The enamel of health dental and caries have almost the same effective atomic number and is difficult to discriminate in principle. However, it is highly possible that the dental caries progress by decalcification and destruction, so the electron density is likely to change. In this experiment, we use sliced teeth of 3 mm thickness (prepared at Tohoku University). From Fig. 14.6, a slight difference is observed between the carious part and the healthy tooth part in the transmission image, but little difference is seen in the effective atomic number image. However, the contrast was observed in the electron density mapping, and the distinction can be made as expected. A quantitative comparison between the observed images and theoretical calculations is the next step of this research.

Figure 14.7 shows an X-ray CT tomographic image of a tooth taken by the photon-counting X-ray imaging device. There is a changing the lower limit discrimination of energy for image reconstruction because gutta-percha cone (GPC), which is a relaxing

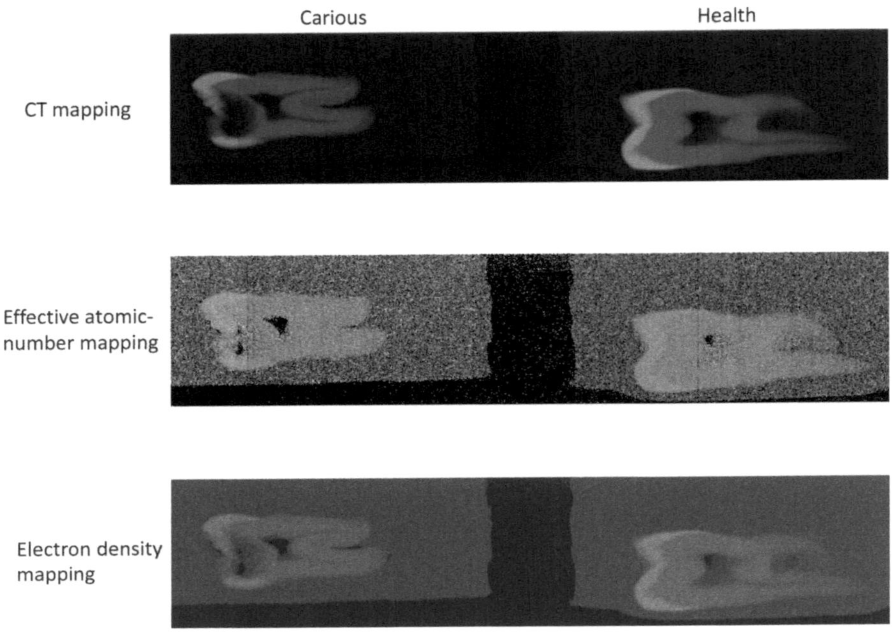

Figure 14.6 X-ray images of healthy-tooth and carious-tooth.

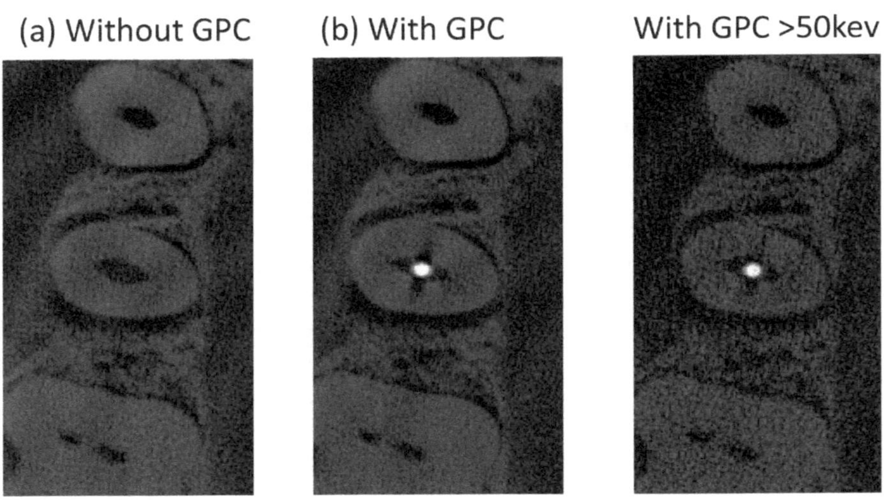

Figure 14.7 X-ray CT images with/without GPC in teeth with energy discrimination by photon-counting X-ray imaging device.

filler, generates large artifacts. Although no tomographic image with little noise was obtained without GPC in Fig. 14.7a, the area around the observed portion is greatly distorted due to the artifacts with GPC as shown in Fig. 14.7b as the small white-dots seen in the center of the middle tooth under the same condition of the energy lower-limit discrimination. When the energy of the lower-limit discriminator is increased to about 50 keV or more, the artifact becomes sufficiently small, but the number of available photons decreases. Therefore, the signal noise (S/N) ratio becomes deteriorated. Although there is a balance with the exposure dose, it is necessary to find the optimal point while observing the reduction of the artifact and the increase of the image noise. However, this is an example in which the artifact can be reduced by using the energy information.

14.6 Summary

In this chapter, the latest X-ray, gamma-ray semiconductor imaging device technology is explained and the examples of their applications in medical-imaging are shown. Although this chapter has been limited to X-ray imaging, this imaging device can also be used for γ-rays and is expected to be applied to SPECT and nuclear medical monitors. We hope that X-ray imaging devices equipped with these advanced technologies will help patients a little.

Acknowledgment

The authors thank Mr. H. Morii, Mr. T. Okunoyama, Mr. T. Takagi and Mr. T. Terao of ANSeeN Inc., as well as Prof. K. Takase, Dr. M. Iikubo, and Dr. H. Ishihata of Tohoku University for preparing tooth samples and imaging. A part of this chapter was supported by Japan Agency for Medical Research and Development.

References

1. H. Mimura, S. Kawahito, N. Hiromoto, K. Hara, and T. Aoki (2009) *Nanovision Science – Evolution of Imaging Technology-*, T. Aoki,

Chapter 4, "Penetration imaging by high-energy beam," (Corona Publishing, Tokyo, Japan) pp. 135–173 (in Japanese).

2. K. Taguchi and J. S. Iwanczyuk (2013). Vision 20/20: Single photon counting x-ray detectors in medical imaging, *Med. Phys.*, **40** (10), 100901.
3. L. A. Kosyachenko, V. M. Sklyarchuk, O. F. Sklyarchuk, O. L. Maslyanchuk, V. A. Gnatyuk, and T. Aoki (2009). Higher Voltage Ni/CdTe Schottky diodes with low leakage current, *IEEE Tans. Nucl. Sci.*, **56**(4), pp. 1827–1834.
4. K. Hiromi, S. Shoji, and I. Keizo (2013). Advances in TlBr detector development, *J. Crystal Growth*, **379**, pp. 93–98.
5. T. Aoki, H. Morii, H. Nakashima, T. Takahashi, Y. Onishi, G. Tomita, T. Neo, and H. Mimura (2008). *X-Ray, Gamma-Ray Detector/Imager by CdTe Semiconductor and Its Applications, Proc. SPIE* ***7008***, R80.
6. K. Takagi, A. Koik, and T. Aoki (2017). *Direct Charge Handling Method for Dead-Time-Less Photon Counting, Proc. SPIE* **10209,** 102091D.
7. K. Takagi, T. Terao, A. Koike, and T. Aoki (2018). Study of an X-ray/Gamma-ray photon counting circuit based on charge injection, *Sens. Mater.*, **30**(7), pp. 1611–1616.
8. Z. Y. Zou, T. Nakashima, Y. Onishi, A. Koike, B. Shinomiya, H. Morii, Y. Neo, H. Mimura, and T. Aoki (2008). Atomic number and electron density measurement using a conventional X-ray tube and a CdTe detector, *Jpn. J. Appl. Phys.*, **47**(9), pp. 7317–7323.

Chapter 15

Deep Learning in Medical Image Processing and Computer-Aided Diagnosis

Kenji Suzuki

Institute of Innovative Research, Tokyo Institute of Technology, 4259 Nagatsuta, Midori, Yokohama, Kanagawa 226-8503, Japan

suzuki.k.di@m.titech.ac.jp

Deep leaning is one of the most active areas of research in the biomedical engineering field, because "learning from examples or data" is crucial to handling a large amount of data ("big data") coming from biomedical informatics or imaging systems. Deep learning is a versatile, powerful framework that can acquire image-processing and analysis functions through training with image examples. We invented ones of the earliest deep-learning models, and studied, developed, and commercialized their applications to medical image processing and computer-aided diagnosis in medical images. These studies include (1) separation of bones from soft tissue in chest radiographs, (2) semantic segmentation of organs in medical images, (3) radiation dose reduction in computed tomography (CT) and x-ray images,

Biomedical Engineering
Edited by Akihiro Miyauchi and Yuji Miyahara

ISBN 978-981-4877-63-3 (Hardcover), 978-1-003-14194-5 (eBook)
www.jennystanford.com

(4) classification between lesions and non-lesions in medical images, and (5) classification among lesion types. Deep learning is a breakthrough technology that plays a major, or often dominant, role and is becoming indispensable in many applications in the biomedical engineering field.

15.1 History of Machine and Deep Learning

Deep learning is a subfield of the field of machine learning (ML). The history of the ML field is shown in Fig. 15.1. Before the popularity of "deep learning" starting in 2013 due to the event when one of deep-learning methods won the ImageNet computer vision competition in late 2012, feature-based ML (or classifiers) was dominant in the field. Before 1980, even when the term "machine learning" did not exist, classical classifiers such as linear discriminant analysis (LDA), quadratic discriminant analysis (QDA), and a k-nearest neighbor classifier (k-NN) were used for classification. In 1986, multilayer perceptron (MLP) was proposed by Rumelhard and Hinton [1]. The MLP created the 2nd neural network (NN) research boom (the first one was in the 1960s). In 1995, Vapnik proposed support vector machines (SVMs) [2] and became the most popular classifier for a while, partially because of publicly available code on the Internet, and because of the beautiful theory in the linear model, although nonlinear models require a "trick" called the kernel trick. Other ML methods were proposed and gained some popularities, including random forests by Ho et al. in 1995 [3], and dictionary learning by Mairal et al. in 2009 [4].

On the other hand, various ML with image input (image-based ML) techniques were proposed before the introduction of the term "deep learning." It started from the Neocognitron by Fukushima in 1980 [5]. In 1989, LeCun et al. simplified the Neocognitron and proposed a convolutional neural network (CNN) [6], but he did not study CNNs much until recently. In 1994, Suzuki et al. applied an MLP to cardiac images in a convolutional way ("convolutional MLP") [7]. Two years later, Suzuki et al. proposed neural filters based on a modified MLP ("MLP regression") to reduce noise in images [8], and in 2000, they proposed neural edge enhancers [9]. Suzuki et al. extended the neural filters and neural edge enhancers to accommodate pattern recognition and classification tasks and proposed massive-training artificial neural networks (MTANNs) in 2003 [10], detection of objects in an "end-to-end" fashion in 2009 [11], separation of specific patters from other patterns ("bone separation") in x-ray images in 2006 [12], multiresolution MTANNs that has a 'U' structure ("U-Net") in 2006 [12], and reduction of noise and artifacts on CT images in 2012 [13] and mammography in 2015 [14].

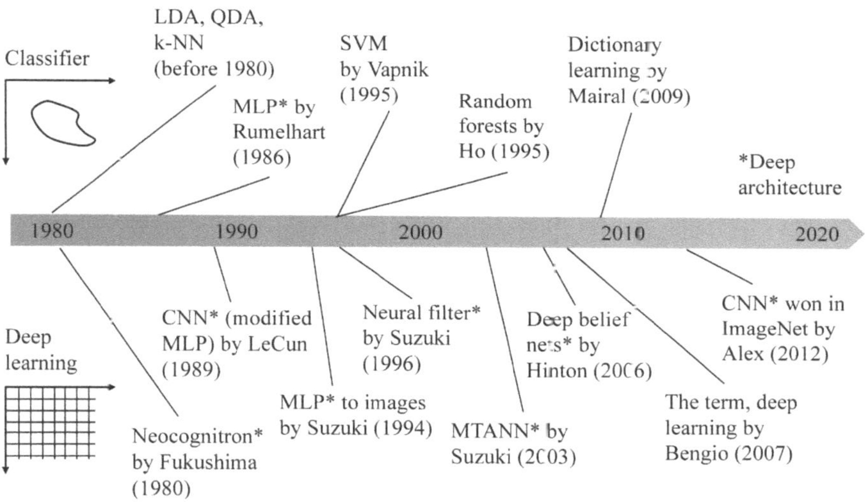

Figure 15.1 History of machine learning.

Hinton et al. proposed a deep brief network (DBN) in 2006 [15], and Bengio and others created the term "deep learning" a year later. Deep learning was not recognized much until late 2012. In late 2012, a CNN won in the ImageNet competition [16]. Among ML models, Neocognitron, MLP, CNN, neural filters, MTANN, and DBN are capable of deep architecture. Thus, at present the term "deep learning," which is ML with image input (image-based ML) with a deep architecture, to be accurate, does not offer new ML models, but rather it is essentially a collection of earlier work on ML (namely, ML with image input) that was reinvented with a different terminology. Since then, variations of image-based ML models have been proposed in the field of deep learning, including some truly new ML methods such as generative adversarial nets (networks) (GAN) [17].

15.2 Massive-Training Artificial Neural Network (MTANN) Deep Learning

In the field of signal and image processing, supervised nonlinear filters based on a modified MLP model ("MLP regression"), called neural filters, have been proposed [8, 18, 19]. The neural filter employs a linear-output-layer NN regression model as the kernel of a convolution filter. The inputs to the neural filter are an object pixel and spatially/spatiotemporally adjacent pixels in a subregion (or local window, image patch, kernel). The output of the neural filter is a single pixel. The neural filter is trained with input images and corresponding "teaching" (desired or ideal) images. The class of neural filters is used for image-processing tasks such as edge-preserving noise reduction in radiographs and other digital pictures [18, 19], edge enhancement from noisy images [20], and enhancement of subjective edges traced by a physician ("semantic segmentation") in left ventriculograms [21, 22].

An MTANN was developed by extending of neural filters to accommodate various pattern-recognition tasks [10], including classification [10, 12, 23–29], pattern enhancement and suppression [12], and object detection [11]. In other words, neural filters are a subclass or a special case of MTANNs. A two-dimensional (2D) MTANN was first developed for distinguishing a specific pattern from other patterns in 2D images [10]. Figure 15.2 summarizes the research activities of our lab that has been actively, continuously studying, developing, applying, and commercializing deep learning since 1996.

A 2D MTANN was applied to reduction of false positives (FPs) in computer-aided diagnosis (CAD) for detection of lung nodules on 2D CT slices [10, 30, 31], and in chest radiographs (chest x-ray: CXR) [27], the separation of bones from soft tissue in CXR [12, 32, 33], and the distinction between benign and malignant lung nodules on 2D CT slices [23]. For processing of three-dimensional (3D) volume data, a 3D MTANN was developed by extending of the structure of the 2D MTANN, and it was applied to 3D CT colonography data [24–26, 28, 29]. Various MTANN architectures were developed, including multiple MTANNs [10, 18, 19, 23, 27, 30], a mixture of expert MTANNs [24, 25], a multi-resolution MTANN [12], a Laplacian eigenfunction MTANN [29], as well as a massive-training support vector regression (MTSVR) and a massive-training nonlinear Gaussian process regression [28].

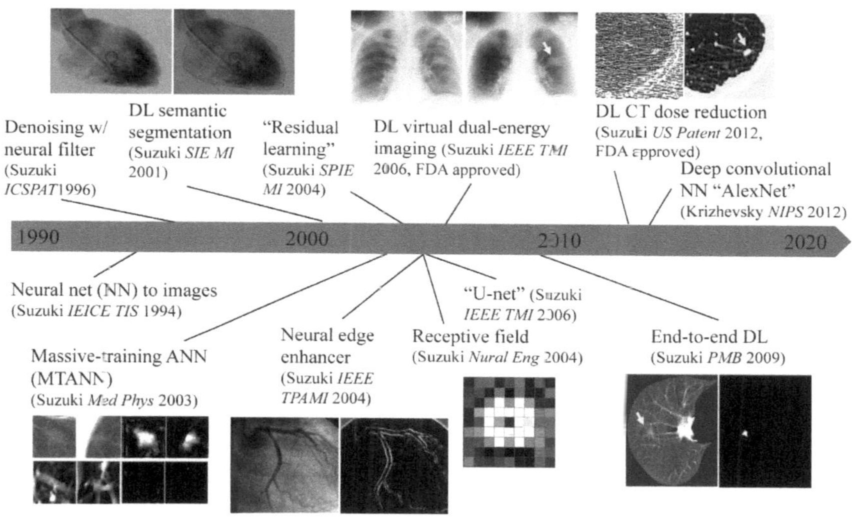

Figure 15.2 History of machine and deep learning research in Suzuki Lab.

The architecture of an MTANN is illustrated in Fig. 15.3. An MTANN consists of an ML model such as linear-output-layer artificial NN (ANN) regression, support vector regression [2, 34], and nonlinear Gaussian process regression, which is capable of operating on pixel data directly [20]. The core part, "machine learning convolution kernel," of the MTANN consists of an input layer, multiple hidden layers, and an output layer, as illustrated in Fig. 15.3. The linear-output-layer ANN regression model employs a linear function instead of a sigmoid function as the activation function of the unit in the output layer because the characteristics of an ANN were improved significantly with a linear function when it was applied to the continuous mapping of values in image processing [20]. Note that the activation functions of the units in the hidden layers are a sigmoid function (or another nonlinear function) for nonlinear processing. The input to the MTANN consists of pixel values in a subregion (image patch), R, extracted from an input image. The output of the MTANN is a continuous scalar value, which is associated with the center pixel in the subregion, represented by

$$O(x,y,z) = ML\{I(x-i, y-j, z-k) \mid (i,j,k) \in R\}, \tag{15.1}$$

where x, y, and z are the coordinate indices, $ML(\cdot)$ is the output of the ML model, and $I(x,y,z)$ is a pixel value of the input image. The structure of input units and the number of hidden units in the ANN may be designed by use of sensitivity-based unit-pruning methods [35, 36]. ML regression models rather than ML classification models would be suited for the MTANN framework, because the output of the MTANN consists of continuous scalar values (as opposed to nominal categories or classes). The entire output image is obtained by scanning with the input subregion of the MTANN in a convolutional manner on the entire input image, as illustrated in Fig. 15.3. This convolutional operation offers a shift-invariant property that is desirable for image classification. The input subregion and the scanning with the MTANN are analogous to the kernel of a convolution filter and the convolutional operation of the filter, respectively. The output of the MTANN is an image that may represent a likelihood map, unlike the class of the original CNNs.

For use of the MTANN as a classifier, a scoring layer is placed at the end to convert the output probability map into a single score that represents a likelihood of being a certain class for a given image, as shown in Fig. 15.3. A score for a given image is defined as

$$S = \sum_{(x,y,z) \in R_E} f_W(x,y,z) \times O(x,y,z), \tag{15.2}$$

where f_W is a weighting function for combining pixel-based output responses from the trained MTANN into a single score, which may often be the same distribution function used in the teaching images, and with its center corresponding to the center of the region for evaluation, R_E. This score represents the weighted sum of the estimates for the likelihood that the image (e.g., a lesion candidate) contains an object of interest (e.g., a lesion) near the center; i.e., a higher score would indicate an object (e.g., a lesion) of interest, and a lower score would indicate other patterns. Thresholding is then performed on the scores for distinction between classes. Thus, conversion of image processing to classification is performed with the scoring layer in this way.

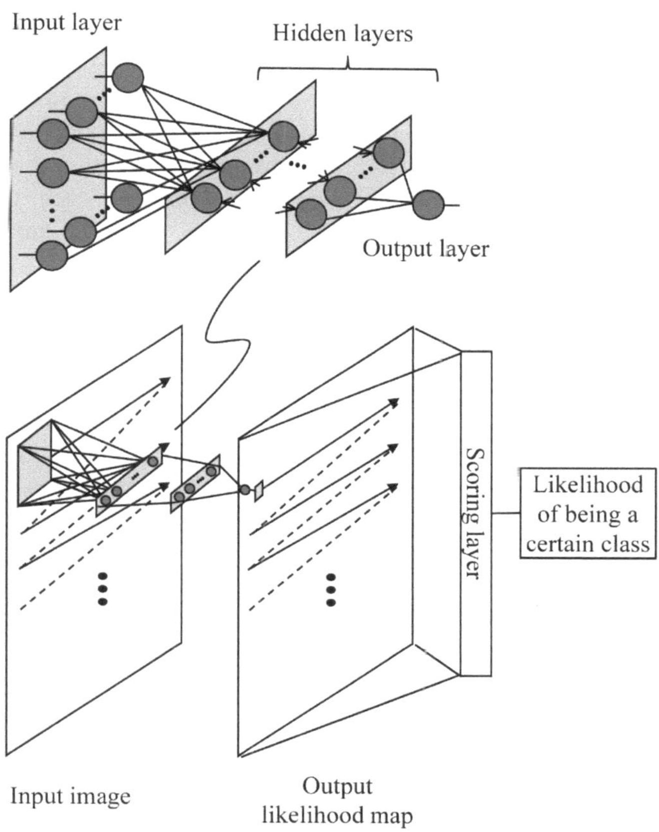

Figure 15.3 Architecture of a massive-training artificial neural network (MTANN).

The MTANN is trained with input images and the corresponding "teaching" (desired or ideal) images for enhancement of specific patterns and suppression of other patterns in images. For enhancement of objects of interest (e.g., lesions), L, and suppression of other patterns (e.g., non-lesions), the teaching image contains a probability map for objects of interest, represented by

$$T(x,y,z)=\begin{cases}\text{a certain distribution} & L \\ 0 & \text{otherwise.}\end{cases} \tag{15.3}$$

For enrichment of training samples, a training region, R_T, extracted from the input images is divided pixel by pixel into a large number of overlapping subregions. Single pixels are extracted from the corresponding teaching images as teaching values. The MTANN is massively trained by use of each of a large number of input subregions together with each of the corresponding teaching single pixels; hence the term "massive-training ANN." The error to be minimized by training of the MTANN is defined as:

$$E=\frac{1}{P}\sum_{(x,y,z)\in R_T}\{T(x,y,z)-O(x,y,z)\}^2, \tag{15.4}$$

where P is the number of total training pixels in the training region, R_T. The MTANN is trained by a linear-output-layer back propagation (BP) algorithm [20] which was derived for the linear-output-layer ANN model by use of the generalized delta rule [1]. After training, the MTANN is expected to output the highest value when an object of interest is located at the center of the subregion of the MTANN, a lower value as the distance from the subregion center increases, and zero when the input subregion contains other patterns.

15.3 Separation of Bones from Soft Tissue in Chest Radiographs

Studies showed that 82% to 95% of the lung cancers missed by radiologists in chest radiographs (chest x-ray: CXR) were partly obscured by overlying bones such as ribs and/or clavicles [37, 38]. To prevent such misses, we developed MTANNs for separation of bones from soft tissue in CXR [12, 32]. To this end, the MTANNs were trained with input CXRs with overlapping bones and the corresponding "teaching" dual-energy bone images acquired with a dual-energy radiography system [39]. Figure 15.4 shows a non-training original CXR and a "virtual" dual-energy soft-tissue image obtained by use of the trained MTANN. The ribs are suppressed substantially in the MTANN soft-tissue image, whereas the conspicuity of the lung nodule is improved, and the contrast of soft tissue such as lung vessels is maintained.

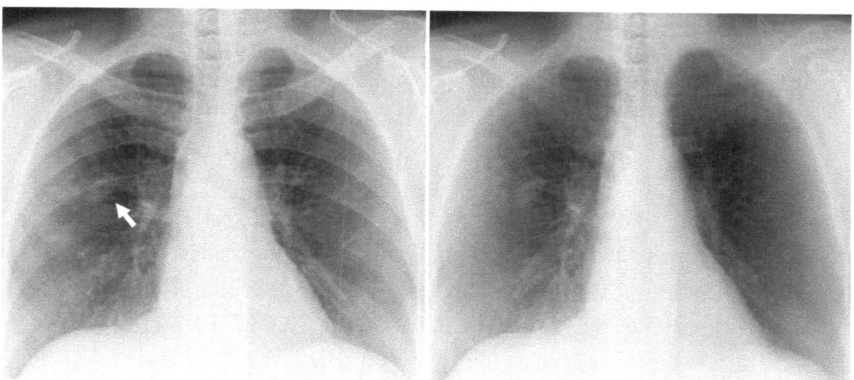

(a) Input chest radiograph with a nodule (arrow)

(b) "Virtual" dual-energy soft-tissue image by MTANN

Figure 15.4 Illustration of bone suppression in a chest radiograph by using our MTANN-based virtual dual-energy technology.

15.4 Radiation Dose Reduction in Computed Tomography

We developed radiation dose reduction technology in CT by using the MTANN. Our technology has a training step and an application step. In the training step, we acquire pairs of lower-dose (LD) CT images (e.g., 0.1 mSv) reconstructed by the filtered back-projection (FBP) algorithm and corresponding "teaching" (or desired) higher-dose (HD) CT images (e.g., 5.7 mSv) reconstructed by FBP of an anthropomorphic chest phantom. Through the training, the MTANN learns the relationship between the input LDCT and teaching HDCT images to convert LDCT images with noise and artifacts due to low radiation exposure into HDCT images. Once trained, the MTANN no longer requires HDCT images. In the application step, the trained MTANN model is applied to unseen new LDCT images of a patient to produce "high-dose-like" CT images where noise and artifacts are substantially reduced, while maintaining lesions and anatomic structures such as lung nodules and lung vessels; thus we term "virtual" HD (VHD) CT.

To train our MTANN, we acquired CT scans of an anthropomorphic chest phantom (Lungman, Kyoto Kagaku, Kyoto, Japan) without motion at LD (0.1 mSv) and HD (5.7 mSv) levels with a CT scanner (LightSpeed VCT with 64 slices, GE, Milwaukee, WI) at Hiroshima University Hospital, Hiroshima, Japan. We changed radiation doses by changing x-ray tube current, while fixing an x-ray tube voltage at 120 kVp. Reconstructed CT size was 512 × 512 pixels, and reconstructed slice thickness was 5 mm. The 5 mm slice thickness was chosen by following the Japanese lung cancer screening guideline. We trained the MTANN with pairs of the ULDCT (0.1 mSv) slices and corresponding "teaching" (desired) HDCT (5.7 mSv) slices.

To validate our radiation dose reduction technology based on our MTANN, we acquired CT scans of the anthropomorphic chest phantom at five more different dose levels, namely, 0.25, 0.5, 1.0, 1.5, and 3.0 mSv. Tube current; tube current time product; and CTDIvol for the CT scans were 25, 50, 100, 150, and 300 mA; 10, 20, 40, 60, and 120 mAs; and 0.60, 1.19, 2.38, 3.57, and 7.14 mGy, respectively. We applied the trained MTANN to reconstructed CT slices. To evaluate the performance of our virtual HD technology, we used the structural similarity (SSIM) index [40], which overcame the limitation of conventional contrast-to-noise-ratio (CNR) with lack of spatial information (e.g., structure) in evaluation, for measuring the image quality of CT. We used the highest dose CT scan (5.7 mSv) as the "gold standard" in the calculation of the SSIM. We used a two-fold cross validation.

In our VHD image, heavy noise and streak and other artifacts in the input ULDCT image (0.1 mSv) was reduced substantially, while maintaining anatomic structures such as pulmonary vessels. We examined the relationship between the image quality in terms of SSIM and effective dose. An average SSIM of our VHD image of 0.94 was equivalent to the image quality of 1.1 mSv CT images, which corresponds to 91% dose reduction, as shown in Fig. 15.5.

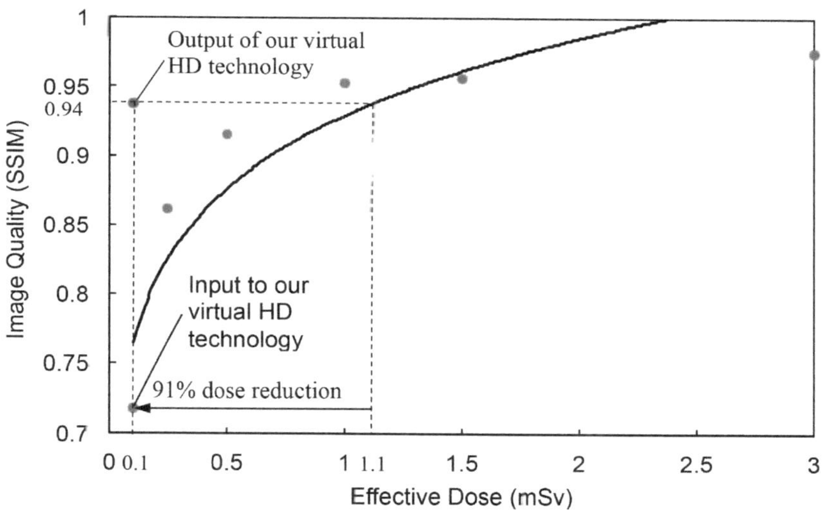

Figure 15.5 Quantitative evaluation of radiation dose reduction by using our MTANN-based virtual high-dose technology.

15.5 "Semantic" Segmentation of Lesions or Organs

Neural edge enhancers (NEEs; predecessor of MTANNs) enhanced subjective edges traced by a physician ("semantic segmentation") in left ventriculograms [21], as illustrated in Fig. 15.6. The edge enhancement performance of the NEE was superior to that of conventional edge detectors in this challenging segmentation problem. The segmentation by the NEE agreed almost perfectly with the "gold-standard" manual segmentation by an experienced cardiologist.

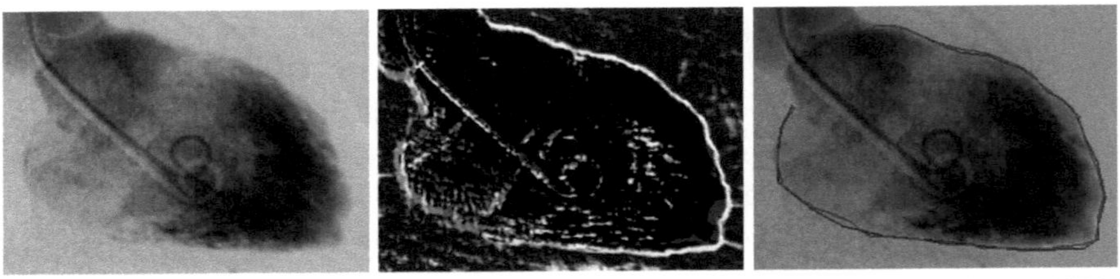

(a) Input left ventriculogram (b) Output image of our trained NEE (c) Segmentation by our NEE (red) and by physician (blue)

Figure 15.6 Semantic segmentation of the left ventricle of the heart in an X-ray image by using our neural edge enhancer (NEE).

15.6 Classification between Lesions and Non-Lesions (Normal Structures)

The class of "deep" MTANNs with 4–7 layers has been used for classification, such as false-positive (FP) reduction in CAD schemes for detection of lung nodules in CXR [27] and CT [10, 30, 31], and FP reduction in a CAD scheme for polyp detection in CT colonography [24–26, 28, 29]. Figure 15.7 shows a schematic diagram of an MTANN for classification between lesions and non-lesions (i.e., normal structures) in medical images. For enhancement of lesions and suppression of non-lesions, the teaching image contains a distribution of values that represent a map for the probability of being a lesion. For example, the teaching volume contains a 3D Gaussian distribution with standard deviation for a lesion and zero (i.e., completely dark) for non-lesions, as illustrated in Fig. 15.7. After training, a scoring method is used for combining of output voxels from the trained MTANNs. Thresholding is then performed on the scores for distinction between lesions and non-lesions.

Figure 15.8 shows the output images of the MTANN trained to enhance lung nodules and suppress various types of non-nodules in CAD for CT. Various lung nodules are enhanced in the MTANN output images, whereas various types of non-nodules are suppressed. Nodules such as a solid nodule, a part-solid (mixed-ground-glass) nodule, and a non-solid (ground-glass) nodule are enhanced, whereas non-nodules such as different-sized lung vessels and soft-tissue opacity are suppressed around

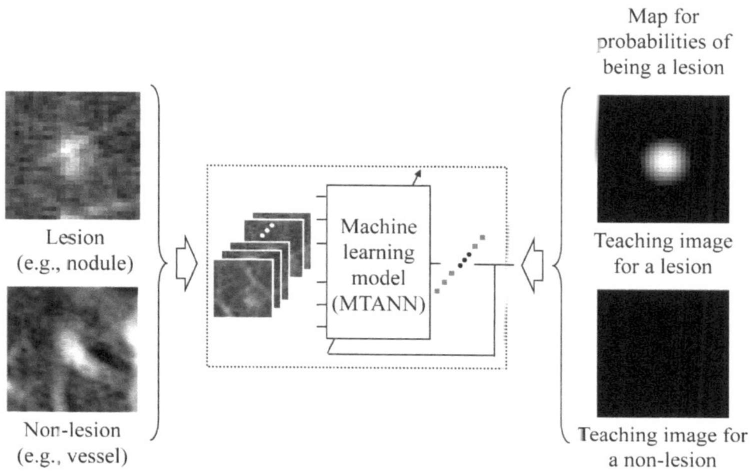

Figure 15.7 Training of an MTANN for distinction between lesions and non-lesions.

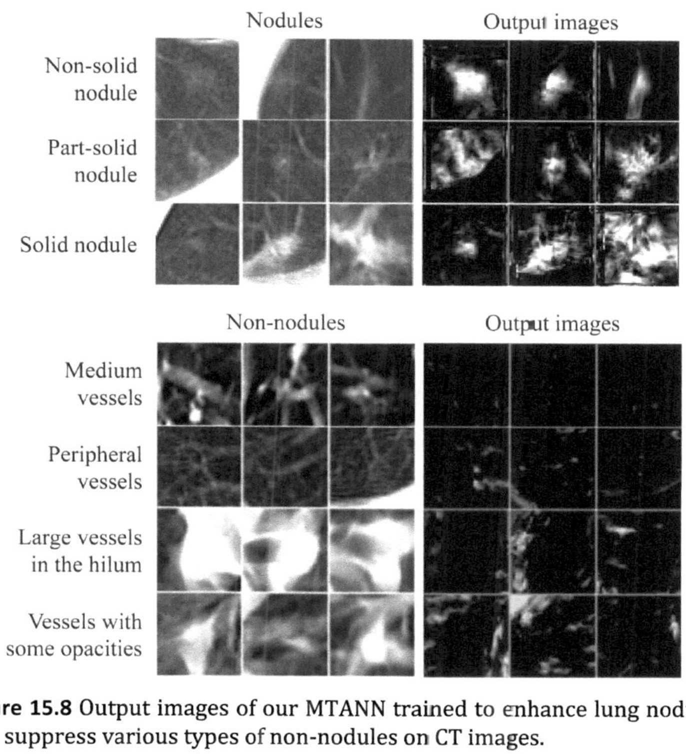

Figure 15.8 Output images of our MTANN trained to enhance lung nodules and suppress various types of non-nodules on CT images.

the centers of ROIs. With those nodule-enhanced images, distinction between nodules and non-nodules is made by use of the scoring method described above. In other words, classification between a particular pattern and other patterns is made by enhancement of the particular pattern, which may be referred to as "classification by enhancement."

15.7 Comparisons of MTANNs with CNNS

The performance of well-known CNNs (including the AlexNet, the LeNet, a relatively deep CNN (rd-CNN), a shallow CNN (sh-CNN), and a fine-tuned AlexNet (FineTuned AlexNet) which used transfer learning from a computer-vision-trained AlexNet) and MTANNs was compared extensively in a focal lesion detection problem in medical imaging [41]. Comparison experiments were done for detection of lung nodules in CT with the same databases. The experiments demonstrated that the performance of MTANNs was substantially higher than that of the best-performing CNN under the same condition, as demonstrated in Fig. 15.9a. With a larger training dataset used only for CNNs, the performance gap became less evident, even though the margin was still significant, as shown in Fig. 15.9b. The MTANNs generated 2.7 FPs per patient at 100% sensitivity, which was significantly ($p < 0.05$) lower than that for the best-performing CNN model (FineTuned AlexNet), with 22.7 FPs per patient at the same level of sensitivity.

15.8 Classification of Lesion Types

Before the introduction of the term "deep learning," "deep" MTANNs with seven layers were applied to the distinction between benign and malignant lung nodules in low-dose screening CT [23]. As shown in Fig. 15.10, the MTANNs were able to enhance various types of malignant nodules, while suppressing benign nodules. The MTANNs achieved an area under the receiver-operating-characteristic curve (AUC) value of 0.882 in the classification between 76 malignant and 413 benign lung nodules, whereas an AUC value for chest radiologists for the same task with a subset of the database was 0.56.

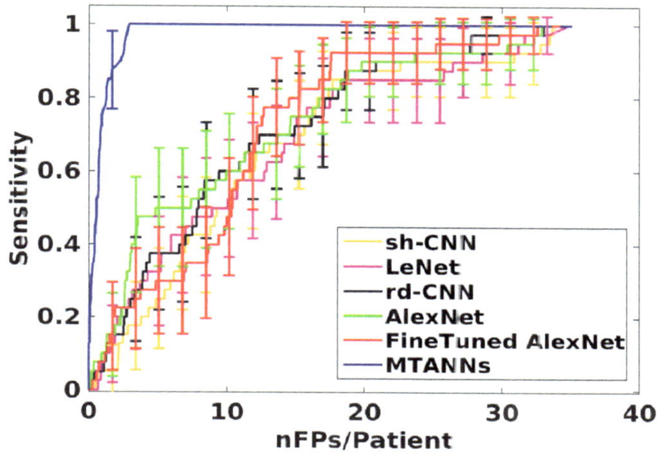

(a) All deep learning models were trained with the same small number of cases (10 positives and 90 negatives)

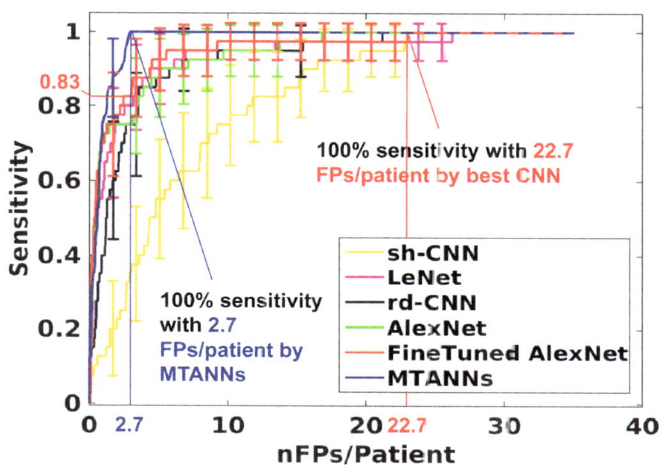

(b) CNN models were trained with all cases in the database (50 positives and 490 negatives)

Figure 15.9 Comparison of the performance of our MTANN with 5 representative CNNs in detection of lung nodules in CT.

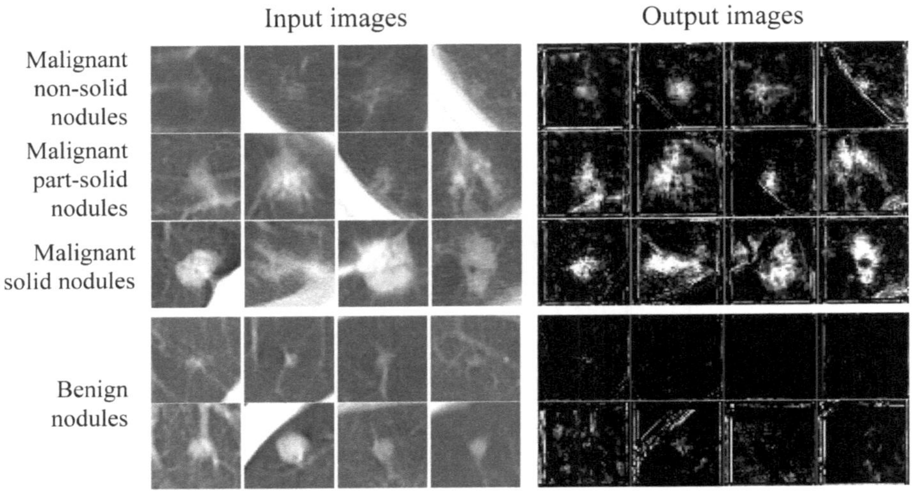

Figure 15.10 Output images of our MTANN trained to distinguish malignant nodules from benign nodules on CT images.

15.9 Advantages and Limitations of MTANNs

Limitations of "deep" CNNs (in ML with image input) include (1) a very high computational cost for training because of the high dimensionality of input data, and (2) the required large number of training images due to a large number of parameters of the model. Because "deep" CNNs use pixel data in images directly, the number of input dimensions is generally large. A CNN requires a huge number of training images (e.g., 1,000,000) for determining a large number of parameters in the CNN. However, an MTANN requires a small number of training images (e.g., 20) because of its simpler, concise architecture. With GPU implementation, an MTANN completes training in a few hours, whereas a deep CNN takes several days.

15.10 Summary

This chapter describes deep learning and its applications to medical image processing and CAD. There is a long history of deep-learning techniques, including the Neocognitron, CNNs, neural filters, and MTANNs in the class of ML with image input (or the new term, "deep learning"). In particular, we introduced ones of the earliest deep-learning models for image processing, semantic segmentation, object enhancement, and classification of patterns in medical images. We have been actively studying on deep learning in medical imaging in the past 23 years. In this talk, medical image processing, pattern recognition, and AI-aided diagnosis with deep learning are introduced, including (1) computer-aided diagnosis for cancer in CT and x-ray images, (2) semantic segmentation of lesions and organs in medical images, (3) separation of bones from soft tissue in chest radiographs, and (4) radiation dose reduction by reducing noise and artifact in CT and mammography. Deep learning is a very powerful, versatile technology with higher performance, which can bring the current state-of-the-art performance level of medical image analysis to the next level. ML including deep learning in medical imaging is an explosively growing, promising field. It is expected that ML with image input including deep learning will be the mainstream technology in medical imaging in the next few decades.

Acknowledgments

The authors are grateful to members in the Suzuki Laboratory at Tokyo Institute of Technology, Illinois Institute of Technology, and University of Chicago for their valuable contributions to machine-learning and deep-learning research in medical imaging over the past 15 years. Some of machine learning and computer-aided diagnosis technologies in these laboratories have been non-exclusively licensed to several companies and have been commercialized.

References

1. Rumelhart, D. E., G. E. Hinton, and R. J. Williams, Learning representations by back-propagating errors. *Nature*, 1986. 323: pp. 533–536.
2. Vapnik, V. N., *The Nature of Statistical Learning Theory*, 1995. Berlin: Springer-Verlag.

3. Ho, T. K. Random decision forests. in *Document Analysis and Recognition, 1995., Proceedings of the Third International Conference on*, 1995. IEEE.
4. Mairal, J., et al., Online dictionary learning for sparse coding, in *Proceedings of the 26th Annual International Conference on Machine Learning*, 2009, ACM: Montreal, Quebec, Canada. pp. 689–696.
5. Fukushima, K., Neocognitron: A self organizing neural network model for a mechanism of pattern recognition unaffected by shift in position. *Biol. Cybern.*, 1980. 36(4): pp. 193–202.
6. LeCun, Y., et al., Backpropagation applied to handwritten zip code recognition. *Neural Comput.*, 1989. 1(4): pp. 541–551.
7. Suzuki, K., et al., Recognition of coronary artery stenosis using neural network on DSA system. *IEICE Trans. Inf. Syst.*, 1994. J77-D-II: pp. 1910–1916.
8. Suzuki, K., et al., Improvement of image quality of x-ray fluoroscopy using spatiotemporal neural filter which learns noise reduction, edge enhancement and motion compensation. in *Proc. Int. Conf. Signal Processing Applications and Technology (ICSPAT)*, 1996. Boston, MA.
9. Suzuki, K., I. Horiba, and S. N., Edge detection from noisy images using a neural edge detector. *Proc. IEEE Int. Workshop Neural Networks Signal Processing (NNSP)*, 2000. 10: pp. 487–496.
10. Suzuki, K., et al., Massive training artificial neural network (MTANN) for reduction of false positives in computerized detection of lung nodules in low-dose computed tomography. *Med. Phys.*, 2003. 30(7): pp. 1602–1617.
11. Grelewicz Z., Suzuki K., Kohlbrenner R., Obajuluwa A. M., Ng E., Tompkins R., Epstein M. L., Hori M., and Baron R. L., Computer-aided diagnostic scheme for detection of hepatocellular carcinoma in contrast-enhanced hepatic CT: Preliminary results. *Med. Phys.*, 2009. 36: p. 2434.
12. Suzuki, K., et al., Image-processing technique for suppressing ribs in chest radiographs by means of massive training artificial neural network (MTANN). *IEEE Trans. Med. Imaging*, 2006. 25(4): pp. 406–416.
13. Suzuki, K., et al. Supervised Massive-Training Artificial Neural Network (MTANN) for reduction of radiation dose in CT in an ultra-low-dose screening setting. in *Program of Scientific Assembly and Annual Meeting of Radiological Society of North America* (RSNA), LL-PHS-SU5B, 2012.

14. Suzuki, K., and R. Smathers. Radiation dose reduction in full-field digital mammography (FFDM) by means of pixel-based trainable nonlinear regression (PTNR). in *Program of Scientific Assembly and Annual Meeting of Radiological Society of North America* (RSNA), PH259-SD-TUB9, 2015.

15. Hinton, G., S. Osindero, and Y.-W. Teh, A fast learning algorithm for deep belief nets. *Neural Comput.*, 2006. 18(7): pp. 1527–1554.

16. Krizhevsky, A., I. Sutskever, and G. E. Hinton. Imagenet classification with deep convolutional neural networks. in *Advances in Neural Information Processing Systems*, 2012.

17. Goodfellow, I., et al., Generative adversarial nets. in *Advances in Neural Information Processing Systems*, 2014.

18. Suzuki, K., et al., Neural filter with selection of input features and its application to image quality improvement of medical image sequences. *IEICE Trans. Inf. Syst.*, 2002. E85-D(10): pp. 1710–1718.

19. Suzuki, K., I. Horiba, and N. Sugie, Efficient approximation of neural filters for removing quantum noise from images. *IEEE Trans. Signal Proc.*, 2002. 50(7): pp. 1787–1799.

20. Suzuki, K., I. Horiba, and N. Sugie, Neural edge enhancer for supervised edge enhancement from noisy images. *IEEE Trans. Pattern Anal. Mach. Intell.*, 2003. 25(12): pp. 1582–1596.

21. Suzuki, K., et al., Extraction of left ventricular contours from left ventriculograms by means of a neural edge detector. *IEEE Trans. Med. Imaging*, 2004. 23(3): pp. 330–339.

22. Suzuki, K., et al., Extraction of the contours of left ventricular cavity, according with those traced by medical doctors, from left ventriculograms using a neural edge detector. in *Proc. SPIE Medical Imaging* (SPIE MI), 2001. San Diego, CA.

23. Suzuki, K., et al., Computer-aided diagnostic scheme for distinction between benign and malignant nodules in thoracic low-dose CT by use of massive training artificial neural network. *IEEE Trans. Med. Imaging*, 2005. 24(9): pp. 1138–1150.

24. Suzuki, K., D. C. Rockey, and A. H. Dachman, CT colonography: Advanced computer-aided detection scheme utilizing MTANNs for detection of "missed" polyps in a multicenter clinical trial. *Med. Phys.*, 2010. 37(1): pp. 12–21.

25. Suzuki, K., Z. Shi, and J. Zhang, Supervised enhancement of lesions by use of a massive-training artificial neural network (MTANN) in computer-aided diagnosis (CAD). in *Proc. Int. Conf. Pattern Recognition* (ICPR), 2008. Tampa, FL.

26. Suzuki, K., et al., Massive-training artificial neural network (MTANN) for reduction of false positives in computer-aided detection of polyps: Suppression of rectal tubes. *Med. Phys.*, 2006. 33(10): pp. 3814–3824.
27. Suzuki, K., et al., False-positive reduction in computer-aided diagnostic scheme for detecting nodules in chest radiographs by means of massive training artificial neural network. *Acad. Radiol.*, 2005. 12(2): pp. 191–201.
28. Xu, J., and K. Suzuki, Massive-training support vector regression and Gaussian process for false-positive reduction in computer-aided detection of polyps in CT colonography. *Med. Phys.*, 2011. 38: pp. 1888–1902.
29. Suzuki, K., J. Zhang, and J. Xu, Massive-training artificial neural network coupled with Laplacian-eigenfunction-based dimensionality reduction for computer-aided detection of polyps in CT colonography. *IEEE Trans. Med. Imaging*, 2010. 29(11): pp. 1907–1917.
30. Arimura, H., et al., Computerized scheme for automated detection of lung nodules in low-dose computed tomography images for lung cancer screening. *Acad. Radiol.*, 2004. 11(6): pp. 617–629.
31. Li, F., et al., Computer-aided detection of peripheral lung cancers missed at CT: ROC analyses without and with localization. *Radiology*, 2005. 237(2): pp. 684–690.
32. Suzuki, K., et al., Suppression of the contrast of ribs in chest radiographs by means of massive training artificial neural network. in *Proc. SPIE Medical Imaging* (SPIE MI), 2004. San Diego, CA.
33. Oda, S., et al., Performance of radiologists in detection of small pulmonary nodules on chest radiographs: Effect of rib suppression with a massive-training artificial neural network. *Am. J. Roentgenol.*, 2009. 193(5): pp. W397–W402.
34. Vapnik, V. N., *Statistical Learning Theory*, 1998, New York: Wiley.
35. Suzuki, K., Determining the receptive field of a neural filter. *J. Neural Eng.*, 2004. 1(4): pp. 228–237.
36. Suzuki, K., I. Horiba, and N. Sugie, A simple neural network pruning algorithm with application to filter synthesis. *Neural Proc. Lett.*, 2001. 13(1): pp. 43–53.
37. Austin, J. H., B. M. Romney, and L. S. Goldsmith, Missed bronchogenic carcinoma: Radiographic findings in 27 patients with a potentially resectable lesion evident in retrospect. *Radiology*, 1992. 182(1): pp. 115–122.

38. Shah, P. K., et al., Missed non-small cell lung cancer: Radiographic findings of potentially resectable lesions evident only in retrospect. *Radiology*, 2003. 226(1): pp. 235–241.

39. Ishigaki, T., et al., One-shot dual-energy subtraction imaging. *Radiology*, 1986. 161(1): pp. 271–273.

40. Wang, Z., et al., Image quality assessment: From error visibility to structural similarity. *IEEE Trans. Image Process*, 2004. 13(4): pp. 600–612.

41. Tajbakhsh, N., and K. Suzuki, Comparing two classes of end-to-end learning machines for lung nodule detection and classification: MTANNs vs. CNNs. *Pattern Recognit.*, 2017. 63: pp. 476–486.

Chapter 16

A Hierarchical Type Segmentation Hardware for Colorectal Endoscopic Images with Narrow-Band Imaging Magnification

Tetsushi Koide,[a] Toru Tamaki,[b] Shigeto Yoshida,[c] and Shinji Tanaka[d]

[a]*Research Institute for Nanodevice and Bio Systems, Hiroshima University, Japan*
[b]*Department of Information Engineering, Graduate School of Engineering, Hiroshima University, Japan*
[c]*Department of Gastroenterology, Hiroshima General Hospital of West Japan Railway Company, Japan*
[d]*Department of Endoscopy, Hiroshima University Hospital, Higashi-Hiroshima, Japan*

koide@hiroshima-u.ac.jp

In this chapter, a hardware design of type classification in the computer-aided diagnosis (CAD) system for colorectal endoscopic images with narrow-band imaging (NBI) magnification is proposed for real-time processing of full high-definition image. A pyramid-style image segmentation with support vector machines (SVMs) for multi-size scan windows, which can be implemented on a

Biomedical Engineering
Edited by Akihiro Miyauchi and Yuji Miyahara

ISBN 978-981-4877-63-3 (Hardcover), 978-1-003-14194-5 (eBook)
www.jennystanford.com

field-programmable gate array (FPGA) with small circuit area and achieve high accuracy, is proposed for actual complex colorectal endoscopic images.

16.1 Introduction

With the increase in the number of colorectal cancer patients, systems which support a doctor's diagnosis have been researched. The CAD system for colorectal endoscopic images with narrow-band imaging (NBI) magnification [1] has already been proposed [2]. The proposed CAD system classifies colorectal endoscopic images obtained by classifying endoscopic diagnosis into three types (Types A, B, and C3) based on the NBI magnification findings (Fig. 16.1).

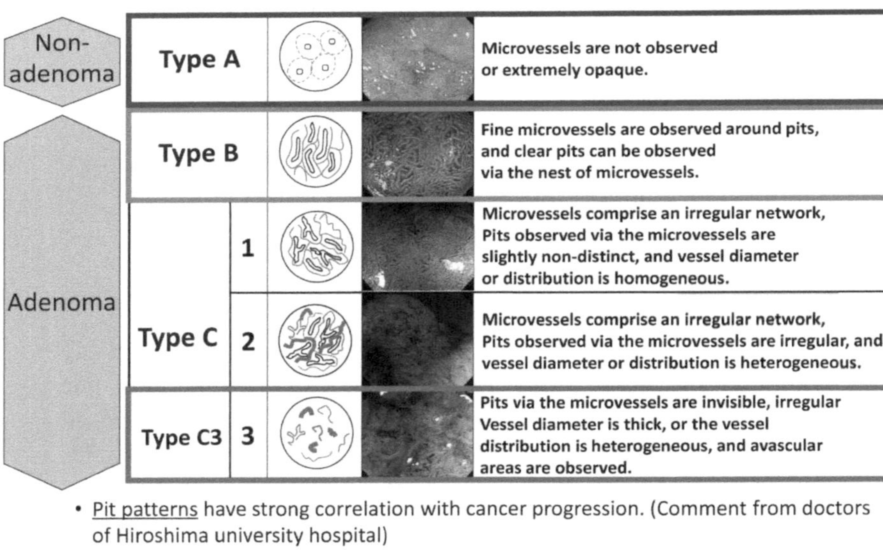

Figure 16.1 Narrow-band imaging (NBI) magnification findings [1].

It can process only the center 120 × 120 pixels of the endoscopic image for diagnosis and achieves 14.7 fps in throughput. In order to diagnosis a full-HD (1920 × 1080 pixels) endoscopic image, which may include several types of NBI magnification findings, that system needs to raster scan the image by scan window (SW). The raster scanning a Full HD image using 120 × 120 pixels SW size at every 10 pixels on software requires (1/14.7 fps) × (17,557 SWs) = 20 min, which is not acceptable in real-time diagnosis. Our proposed system processes Full HD images and shows the diagnosis results at the same time with the original input image for comparison. Hence, the processing time should be shorter than 1 sec to synchronize the original image and result.

The computation time of software implementation is exponentially increased with the increase of image size; therefore, a hardware realization is indispensable for further speed improvement of high-resolution image. As a demand on clinical doctors, the proposed CAD system satisfies the throughput of 1–5 fps (frame per second) and the latency is at least 1 sec for on-the-fly diagnostic supporting.

16.2 Overview of Computer-Aided Diagnosis System

Outline of the proposed CAD system is shown in Fig. 16.2. The system is based on a Bag-of-Features (BoF) representation [3] of local features in the endoscopy image. The system has two phases, learning and testing. The overview of processing flow of the system is as follows.

First, the local feature quantities of the endoscopy images in each type are extracted based on Dense Scale-Invariant Feature Transform (D-SIFT) algorithm [3] because the pit patterns of endoscopic images (Fig. 16.1) are very complex and irregular comparing with object recognition such as face and pedestrian recognitions.

Then the features obtained from the learning phase are clustered and the center of each cluster is saved as a visual-word (VW) for each type, which are used for feature representation using k-means clustering [3]. In the classification module, support vector for SVM is obtained at the learning phase using the type information of leaning image which is judged by clinical expert doctors.

Next, in the testing phase, the D-SIFT based feature extraction is performed for a whole input image and a visual-words histogram is created by voting for the nearest VW. Then the CAD system classifies the testing image within an endoscopy movie (frame) by the pre-learned SVM.

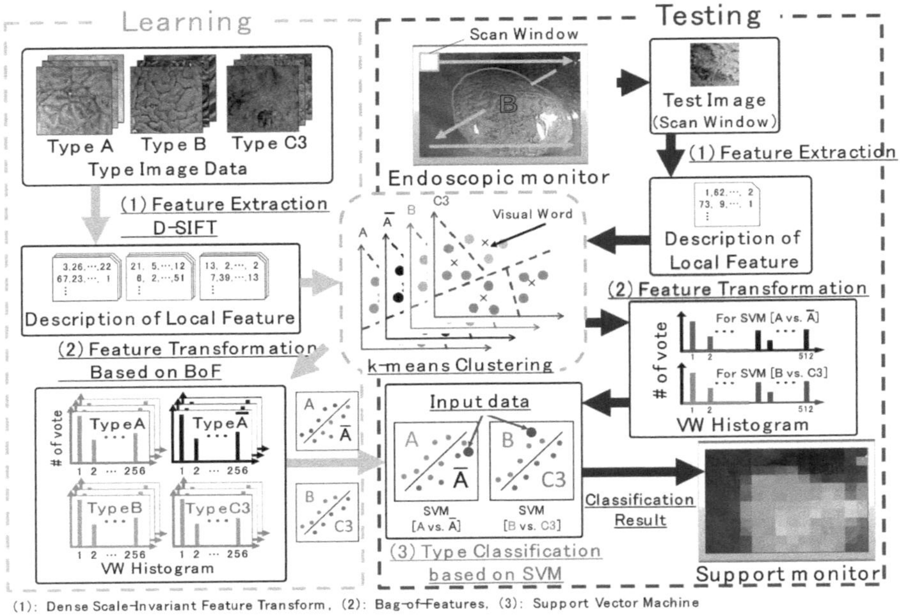

Figure 16.2 Overview of the proposed computer-aided diagnosis (CAD) system for endoscopic images.

Finally, a color gradation map which is converted from the result of classifier for each SW displays for doctor as a "second opinion" (Fig. 16.3). In our software implementation, D-SIFT of Library VLFeat [3] is used for the feature extraction and SVM of LIBSVM [5] is used for type classification.

Also, as a utility of the real-time image recognition system, our research group applied the system to real clinical test. In the learning phase, a set of 2,247 cutout endoscopic images which were collected by clinical export doctors are used. The learning images are separable into 504 Type A images and 1,743 Type B and C3 images, so in this experiment, the system identifies into

Type A or B&C3, that is, non-neoplastic lesions or neoplastic lesions, respectively. The feature quantities extracted from D-SIFT algorithm are 128-dimensional vectors. Then, an output of the system is the SVM output value, and a cutoff value of the SVM output value is 0.5. Figure 16.4 shows that the result of evaluation and from this result, our group verified that the SVM output value of neoplastic lesions could identify the non-neoplastic lesions or neoplastic lesions [6].

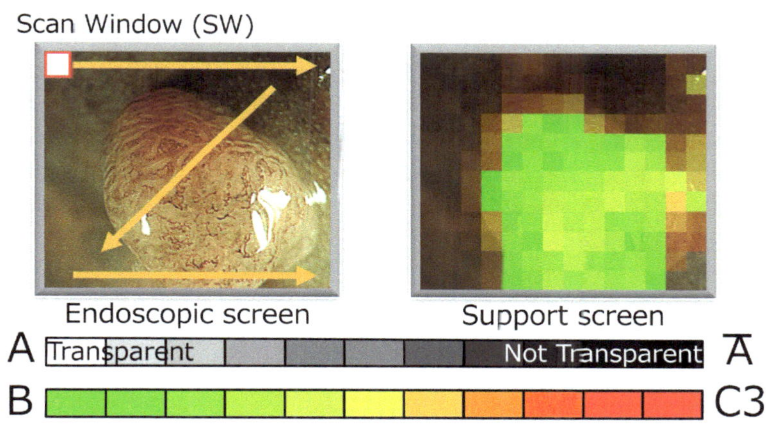

Figure 16.3 A classification result for Type B NBI endoscopic image.

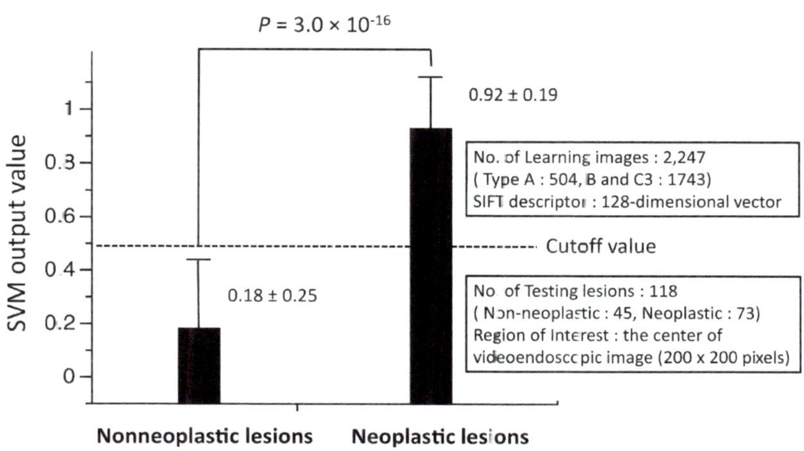

Figure 16.4 Support vector machine (SVM) output values for the images of non-neoplastic and neoplastic lesions [6].

16.3 Type Classifier Based on Support Vector Machine

16.3.1 Support Vector Machine

Support vector machine (SVM) is a technique of binary classification introduced in 1990s by Vapnik [4]. There are several kernels of SVM, which generate classification hyper-plane that maximizes a margin between a class Y and a class Z, allows the SVM to achieve high classification performance to an unlearned image. The accuracy difference in SVM computation using those different kernels is only 1% in our previous experiments [1]. Hence, the simplest one, the linear kernel is selected in our work. The linear kernel is also the best suitable for hardware implementation. Equation (16.1) shows a decision function of SVM with linear kernel in this work.

$$d_{\mathrm{Y:Z}}(\vec{x}) = \sum_{i=1}^{N_Y+N_Z} \mathrm{coef}_i \times \vec{sv_i} \cdot \vec{x} + \rho_{Y:Z} \quad (16.1)$$

In which, $\boldsymbol{x}$ is a test data, $\boldsymbol{sv}_i$ is support vector (SV), which is obtained at the learning step for hyper plane classification between two corresponding classes Y and Z. coef_i is a coefficient of each $\boldsymbol{sv}_i$, and $\rho_{Y:Z}$ is a coefficient of a decision function. If the classification function $d_{Y:Z}(\boldsymbol{x})$ is a positive value (>0), an input data $\boldsymbol{x}$ is determined as the class Y.

In this work, it is better for the hardware implementation to calculate the decision function by fixed-point number rather than floating point one. It is verified from the simulation that using 18-bit fixed-point numbers with 1-bit sign, 1-bit exponent and 16-bit mantissae does not degrade the classification accuracy compared with the results of classification using 32-bit floating-point numbers [7]. The prediction rate shows that a result of classification from input data (image) x is represented as a percentage each classification type (such as Type A, Type B, and Type C3 in our case). [8]. The prediction rate is computed from the result of decision function as shown in Eq. (16.1), and its distribution map with decision function values draws as sigmoid curve.

16.3.2 3-Type Classification for Computer-Aided Diagnosis

In order to realize 3-type classification, the one-versus-one technique [9] is taken. In our work, $f(x)$ is a 2-class identifier with SVM. There are two methods in combining binary classifier. The first method uses majority vote of three binary classifiers, and the second method uses probability estimation technique [5]. As shown in Fig. 16.5, our proposed system receives the original endoscopic image online, extracts feature of each SW before classifying the probability for each type (Type A, B and C3). Then, a color gradation map, which is converted from probabilities of all three types for each SW in the original endoscopic image is displayed on a support screen. It helps doctors to diagnose the type of each region of colorectal endoscopic images. In this work, we use the probability estimation technique among the results of 2-type classifiers (Fig. 16.6).

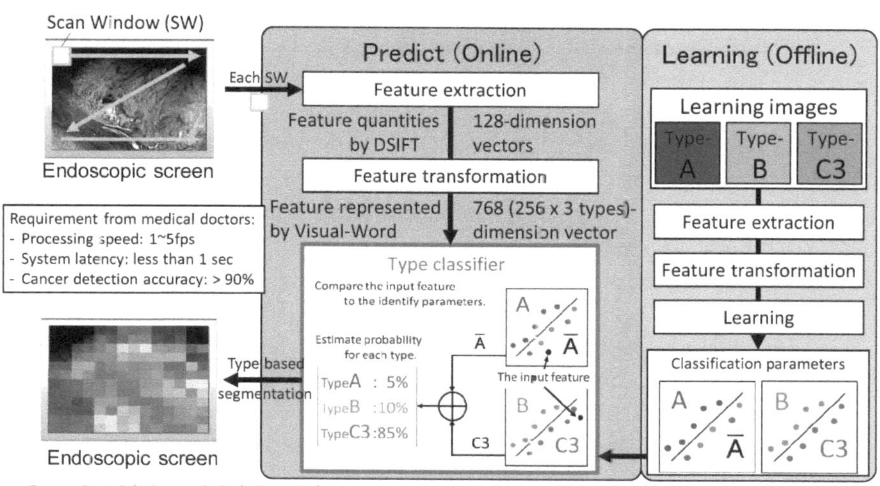

Figure 16.5 The proposed real-time processing for three-type classification and segmentation for CAD system with colorectal endoscopic image.

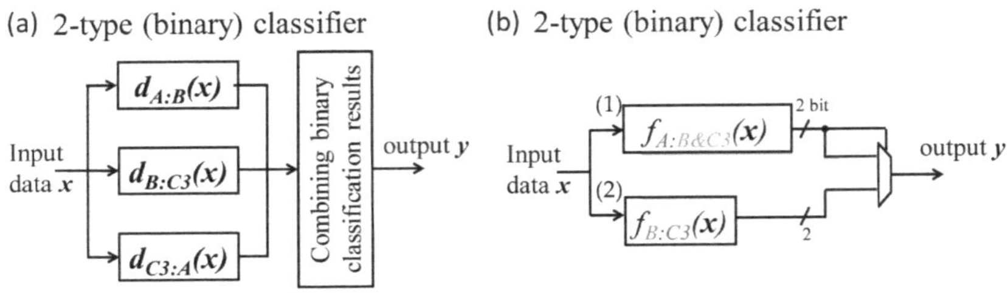

Figure 16.6 3-type classification techniques. (a) one-versus-one (1-step) classification, and (b) 2-step classification.

16.4 Simulation Result for Real Endoscopic Images

Since high dimension feature quantity (768 dimensions) is processed in our medical application, it is necessary to perform the sum-of-product (multiply-accumulate: MAC) operations in parallel. Hence, there is a subject that how to reduce hardware resources while increasing parallel degree. Therefore, we implement the SVM classification module by a fixed-point number instead of floating point number. The bit length reduces from 64 bits to around 16 bits for reducing hardware resources. Then, we suggest an algorithm of 3-type classifier which has efficient processing and high accuracy.

The simple Gaussian filter (GF) [10] which is reported as a simplified hardware implementation is used for feature extraction. We use LIBSVM [5] to create SVM classifiers in simulation. In order to implement the SVM classifier by fixed-point number, Eq. (16.1), which contains floating-point number arithmetic, is changed into fixed-point number arithmetic based on LIBSVM. The *linear kernel* (inner product) is used as a kernel of SVM, and the number of visual-word (VW) is set to 768. 1260 real endoscopic images in Table 16.1, which are taken by Hiroshima University Hospital Department of Endoscopy, are used as the learning and testing data set as shown in Fig 16.7. These images are classified based on the NBI magnification findings [1] by at least two professional doctors in six years. Equation (16.2) is used for accuracy evaluation. The True Positive is used to determine whether classification of each type is carried out precisely.

$$\text{True Positive}(i) = \frac{\text{Posi\_Num}(i)}{\text{Img\_Num}(i)} \times 100\ [\%]$$

i : Type A, Type B, Type C3

Posi_Num(i) : Number of images identified correctly.

Img_Num(i) : Total number of image data of i. (16.2)

Table 16.1 Endoscopic image data of narrow-band imaging (NBI) magnification findings

Type	A	B	C3	Total
Number of images	420	420	420	1,260

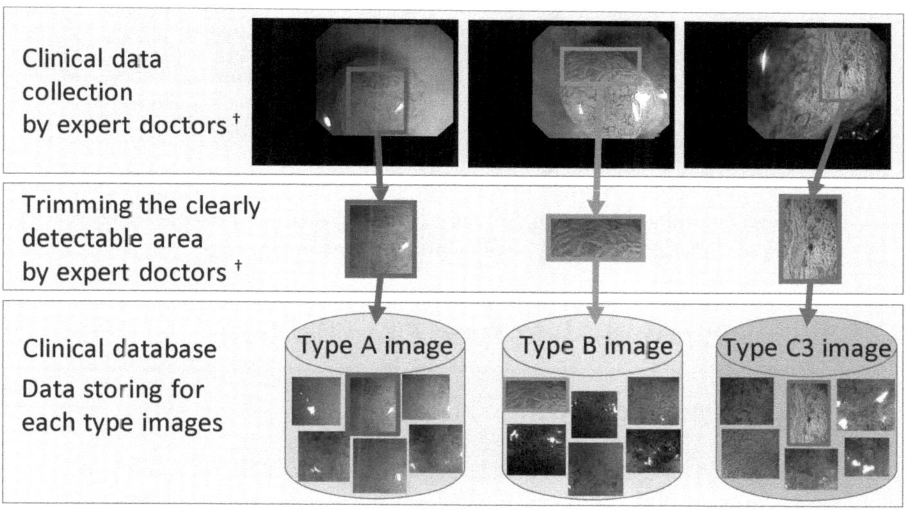

† co-researchers: Hiroshima Univ. Hospital

Figure 16.7 Example of the learning and testing data set.

The simulation results of true positive in Eq. (16.2) for 3-type 1-step and 2-step classifications of Fig. 16.6 with 10 times 10-fold cross validation are shown in Fig. 16.8. Since the 2-step classifier [A : $\bar{\text{A}}$] has been shown the sufficient classification performance of 98% in our previous experimental results, we consider a configuration in which 3-type classifier can be performed by 2-step classification. The first step performs with types [A : $\bar{\text{A}}$] classification and the second step performs by types [B : C3] classification as shown in Fig. 16.6b. Figure 16.8 also shows the number of support vectors (SVs) of each classifier in these experiments. By employing 2-step classifier, it is possible to reduce by about 10% SVs without losing most of the classification performance, and also can reduce the hardware cost, namely the number of classifiers.

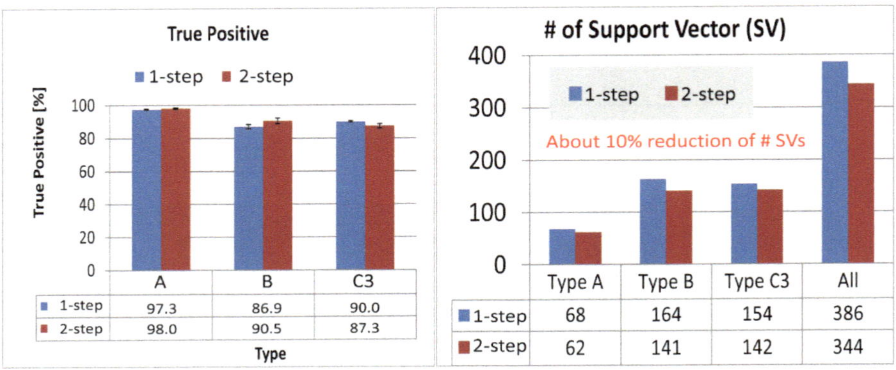

Figure 16.8 Simulation results of true positive and the number of support vectors for 3-type 1-step and 2-step classifications in Fig. 16.6.

16.5 Pyramid-Style Type Classification

16.5.1 Basic Concept

Accordingly, due to the complexity of the boundary of each type as shown in Fig. 16.9, it is difficult to catch the boundary of each type only by performing classification using single-size scan windows, and to determine the image segmentation from the results. Thus, we proposed a pyramid-style classification method using multiple-size SWs in Fig. 16.10 [11].

In this example, four multi-level scan window sizes, such as 60 × 60, 120 × 120, 180 × 180, and 240 × 240 pixel, are used. In general, the multi-level scan window method does not necessarily need to process simultaneously. Since the sequential processing is suitable in software implementation, if the type classification result does not clearly determine in the current level scan window (for example, 240 × 240), then the scan window will be broken down to the lower level scan window size (such as 120 × 120, 60 × 60 and so on). This multi-level scan window method is a top-down hierarchical classification. In our approach, a bottom-up hierarchical classification method is used. We call this bottom-up method as a pyramid-style classification. In this method, the type classification results of all levels are accumulated, and the probability of each type of each unit region (unit scan window, e.g., 60 × 60 pixel) is calculated. Finally, an image segmentation result is obtained based on the grid prediction rate of each unit scan window.

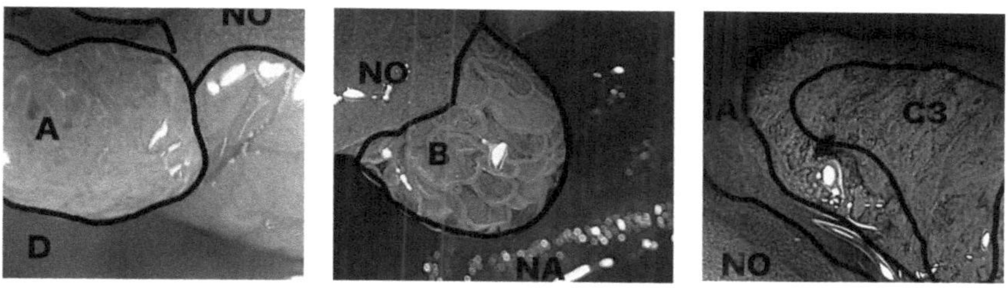

(a) Type A (b) Type B (C) Type C3

Figure 16.9 Examples of segmentation of the real endoscopic images (A: Type A, B: Type B, C3: Type C3, D: Defocus, NO: Normal).

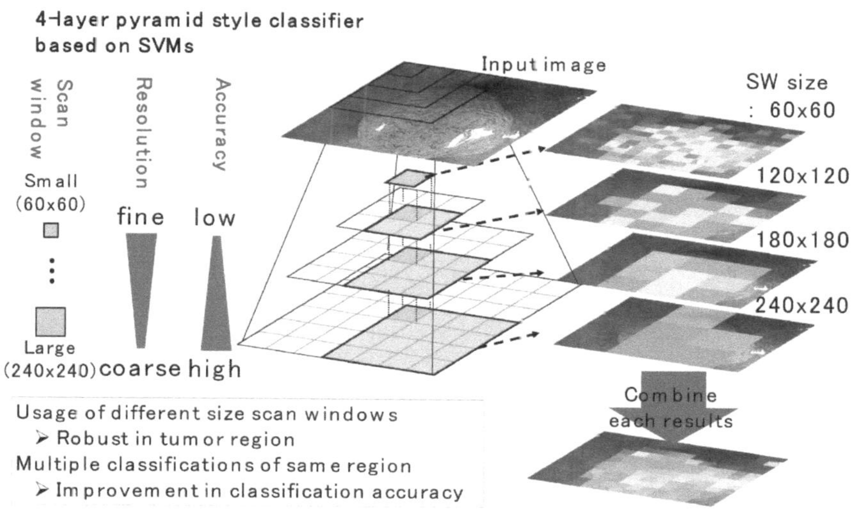

Figure 16.10 Concept of the image segmentation with four-layered pyramid-style SVM.

In this method, the probability of each unit is calculated using SVMs by learning each scan window. Therefore, compared with the case of SVM learning in single scan window, the whole number of scanning windows is substantially reduced to 1/10 (the number of SWs: 17555 to 1901). This simplification makes this method suitable for hardware implementation. Moreover, it is possible to improve the resolution of image segmentation by combining multi-level scan windows.

In general, the classification accuracy of a small scan window becomes low. However, the pyramid-style hierarchical classification can suppress the decrease of classification accuracy by considering the classification results of scan window for each level. Since the multi-level SVMs in the bottom-up method can be calculated by one image scan and does not require random access to an external memory, it is suitable for the hardware implementation of the streaming image data processing.

16.5.2 Calculation of Type Probabilities with Multiple SVMs

The outline of the pyramid-style hierarchical classification method which is suitable for hardware implementation is shown in Figs. 16.11 and 16.12, in which the level number is assumed as 3. We can obtain all input features for each level SVM by only one streaming scan using the hardware oriented feature extraction method which we have been proposed in [12, 13].

First, the type classifications are performed by each SVM for the three scan-size windows which are contained the same reference grid (60 × 60) (Fig. 16.11). Next, the obtained type probabilities for overlapped grid (60 × 60) in each level are combined by averaging with different weights for each levels. The weight of each level SVM are determined by the true positive score (accuracy) in previous learning and testing experiments. In Fig. 16.12, the weights of three SVMs, SVM60 × 60, SVM120 × 120, and SVM180 × 180 are 28%, 34%, and 37%, respectively. Then the final estimation probability of the upper-left corner grid became $P_A = 0.75$, $P_B = 0.22$, $P_{C3} = 0.07$. Therefore, this grid seems to be Type A and the gradation of the grid is calculated based on the above probability.

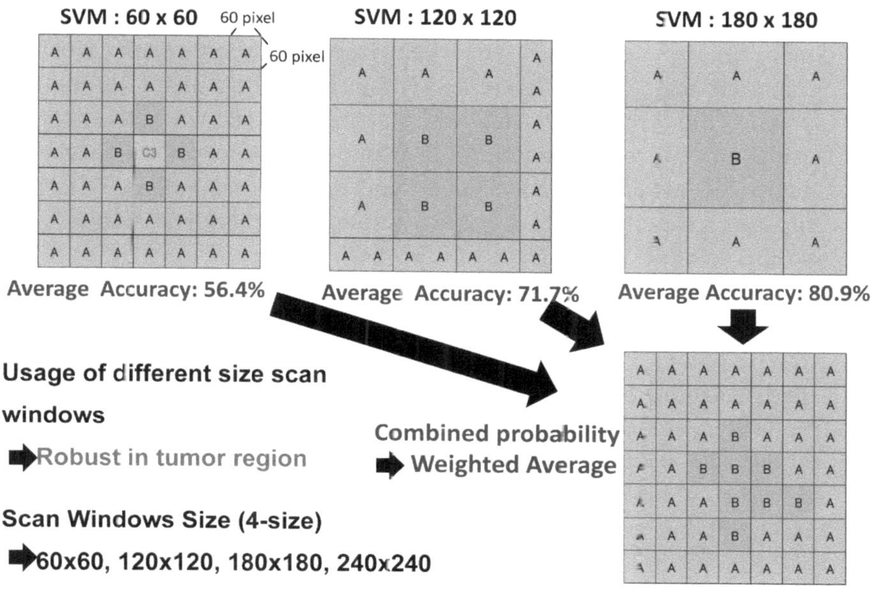

Figure 16.11 An example of three-level pyramid-style classification.

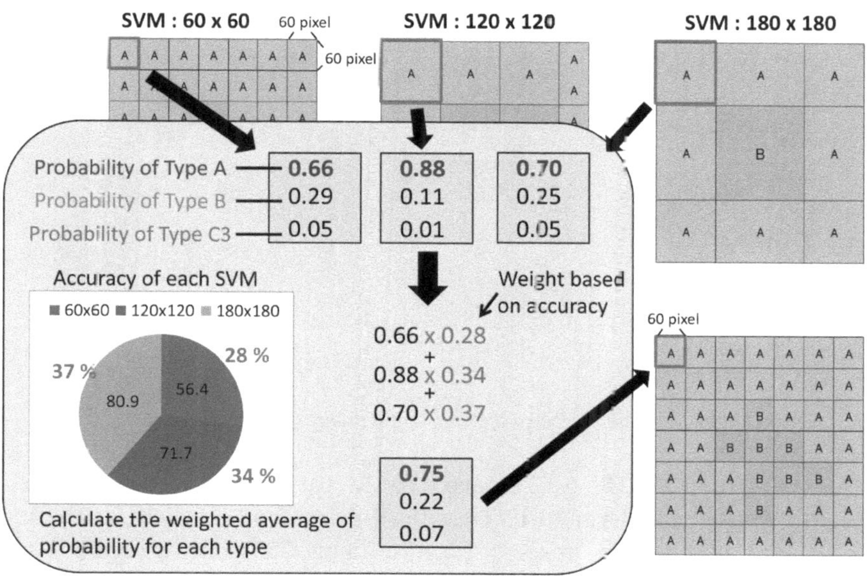

Figure 16.12 Calculation of probability of each gradation of grid (60 × 60) in pyramid-style classification.

In this way, all grids (unit scan windows) of the input image are processed, and the image segmentation result with gradation map can be obtained. Although in this example, the scan window size of each level is a multiple size of reference grid (60 × 60) and scan step (scan window displacement) of each level is 60 pixels, we can change them to arbitrary values. Then this can extend to obtain more complex and highly resolution gradation map.

These gradation maps are generated based on the classification results. In these figures, if $P_A = 1.0$ (Type A) then the grid (unit scan window) is transparent, otherwise the grid is painted by specified colors based on Alpha blending. If $P_B = 1.0$ (Type B) then the grid is colored by green (G), and if $P_{C3} = 1.0$ (Type C) then the grid is colored by red (R). So each gradation map is created by the combination of Alpha blending RGB colors based on the probability of each grid.

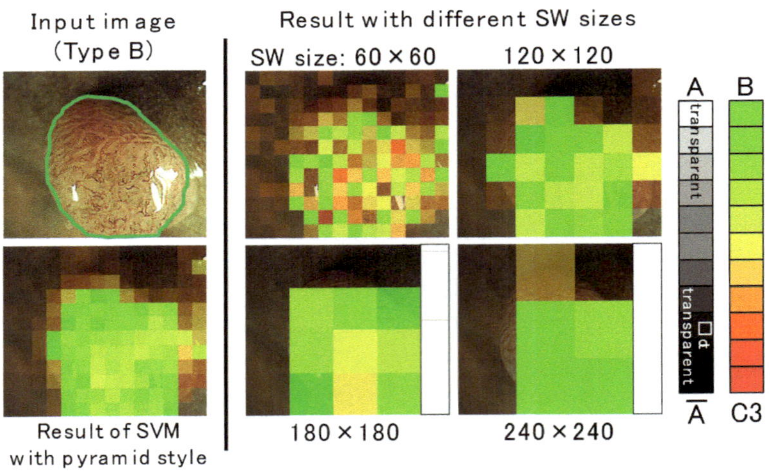

Figure 16.13 A result of the real endoscopic image (Type B).

Figures 16.13, 16.14, and 16.15 are the results of the pyramid-style hierarchical classification method applied to the actual endoscopic images, Type B, and C3 (that is tumor), respectively. In each figure, the top-left image is an input image and the bottom-left image is the gradation map of the result of pyramid-style SVM classification. The right-hand-side images are the gradation maps of scan windows 60 × 60, 120 × 120, 180 × 180, and 240 × 240, respectively.

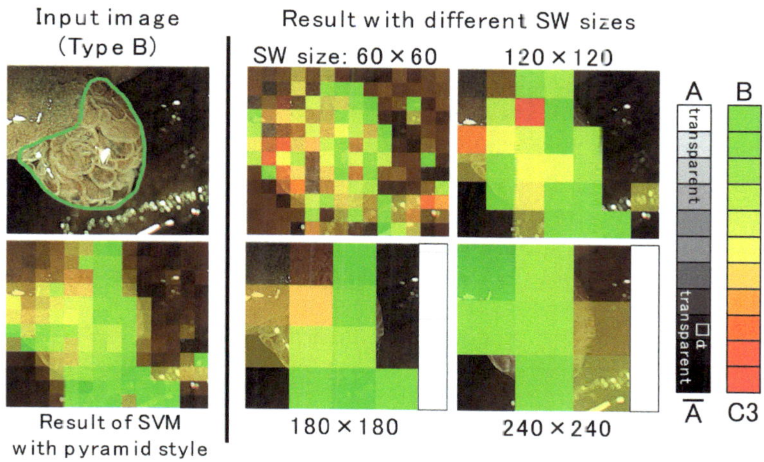

Figure 16.14 A result of Type B image which is difficult due to light reflection in the background.

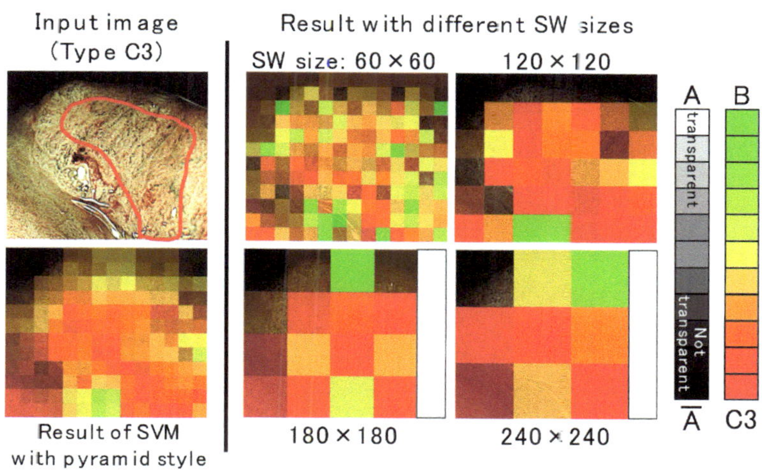

Figure 16.15 A result of the real endoscopic image (Type C3).

From these results, we have succeeded in catching the great portion of tumor in the real endoscopic images.

16.6 An Architecture of Decision Function Calculator

Figure 16.16 shows the block diagram of the decision function module in our type classification module. In the case of the 2-step evaluation method, we calculate two decision function, $d_{A:\bar{A}}(\vec{x})$ and $d_{B:C3}(\vec{x})$, and we need two decision function calculation modules. Since high dimension feature quantity (512 dimensions in 2-step case) is processed in our medical application, it is necessary to use multiple-processing units for calculating the sum-of-product (multiply-accumulate : MAC) operations, which are included the decision function (Eq. (16.1)), in parallel.

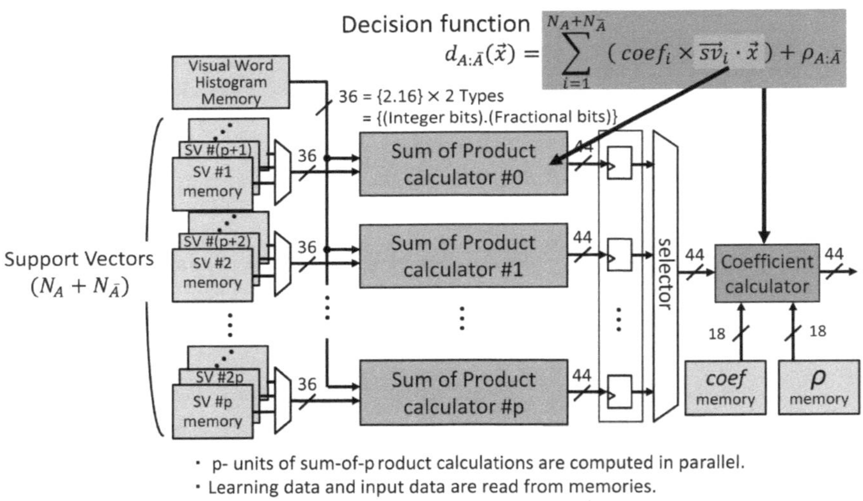

Figure 16.16 Decision function calculation architecture.

Hence, there is a subject that how to reduce hardware resources while increasing parallel degree. The decision function calculation module is implemented using 2-pipelined stage architecture. The first stage is used for sum-of-product computation and the second stage is used for summation. Support vector (SV) and coefficients obtained by learning step are read from memories. The timing chart of the calculation for one scan window is shown in Fig. 16.17. The sum-of-product calculation in the decision function is computed by sum-of-product calculator blocks which are orange-color in parallel. When the first sum-of-product calculation is finish, the other support vectors are read from *sv* memory for the next sum-of-product calculation. At the same time, coefficient calculator reads the result of each sum-of-product, multiplies it with $coef_i$ before summing them up for summation. Finally, the coefficient $\rho_{A:\bar{A}}$ is added to compute the calculation of the decision function.

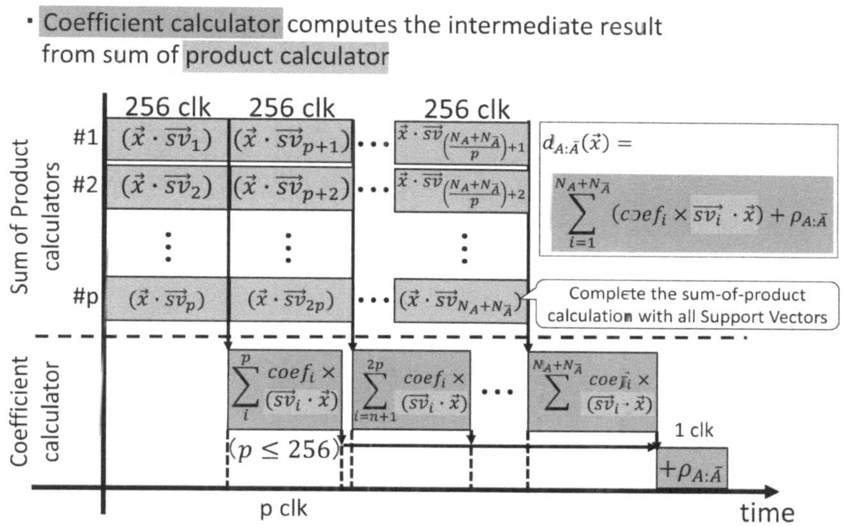

Figure 16.17 Timing chart of calculating the decision function.

16.7 Performance Verification of CAD System

We have implemented the decision function calculation architecture on FPGA, Altera Stratix IV (EP4SE530H35C2) device. Table 16.2 shows the resource utilization of the decision function on FPGA(Altera Stratix IV)for the case that the parallel multiplier digital-signal-processing units (DSPs) are 32, 64 and 128. Also, we verified that a performance of the whole CAD system which computes one Full-HD (1920 × 1080 pixels) endoscopic image from input of the image data into (1) the feature extraction module [12] to output the results from (3) the type classification module via (2) the feature transformation module [13] as shown in Fig. 16.18.

Table 16.2 Resource utilization of the decision function on FPGA

Altera Stratix VI Available (EP4SE530)		No. of parallel multiplier DSPs					
		32		64		128	
# ALUTs	424,960	2,154	1%	2,992	1%	8,079	2%
# registers	424,960	2,256	1%	3,759	1%	7,200	2%
# Logic Array Blocks	21,248	207	1%	299	1%	795	4%
# M9K RAM Blocks	1,280	512	40%	520	41%	512	40%
# M144K RAM Blocks	64	64	100%	64	100%	64	100%
# 18 × 18 DSPs	1,024	288	28%	544	53%	1024	100%
Max Frequency [MHz]		*163.9 MHz*		*133.0 MHz*		*122.61 MHz*	
Processing time (a Full-HD image)		*15,368 clocks*		*7,696 clocks*		*3,872 clocks*	

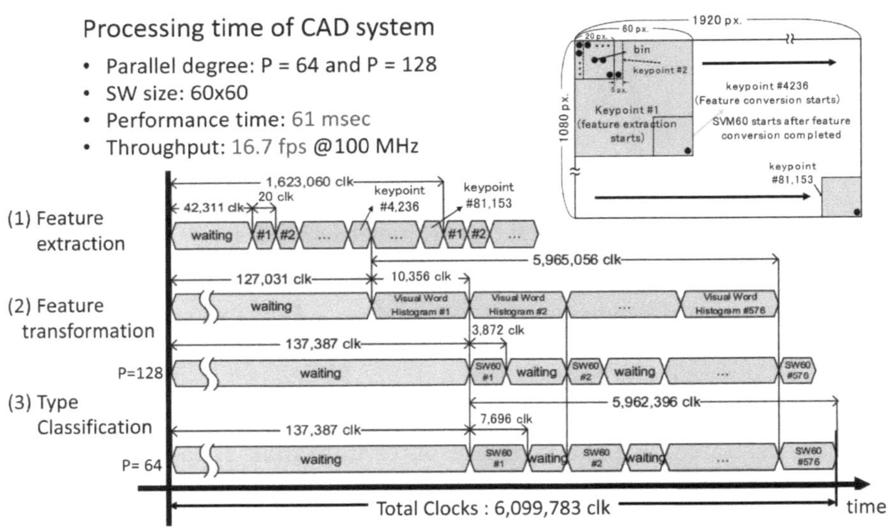

Figure 16.18 A processing time estimation to compute one full-HD (1920 × 1080 pixels) frame.

The processing time of feature transformation module (2) in Fig. 16.18 is the critical path in our system. Therefore, the number of parallel processing multipliers in the type classification module (3) can reduce to 64 (P = 64) from 128 (P = 128) within almost the same processing time as shown in Fig. 16.18. From this performance verification results, throughput is 16.7 fps and latency is 60 msec at 100 MHz. Thus, it is achievable about the real time and on-the-fly diagnostic support for clinical doctor (demand throughput: > 5 fps, latency: < 1 sec).

16.8 Summary

In this chapter, we present the hardware design of type classification in CAD system for colorectal endoscopic images with NBI magnification for real-time processing of Full HD (1920 × 1080 pixels) images. The proposed pyramid-style classifier with SVMs for multi-size and multi-layer scan windows enables smaller circuit area and higher throughput with higher classification accuracy than the conventional methods for actual complex colorectal endoscopic images. We verified the increase of the classification accuracy of pyramid-style classification method by simulation. The proposed method also could achieve high accuracy in type segmentation even if individual SW sizes could not classify correctly by combining segmentation results from other SW sizes. The proposed CAD system with the gradation map for the corresponding colorectal endoscopic image could be very effective as a diagnostic support system for both non-expert and expert doctors. Finally, we propose the hardware architecture of type classification module with SVM for endoscopic images. The estimated processing time shows the system can process one frame in 61 msec@100 MHz (with 64 parallel multiplier DSPs).

Acknowledgments

The author thanks Dr. Hirakawa, Dr. Kominami, Dr. Miyaki, Mr. Okamoto, Mr. Shimizu, Mr. Sugi, Mr. Shigemi, and Mr. Mishima for simulations, experiments and discussions for the CAD system.

Part of this work was supported by Grant-in-Aid for Scientific Researches (B) JSPS KAKENHI, Grant Number 17H01714, JSPS Fellows, Grant Number 16J06130, and collaborative research of the Research Center for Biomedical Engineering, respectively.

The FPGA design tools in this work have been supported by the Altera University Program, the Mentor Graphics Higher Education Program, and Cadence Design Systems, respectively.

References

1. Kanao, H., et al. (2009). Narrow–band imaging magnification predicts the histology and invasion depth of colorectal tumors, *Journal of Gastrointestinal Endoscopy*, vol. 69, no. 3, pp. 631–636.
2. Tamaki, T., et al. (2013). Computer-aided colorectal tumor classification in NBI endoscopy using local features, *Medical Image Analysis*, vol. 17, no. 1, pp. 78–100.
3. Vedaldi, A., Fulkerson, B., Vlfeat: An open and portable library of computer vision algorithms, URL: http://www.vlfeat.org/.
4. Vapnik, V. (1998). *Statistical Learning Theory*, John Wiley & Sons Inc., New York.
5. LIBSVM : A Library for Support Vector Machines, URL: http://www.csie.ntu.edu.tw/~cjlin/libsvm/.
6. Kominami, Y., et al. (2016). Computer-aided diagnosis of colorectal polyp histology by using a real-time image recognition system and narrow-band imaging magnifying colonoscopy, *Gastrointestinal Endoscopy*, vol. 83, no. 3, pp. 643–649.
7. Shigemi, S., et al. (2013). An FPGA implementation of support vector machine identifier for colorectal endoscopic images with NBI magnification, *Proceedings of the 28th Intl. Conference on Circuits/Systems, Computers and Communications*, pp. 571–572.
8. Wu, T.-F., Lin, C.-J., Weng, R. C. (2004). Probability estimates for multi-class classification by pairwise coupling, *Journal of Machine Learning Research*, vol. 5, pp. 975–1005.
9. John, C. Platt., et al. (1999). Large margin DAGs for multiclass classification, *Neural Information Processing Systems 12 (NIPS1999)*, pp. 547–553.
10. Mishima, T., et al. (2013). A simple and effective hardware oriented feature extraction algorithm for colorectal endoscopic images with NBI magnification, *Proceedings of the 28th International Conference on Circuits/Systems, Computers and Communications (ITC-CSCC2013)*, pp. 567–570.
11. Koide, T., et al. (2014). FPGA implementation of type identifier for colorectal endoscopic images with NBI magnification, *Proceedings*

of the 12th IEEE Asia Pacific Conference on Circuits and Systems (APCCAS 2014), pp. 651–654.

12. Koide, T., et al. (2016). A hardware accelerator for bag-of-features based visual word transformation in computer aided diagnosis for colorectal endoscopic images, *Proceedings of the 31th International Technical Conference on Circuits/Systems, Computers and Communications 2016*, pp. 233–236.
13. Koide, T., et al. (2016). Compact and high-speed hardware feature extraction accelerator for dense scale-invariant feature transform, *Proceedings of the International Technical Conference on Circuits/ Systems, Computers and Communications 2016*, pp. 387–390.

Chapter 17

Robotics in Minimally Invasive Surgery

Kenji Kawashima and Takahiro Kanno

Institute of Biomaterials and Bioengineering,
Tokyo Medical and Dental University,
2-3-10 Kanda-Surugadai, Chiyoda-ku, Tokyo 101-0062, Japan

kkawa.bmc@tmd.ac.jp

In this chapter, we focus on robots used for minimally invasive surgery, which is one of the most active areas for research and development of surgical robots. First, we briefly introduce the history of surgical robots. Second, we explain robot control by electric and pneumatic actuators. Then, we introduce research and development of master-slave robots with pneumatic drive. Finally, we discuss future directions for surgical robots.

17.1 History of Surgical Robot Research

In recent years, robotic-assisted surgery has been widely performed. Surgical robots are actively studied just a few decades after their introduction. The first robot used in surgery was PUMA 200 about 25 years ago. The robot was used for needle

Biomedical Engineering
Edited by Akihiro Miyauchi and Yuji Miyahara

ISBN 978-981-4877-63-3 (Hardcover), 978-1-003-14194-5 (eBook)
www.jennystanford.com

placement in a CT-guided brain biopsy [1]. Since the 1990s, research and development of surgical robots have been increasingly active. An orthopedic surgery robot, ROBODOC, was used during a total hip replacement in 1992 [2]. In the early 2000s, as a surgical robot for minimally invasive surgery (MIS), Intuitive Surgical launched the da Vinci system. Recently, as shown in Fig. 17.1, surgical robots are being developed for use in many types of surgery [3–6].

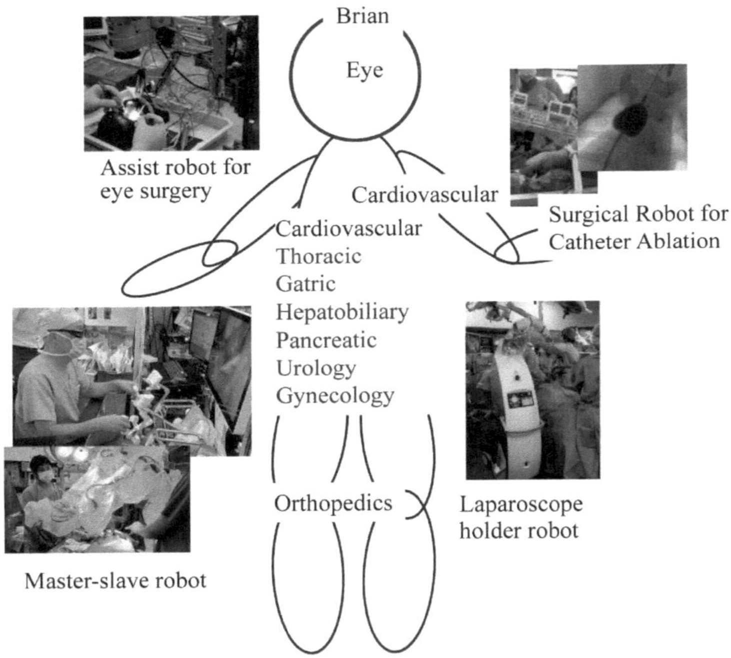

Figure 17.1 Application of robots in surgery.

17.2 Robot Control

Actuators are needed to control surgical robots. DC (direct current) electric motors are widely used in robots. For example, permanent magnet DC motors with coreless winding are used in the da Vinci system. A reduction gear is required to generate enough torque for the motor to rotate the robot's joint. DC motors are suitable for precise control. On the other hand, the reduction gear reduces the back drivability. Pneumatic actuators such as cylinders can generate linear motions with high power to ratio without using reduction mechanisms. Therefore, cylinders have high back drivability. However, the position control performance of pneumatic actuators is inferior to that of DC motors. In the following section, the control method of both actuators is explained.

17.2.1 Control of DC Motor

The dynamics of a permanent magnet DC motor shown in Fig. 17.2 can be given as follows.

The voltage equation of a motor is written as

$$V_a(t) = R_a i_a(t) + L_a \frac{di_a(t)}{dt} + K_b \omega(t), \tag{17.1}$$

where $V_a(t)$ is the applied voltage, $i_a(t)$ is the armature current, R_a is the armature resistance, L_a is the armature inductance, K_b is the electromotive-force constant, and $\omega(t)$ is the angular velocity output of the motor. The relation between the torque and speed is given as

$$\tau_M(t) - \tau_L(t) = J\frac{d\omega(t)}{dt} + b\omega(t), \tag{17.2}$$

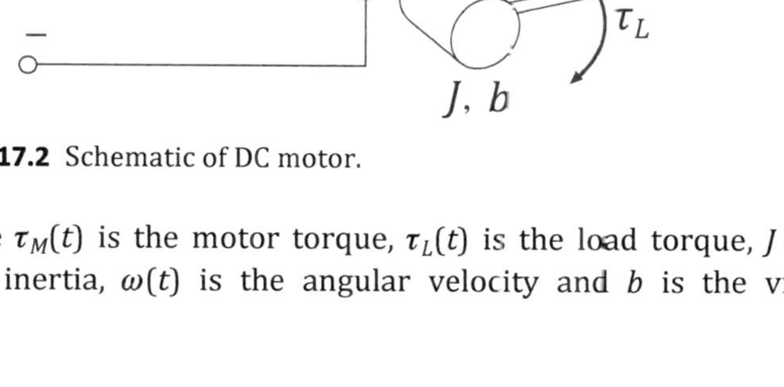

Figure 17.2 Schematic of DC motor.

where $\tau_M(t)$ is the motor torque, $\tau_L(t)$ is the load torque, J is the rotor inertia, $\omega(t)$ is the angular velocity and b is the viscous damping coefficient. The dynamics of a DC motor can be expressed using a block diagram as shown in Fig. 17.3, where K_m is the torque constant.

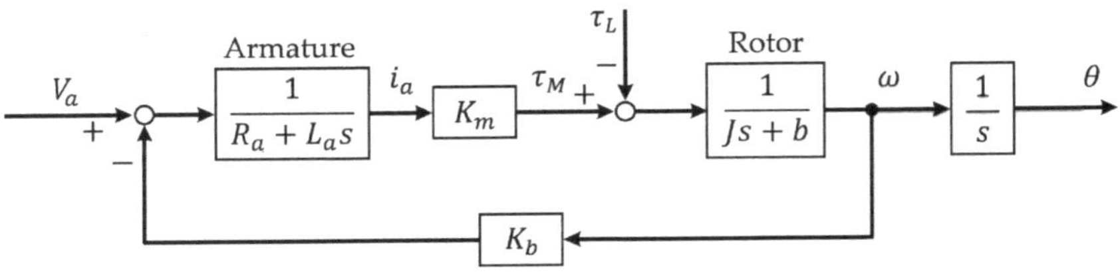

Figure 17.3 Block diagram of DC motor.

The transfer function from the input voltage to the output speed can be given as

$$G(s) = \frac{\omega}{V_a} = \frac{K_m}{L_a J s^2 + (R_a J + bL_a)s + (K_m K_e + R_a b)}. \tag{17.3}$$

Here we define motor time constants

$$T_m = \frac{J}{b},\ T_e = \frac{L_a}{R_a}.$$

T_m is mechanical time constant and T_s is electrical time constant. The electrical time constant is negligibly smaller than the mechanical time constant. Then, the reduced transfer function becomes

$$G(s) = \frac{\omega}{V_a} = \frac{K_s}{T_s s + 1} \tag{17.4}$$

where $T_m = \dfrac{R_a J}{K_b K_m + R_a b},\ K_s = \dfrac{K_m}{K_b K_m + R_a b}.$

As a result, the transfer function from the input voltage to the position of the motor is given as second-order lag system.

$$G_m(s) = \frac{\theta}{V_a} = \frac{K_s}{s(T_s s + 1)} \tag{17.5}$$

Therefore, a proportional-derivative (PD) controller is effective in designing a motor control to determine two poles.

17.2.2 Control of Pneumatic Cylinder

Pneumatic actuators have many safety advantages such as low heat generation, compressibility, the ability to control the maximum force by regulating the supply pressure, ease of releasing the acting force by discharging the compressed air in the actuator, and the ability to develop a robotic arm that is both compact and lightweight.

Pneumatic servo systems, which control pneumatic cylinders using servo valves, have been studied since the 1950s [7, 8]. The performance of the system improved greatly as the pneumatic servo valve became commercially available in the late 1980s. The pneumatic servo valve is the key element in the system [9].

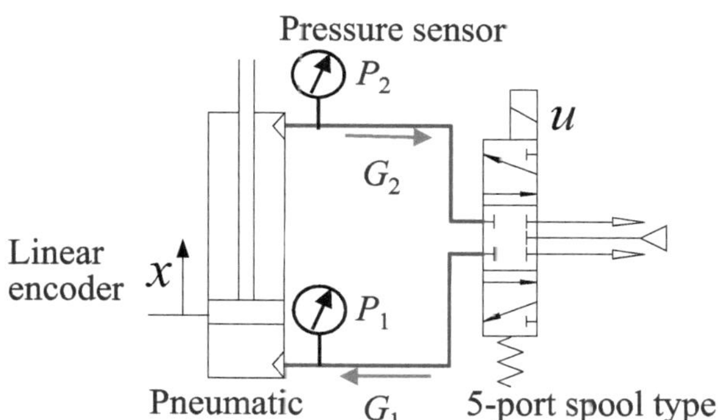

Figure 17.4 Schematic of pneumatic servo system.

The pneumatic servo system is shown in Fig. 17.4. As shown in the figure, the system usually consists of a pneumatic cylinder, a position sensor, two pressure sensors, and a five-port servo valve. The dynamics of a pneumatic servo system can be given as follows. If the friction force is negligibly small, the equation of motion is given as

$$m\ddot{x} = A(P_1 - P_2), \tag{17.6}$$

where m is the mass, x is the position, A is the pressured area, P_1 and P_2 are inner pressures of right and left chambers, respectively. The state change of the gas is assumed to be an isothermal condition when the motion is not so fast. The total difference of the state equation of ideal gas linearized around the equilibrium point is given as

$$V_0 \frac{dP_1(t)}{dt} = R\theta G_1(t) - P_c A \frac{dx(t)}{dt} \tag{17.7}$$

$$V_0 \frac{dP_2(t)}{dt} = R\theta G_2(t) + P_c A \frac{dx(t)}{dt}. \tag{17.8}$$

Here, R is gas constant, θ is atmospheric temperature, V_0 is the volume of the chamber at the initial state, P_c is equilibrium pressure, G_1 and G_2 are the mass flow rates of the right and left chambers, respectively. Since the dynamics of the servo valve is much higher than that of the cylinder, it is assumed as a proportional gain. The characteristic between the effective area of the valve and input voltage can be assumed as linear. Since inner pressures of the chambers, P_1 and P_2, are lower than half of the supply pressure, the charge flow G_1 is choked and the discharge flow G_2 is non-choked.

$$G_1 = K_f K_{SV} P_s u(t) \tag{17.9}$$

$$G_2 = -\delta K_f K_{sv} P_s u(t) \tag{17.10}$$

$$K_f = \sqrt{\frac{\kappa}{R\theta}\left(\frac{2}{\kappa+1}\right)^{(\kappa+1)/(\kappa-1)}}, \quad \delta = \sqrt{1-\left(\frac{P_a/P_c - b}{1-b}\right)^2 \frac{P_c}{P_s}}$$

Here, P_s is supply pressure, $u(t)$ is input voltage, K_{sv} is the proportional gain of the servo valve, κ is specific heat ratio, b is critical pressure ratio and P_a is atmospheric pressure. From Eqs. (17.6–17.10), the open-loop transfer function is given as

$$G(s) = \frac{u}{x} = \frac{K_n K_{sv} \omega_n^2}{s(s^2 + \omega_n^2)} \tag{17.11}$$

$$K_n = \frac{(1+\delta)K_f P_s R\theta}{2A_c P_c}, \qquad \omega_n = \sqrt{\frac{2A^2 P_c}{mV_0}},$$

where, K_n [m/kg s] is the gain and ω_n [rad/s] is the natural frequency of the system. The transfer function becomes a third-order delay system which is different from that of a DC motor as shown in Eq. (17.5). To decide all of three poles, position, velocity and acceleration or pressure feedback is necessary [10]. A cascade controller that includes a minor loop of a force controller as shown in Fig. 17.5 is effective in pneumatic servo systems [11]. A PD controller is used for the main position feedback control.

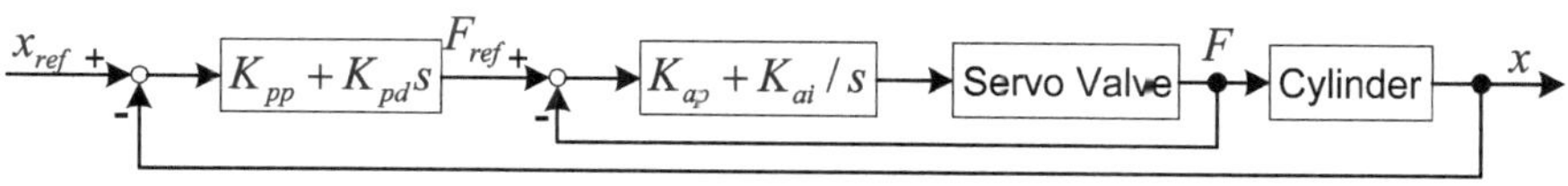

Figure 17.5 Feedback control of pneumatic servo system.

17.3 Forceps Driven by Pneumatic Servo Control

We have developed a pneumatically driven forceps manipulator having a wrist joint and a gripper [12]. Pneumatic servo control introduced in Section 17.2 was used. Figure 17.6 shows the driving mechanism of the forceps. On a plane orthogonal to this plane, the other one-degree of freedom (DOF) joint is installed. Two-DOF bending motion is achieved with only one spring joint. A thin spring is inserted as a backbone to prevent the expansion and contraction of the spring.

The actuation force by the cylinders is transmitted to the tip part via wires. Three wires pass through the forceps shaft and the flexible joint. The cylinder displacements are measured by the linear potentiometers. Another wire passes through the thin spring for the grasper actuation. When the wire is pushed, the grasper is opened, and when it is pulled, the grasper is closed. Two wires transmit the force to the joint for Two-DOF bending. These wires are guided by the pulleys and are attached to the tip of the joint. The wires can be pulled by the cylinders. Since pneumatic actuators have high backdrivability, the grasping and pulling force can be estimated from the pressure difference in the cylinders [12, 13].

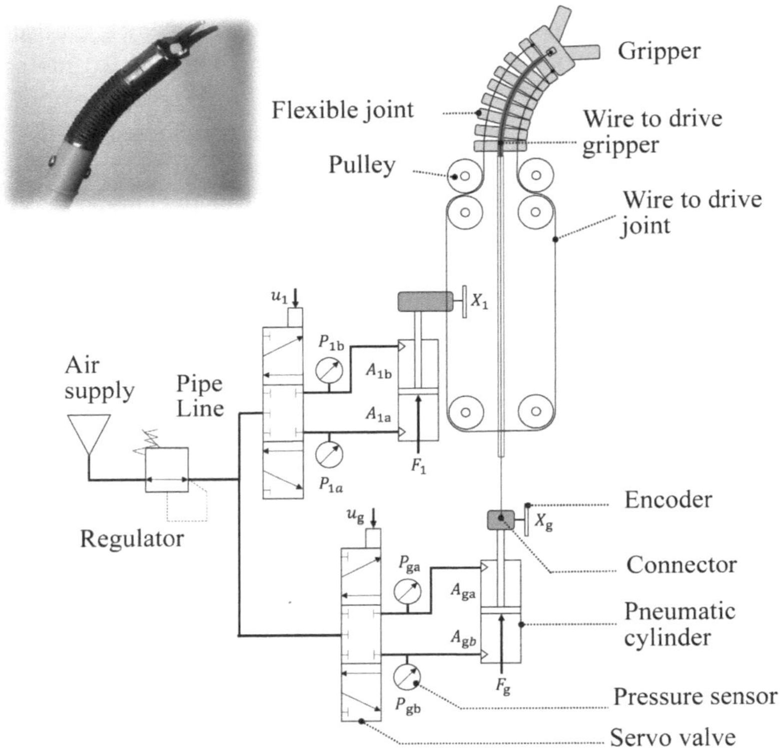

Figure 17.6 Driving mechanism forceps manipulator with pneumatic servo control.

17.4 Master-Slave Robots

Master-slave surgical robots for MIS enable an intuitive operation since the slave arms in the abdomen reproduces the surgeon's hand motion at the console. In addition, robots enable telesurgery over computer networks and microsurgery using motion scaling between the master and the slave.

Generally, the master-slave surgical robot for MIS has 6-DOF of motion, with a 4-DOF arm outside the abdominal cavity and an additional 2-DOF wrist joint. Therefore, the robot allows the instrument tip to approach the target from an arbitrary position and posture in the abdomen. The surgeon operates the remote slave arms with the wrist joint via the master console. The da Vinci surgical system is commercially successful, already introduced in thousands of hospitals around the world.

The problems in the master-slave robots are a lack of haptics (haptesthai, from Greek for "to touch"), large size, and high cost. The importance of haptic feedback is widely recognized, as numbing fingers with a local anesthetic significantly reduces grasping ability. Senhanse (TransEnterix Corp.) is a system with a force sense presentation function and has been put into practical use [14].

We are developing a master-slave surgical robot as shown in Fig. 17.7. The pneumatically-driven robotic forceps shown in Fig. 17.6 was used on the slave side to provide haptic feedback to the master.

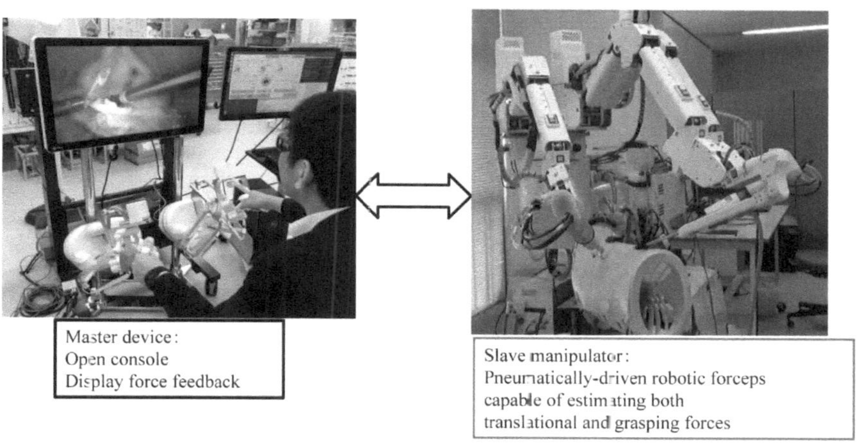

Figure 17.7 Master-slave system using pneumatically-driven forceps on the slave side.

Precise position control at the tip of forceps was achieved with the pneumatic servo control system. Figure 17.8 shows the joint positioning performance with the input references of [−60, 60] deg at 0.2 Hz and a grasping cylinder force 0 N. The results show good positioning performance. The maximum error was less than 1.2 deg.

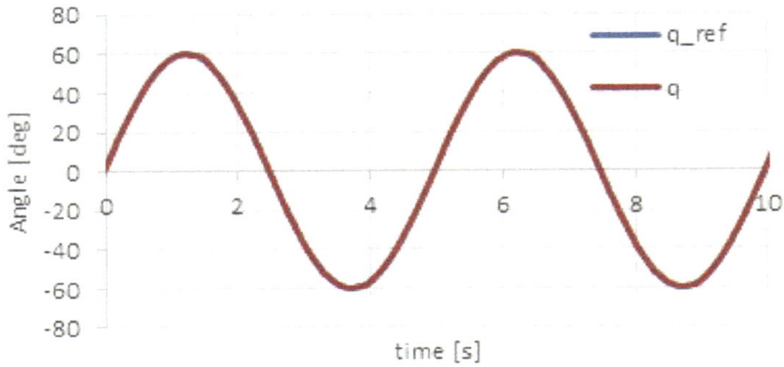

Figure 17.8 Experimental results of joint motion.

Figure 17.9 shows the results of the grasping force estimation. The blue line shows the measured force using a force sensor and the red line shows the estimated force from the pressure difference and the position of the cylinder. The difference can be seen with the force less than 0.2 N. The frictional force at the wire and the cylinder causes small force estimation error. However, the results show that the accuracy is high at 0.2 N and above.

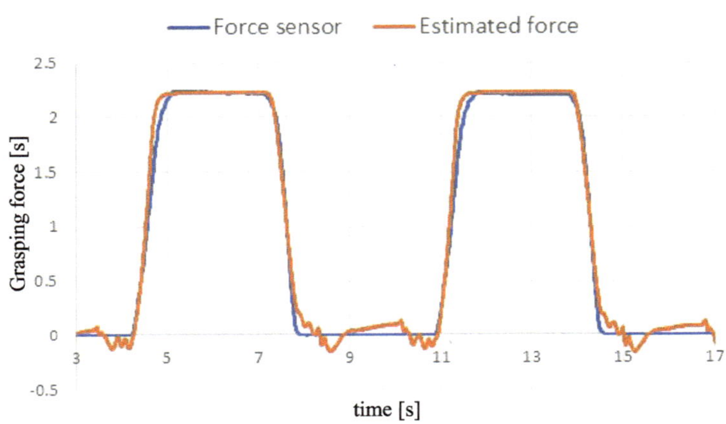

Figure 17.9 Experimental results of grasping force estimation.

17.5 Future Direction of Surgical Robots

For minimally invasive surgery, three to five ports are required. In order to further reduce postoperative pain, risk of hernia, scarring, and formation of adhesions, surgical robots for single-port access surgery (SPA) and NOTES (Natural Orifice Transluminal Endoscopic Surgery) have been actively developed. In both types of procedures, the operation of multiple instruments in a confined space is required. Therefore, a snake-like flexible mechanism is useful for SPA and NOTES. Details can be found in ref. [6, 15].

Surgical robots effectively augment a surgeon's skills to achieve accuracy and high precision during complex procedures. Use of a robot contributes to improved patient quality of life. Therefore, research and development of surgical robots will become more active.

The challenges for surgical robots are as follows:

1. Haptic feedback to the operator
2. Telesurgery
3. Applications of augmented reality
4. SPA and NOTES
5. Automation of surgical tasks
6. Cyber-physical system coupled with robots

Stable control in teleoperation with haptic perception (bilateral control) is being studied by many investigators [16]. It is suggested in ref. [17] that image guidance with robotic surgery using augmented reality represents a major revolution to increase safety and deal with difficulties associated with minimally invasive approaches. To contribute less invasive, on the hardware side, snake-like flexible and soft mechanisms for SPA and NOTES are useful. New surgical robots for SPA and NOTES will be launched in the near future.

On the software side, automation of surgical tasks has the potential to reduce surgeon fatigue and is being actively studied. In ref. [18], levels of autonomy according to the context for use are defined (No autonomy, Robot assistance, Task autonomy, Conditional autonomy, High autonomy, Full autonomy). One of the challenges in autonomous surgery is suturing, which requires precise handling of an arc-shaped needle.

We proposed a single-master dual-slave system. In this system, one of the slave robots is operated manually and the other automatically [19]. The operator inserts the needle to a phantom manually using one of the slaves. Then, the other slave automatically approaches and grasps the needle. We confirmed that the completion time was decreased by 60% by average in gasping and pulling-out phase by the proposed control compared with that of operated by the master-slave system with both hands.

In the future, surgical robotics will bring surgery to the next level with the combination of robots and artificial intelligence. The existing master-slave surgical support robot is positioned as Surgery 3.0, and the next generation will be Surgery 4.0 [20]. Surgery 4.0 will help make surgery less expensive, evidence-based, easier and safer.

References

1. Kwoh Y. S., et al. (1988). A robot with improved absolute positioning accuracy for CT guided stereotactic brain surgery. *IEEE Trans. Biomed. Eng.*, 35(2), pp. 153–161.
2. Pransky J. (1997). ROBODOC - surgical robot success story, *Indus. Robot*, 24(3), pp. 231–233.
3. Davies B. (2000). A review of robotics in surgery, *Proc. Inst. Mech. Eng. H.*, 214(1), pp. 129–140.
4. Bergeles C., and Yang G.-Z. (2014). From passive tool holders to microsurgeons: Safer, smaller, smarter surgical robots, *IEEE Trans. Bioeng. Biomed. Eng.*, 61(5), pp. 1565–1576.
5. Valentina V., et al. (2013). Emerging robotic platforms for minimally invasive surgery, *IEEE Rev. Biomed. Eng.*, 6, pp. 111–126.
6. Simaan N., et al. (2018). Medical technologies and challenges of robot-assisted minimally invasive intervention and diagnostics, *Ann. Rev. Control. Robotics Autonomous Syst.*, 1, pp. 465–490.
7. Shearer J. L. (1956). Study of pneumatic processes in the continuous control of motion with compressed air-I, II. *Trans. ASME*, 2, pp. 233–249.
8. Burrows C. R., and Webb C. R. (1966). Use of the root loci in design of pneumatic servo-motors, *Control*, 8, pp. 423–427.

9. Miyajima T., et al. (2007). Development of a digital control system for high-performance pneumatic Servo valve, *Precision Eng.*, 31, pp. 156–161.

10. Kawashima K., et al. (2010). Development of coarse/fine dual stages using pneumatically driven bellows actuator and cylinder with air bearings, *Precision Eng.*, 34, pp. 526–533.

11. Tadano K., and Kawashima K. (2010). Development of a master slave system with force-sensing abilities using pneumatic actuators for laparoscopic surgery, *Adv. Robotics*, 24(12), pp. 1763–1783.

12. Miyazaki R., et al. (2019). Pneumatically driven surgical instrument capable of estimating translational force and grasping force, *Int. J. Med. Robotics Comput. Assist. Surg.*, 15(3), e1983, pp. 1–9.

13. Haraguchi D., et al. (2015). A pneumatically-driven surgical manipulator with a flexible distal joint capable of force sensing, *IEEE/ASME Trans. Mechatronics*, 20(6), pp. 2950–2961.

14. Fanfani F., et al. (2015). The new robotic TELELAP ALF-X in gynecological surgery: Single-center experience, *Surg. Endosc.*, 30(1), pp. 215–221.

15. Burgner-Kahrs J., et al. (2015). Continuum robots for medical applications: A survey, *IEEE Trans. Robotics*, 31(6), pp. 1261–1280.

16. Li H., et al. (2018). Operator dynamics for stability condition in haptic and teleoperation system: A survey, *Int. J. Med. Robotics Comput. Assist. Surg.*, 14(2), pp. 1–10.

17. Daiana M., and Marescaux J. (2015). Robotic srugery, *Br. J. Surg.*, 102(2), e15–e28.

18. Yang G.-Z. et al. (2017). Medical robotics-Regulatory, ethical, and legal considerations for increasing levels of autonomy, *Sci. Robotics*, 2, pp. 1–2.

19. Watanabe K., et al. (2018). Single master dual slave surgical robot with automated relay of suture needle, *IEEE Trans. Ind. Electronics*, 65(8), pp. 6343–6351.

20. Feuner H., and Park A (2017). Surgery 4.0: The natural culmination of the industrial revolution?, *Innovation Surg. Sci.* 2(3), pp. 105–108.

Chapter 18

Ventricular Assist Devices Utilizing Magnetic Bearing Systems

Tadahiko Shinshi

Tokyo Institute of Technology, 4259 Nagatsuda-cho, Midori-ku, Yokohama 226-8503, Japan

shinshi.t.ab@m.titech.ac.jp

The third generation of artificial hearts (ventricular assist devices (VADs)), continuous flow blood pumps, are characterized by non-contact bearings. Of the non-contact bearings being used, magnetic bearings have advantages over hydrodynamic ones. Impellers supported by magnetic bearings are completely non-contact from the stationary state to high rotational speeds; moreover, magnetic bearings allow a larger fluid gap. This chapter introduces the principles of magnetic bearings, which are key components for third-generation VADs. Furthermore, prototypes of implantable magnetically levitated (maglev) VADs and disposable VADs for extracorporeal circulation are shown.

18.1 Introduction

Heart disease is the first and second cause of death in the USA and Japan, respectively. Heart transplantation is the final treatment

---

Biomedical Engineering
Edited by Akihiro Miyauchi and Yuji Miyahara

ISBN 978-981-4877-63-3 (Hardcover), 978-1-003-14194-5 (eBook)
www.jennystanford.com

for heart disease; however, heart transplants are limited to the number of donors, which is not expected to increase in the future. Thus, for decades, artificial hearts [1] have been anticipated as an alternative to living heart transplants.

From the early stages of development, the final goal for artificial hearts has been to realize total artificial hearts (THA) that can completely replace natural hearts. However, THAs have the problems of durability, compactness, and control of the flow balance between the left and right side of the heart, and they are not yet ready to be used as a reliable replacement for a natural heart. The current mainstream use of artificial hearts is to assist a living heart, with left and right ventricular assist devices (VAD) and bi-VADs being employed.

First, as shown in Fig. 18.1a, pulsatile pumps simulating the behavior of a living heart were developed as ventricular assist devices. However, the development of these has not progressed due to the large size, the low durability of the membrane, and clots generated in the artificial valves. The use of continuous flow pumps as ventricular VADs, as shown in Fig. 18.1b, has been studied to overcome these problems.

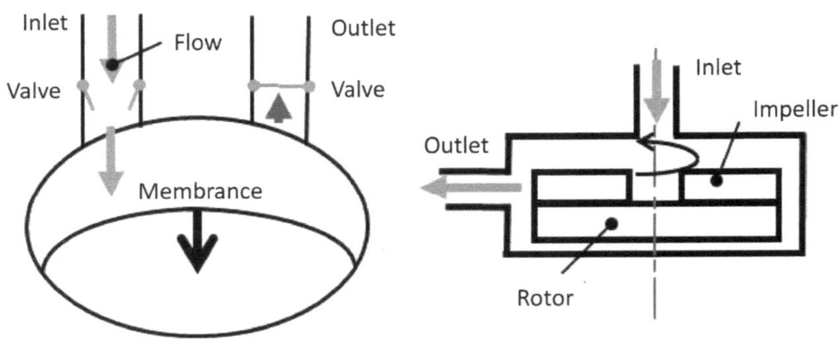

(a) Pulsatile-flow (b) continuous-flow

Figure 18.1 Pulsatile-flow and continuous-flow pumps.

In the early stages of development of continuous flow VADs, problems with durability, hemolysis, and thrombus formation also occurred. As shown in Fig. 18.2a, the use of contact bearings for supporting the impeller/rotors was the main reason for these problems, which were solved by using hydrodynamic bearings that support the rotor without contact. Furthermore, the use of magnetic bearings, as shown in Fig. 18.2b, with which a larger fluid gap can be realized, is more effective in reducing hemolysis and thrombus formation [2]. In this chapter, the principles, configurations, and prototypes of magnetic bearings for VADs are introduced.

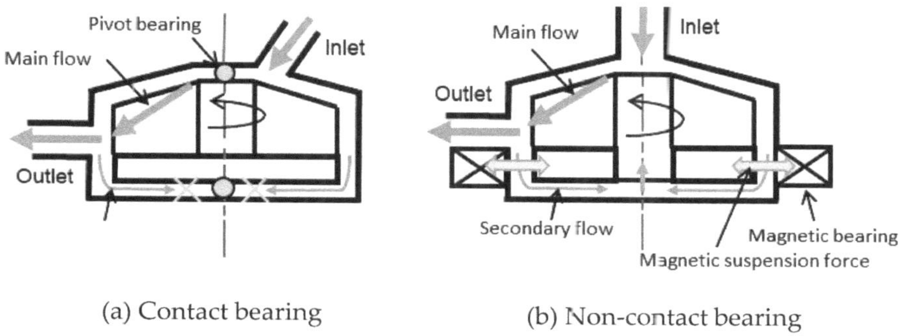

Figure 18.2 Contact and non-contact bearings.

18.2 Principles of Magnetic Bearings for VADs

18.2.1 Combinations of Magnetic Bearings and Motors

There have been two types of maglev continuous VADs: axial flow and centrifugal types. The axial flow type has the advantage of downsizing but requires high-speed rotation of the impeller. The centrifugal type is inferior with regard to downsizing but has the advantage of a relatively low rotation speed. This chapter concentrates on the centrifugal type. In centrifugal-type VADs, a magnetic bearing and a motor are combined in various ways, and the different combinations result in different sizes and control methods.

In the first configuration, power is transmitted to the impeller/rotor, which is supported by magnetic bearings, from a motor via a magnetic coupling, as shown in Fig. 18.3a. This structure could be adopted in maglev VADs for both implantable and disposable use. Although the size is large, the design margin and choice of motor are high, and the motor efficiency is high. Furthermore, cooling of the motor becomes simple because the pump housing and the motor, which is the heat source, can be separated. Moreover, this combination is useful for extracorporeal circulation because the structure of the disposable impeller/rotor can be simplified.

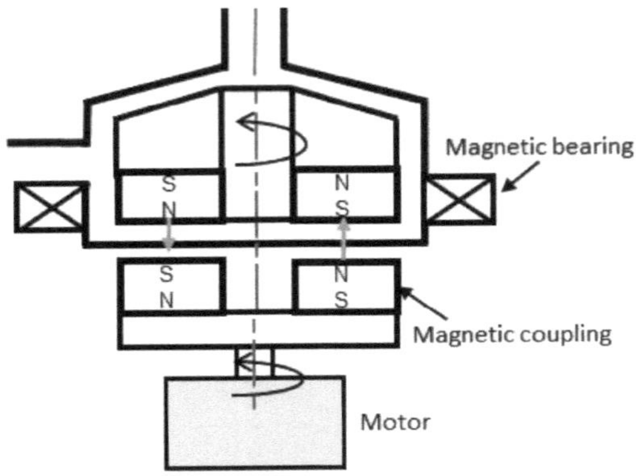

(a) Magnetic coupling + motor

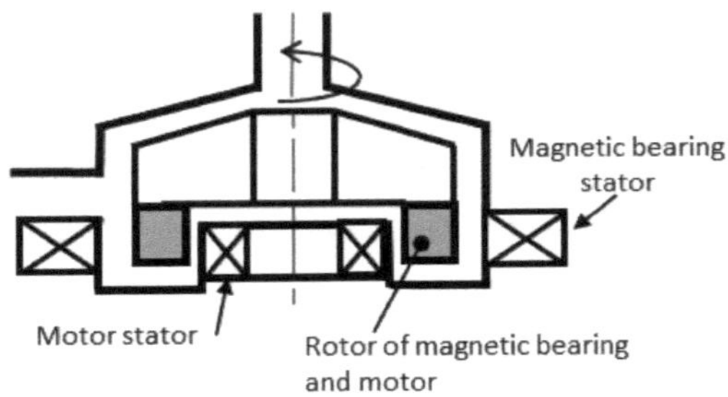

(b) Magnetic bearing and built-in motor

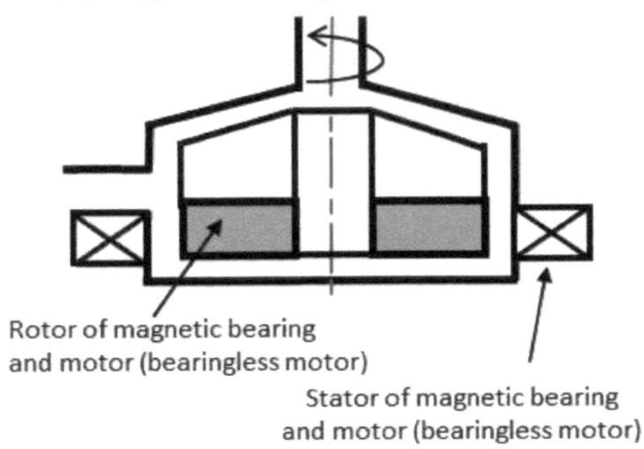

(c) Bearingless motor

Figure 18.3 Locations of magnetic bearing and motor.

In the second configuration, the motor is combined with a magnetic bearing, as shown in Fig. 18.3b. The motor and the magnetic bearing can be designed individually to satisfy the pump requirements.

This structure eliminates the magnetic coupling and is useful for miniaturization of VADs. However, having two sets of stators and permanent magnets for both the magnetic bearing and the motor drive in the impeller/rotor make these VADs complicated. From the viewpoint of cost, it is unlikely that such a structure would be adopted as a disposable pump for extracorporeal circulation.

The third configuration is to use a bearingless motor [3] in which a common stator is used for magnetic levitation and rotation, as shown in Fig. 18.3c. Using a bearingless motor enables miniaturization of the VAD. The design of the bearingless motor satisfying the pump requirements and the control of the magnetic flux for rotation and levitation is complicated. Nevertheless, this technology is being used in state-of-art maglev VADs by the progress of bearingless motor technology.

18.2.2 Active and Passive Magnetic Bearings

In addition to rotating the impeller/rotor with a magnetic force, the impeller/rotor has five degrees of freedom which need to be controlled for stable and contactless levitation. Industrial magnetic bearing systems usually adopt two sets of active radial magnetic bearings and an active thrust magnetic bearing. Therefore, simplifying the magnetic bearing system is essential to reduce the size of the maglev VAD. The use of passive magnetic bearings is known for reducing the number of controlled degrees of freedom, and thus reducing the number of displacement sensors and electromagnets for feedback control. From Earnshaw's theorem [4], at least one degree of freedom control is required to stabilize the system without contact. Some magnetic bearing structures that combine active and passive magnetic bearings have been proposed in order to minimize the number of controlled degrees of freedom and simplify the magnetic bearing system.

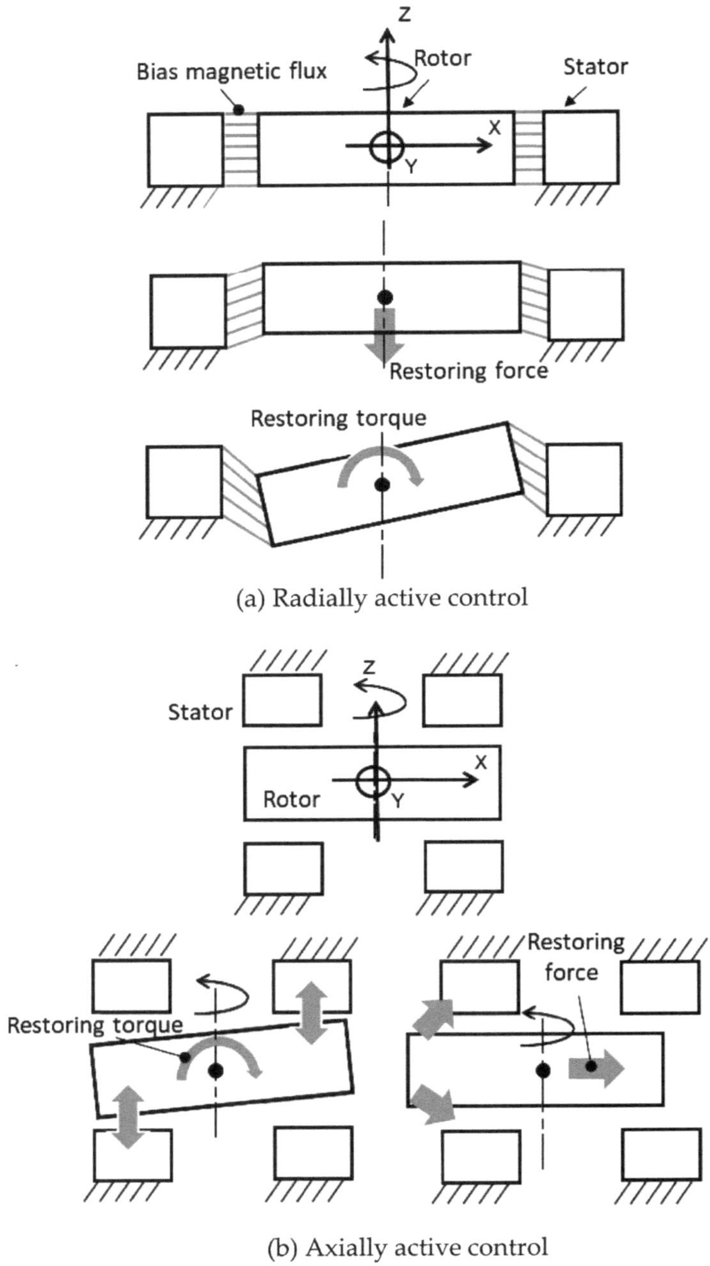

Figure 18.4 Combination of active and passive magnetic bearings.

Figure 18.4a shows a radially (two degrees of freedom) controlled magnetic bearing system combined with passive magnetic bearings. A bias magnetic flux is generated between the stator and the rotor by permanent magnets. The bias magnetic flux generates the restoring force and a torque proportional to the displacement and the angle from the balance point, respectively. The restoring force in the radial direction is generated by the flux obtained by passing currents through the coils. The radial displacement of the rotor is usually measured by non-contact displacement sensors such as eddy current type or inductance type sensors. The radial displacement is fed back to the positioning controller to calculate the references of coil currents, and the magnetic bearing system is stabilized. This basic principle is adopted in many types of centrifugal blood pumps, not only using magnetic bearings but also bearingless motors [2].

Figure 18.4b shows an axially (one degree of freedom) controlled magnetic bearing system combined with passive magnetic bearings [5]. The axial displacement of the rotor is measured by a non-contact displacement sensor and fed back to the controller. An axial electromagnet generates an axial force to stabilize the system. In this magnetic bearing system, passive magnetic bearings generating attractive and repulsive forces are combined to make the bearing stiffness positive in the translational and tilt directions, but not the axial direction. This structure has the minimum number of degrees of freedom required to control a magnetic bearing system.

The stiffness of passive magnetic bearings is generally smaller than that of active magnetic bearings. In this configuration, the stiffness in the radial direction is small. When a magnetic bearing system is adopted in a centrifugal pump, it is necessary to consider the eccentricity of the impeller due to the imbalance generated by the flow inside the pump. Reduction of the local fluid gap has a significant effect on blood damage. It is essential to design a pump that reduces the radial fluid force.

Instead of a magnetic bearing with axial control, a hydrodynamic bearing can be used, and the passive magnetic bearing system can be stabilized without feedback control. However, the clearance with a hydrodynamic bearing is narrower than that with magnetic bearings, which causes the increase of stress on the blood.

18.3 Centrifugal VADs Using Magnetic Bearings

18.3.1 Implantable VADs

This section introduces some prototypes of VADs with magnetic bearings. The development targets of implantable VADs are to realize a pump with high efficiency and compact body size. A higher efficiency pump generates less heat, which reduces the rise in temperature. The temperature of the VAD is closely related to thrombus formation. Furthermore, higher efficiency enables the battery life to be extended.

The first generation of implantable pulsatile-type VADs had a problem in large size to implant into children and small females. Even with early third-generation implantable VADs with magnetic bearings, it was necessary to provide a pocket inside the body to install the pump housing. The latest VADs require further miniaturization so that the pump can be fixed directly to the ventricle without a pocket.

Implantable VADs need to have a minimum flow rate of 5 L/min and a pressure of 100 mmHg. DuraHeart® [2] is Japan's first maglev implantable VAD. This has a three-degrees-of-freedom-controlled magnetic bearing and a mechanism to transmit torque from the motor to the impeller via a magnetic coupling, which means the size of the VAD is not compact.

Figure 18.5a shows the configuration of an implantable maglev VAD utilizing a radially controlled magnetic bearing and a built-in motor [6]. In the prototype of this VAD, the permanent magnet for the magnetic bearing is arranged on the outer periphery of the rotor, and the permanent magnet for the built-in motor is arranged on the inner periphery of the rotor. The permanent magnet ring in the rotor generates a bias flux between the outer magnetic cores and the rotor. The bias magnet flux generates a torque to restore the tilting motion of the rotor and a restoring force in the axial direction. The system is stabilized by generating radial forces by supplying currents to the coils wound around the outer core.

Inside the rotor, a Halbach magnet array is formed on the inner surface of the rotor to generate a strong magnetic field toward the inner surface of the rotor. The current through the motor stator generates a torque due to the interaction with the magnetic flux.

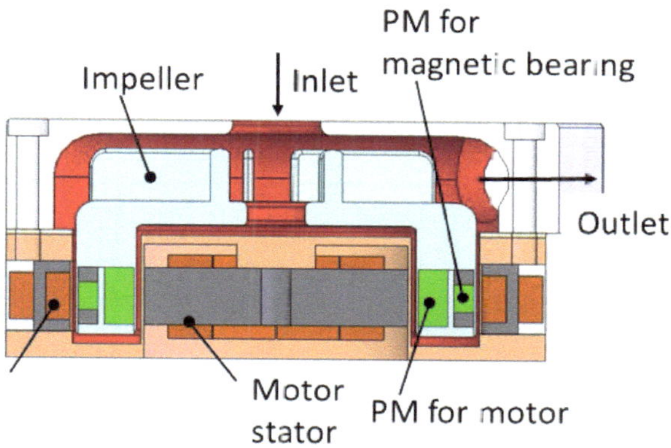

(a) Configuration of an implantable pump

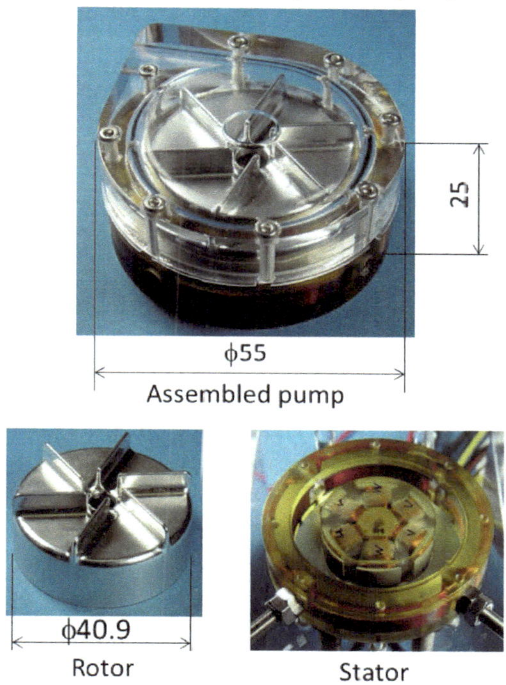

(b) Prototype photograph

Figure 18.5 A prototype of implantable maglev blood pump using radially-controlled magnetic bearing.

In this prototype, shown in Fig. 18.5b, the radial displacement is measured by eddy current displacement sensors, and feedback control is realized. This prototype has a 41 mm diameter impeller, and achieves stable non-contact levitation and rotation from 0 to 2500 rpm, as shown in Fig. 18.6. It also achieves the flow rate and pressure required for blood circulation.

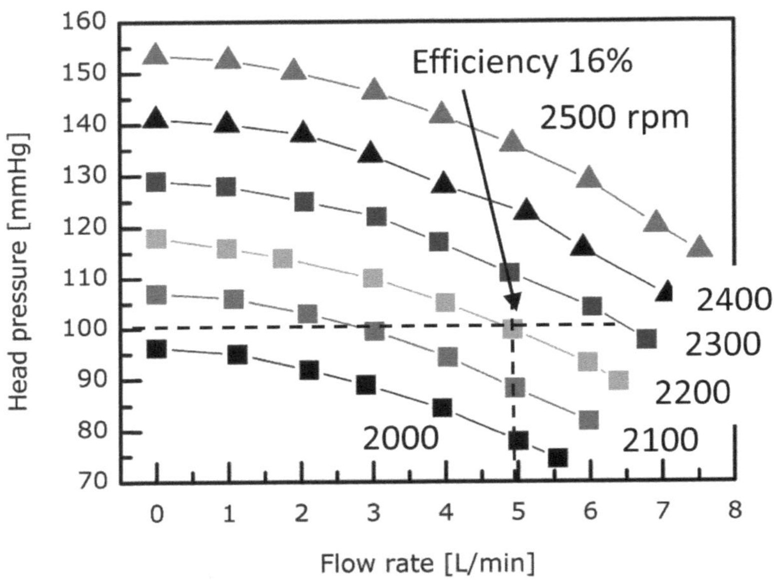

Figure 18.6 Head pressure-flow rate curves of an implantable maglev blood pump using radially-controlled magnetic bearing.

Figure 18.7a also shows a prototype of a maglev VAD using a one degree of freedom controlled magnetic bearing [7]. The rotor/stator of the magnetic bearing has three pairs of permanent magnets. The outer permanent magnet pair forms a repulsion system and generates a restoring force against inclination of the rotor. The permanent magnet ring on the inner perimeter forms an attraction system. This generates a restoring force against displacement in the radial direction. A central electromagnet adjusts the attractive force in the axial direction, and the bearing system is stabilized using the axial displacement measured by an eddy current sensor.

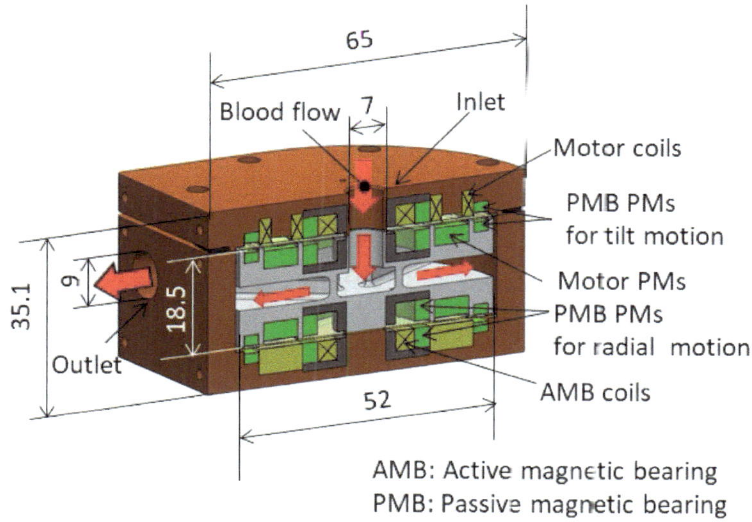

(a) Configuration of an implantable pump using one degree of freedom controlled magnetic bearing

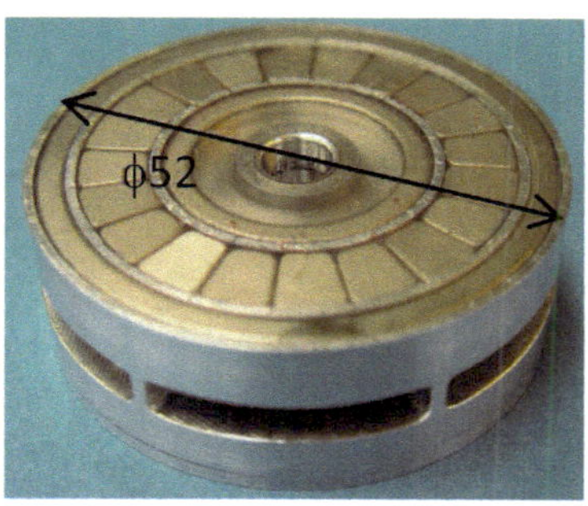

(b) Rotor

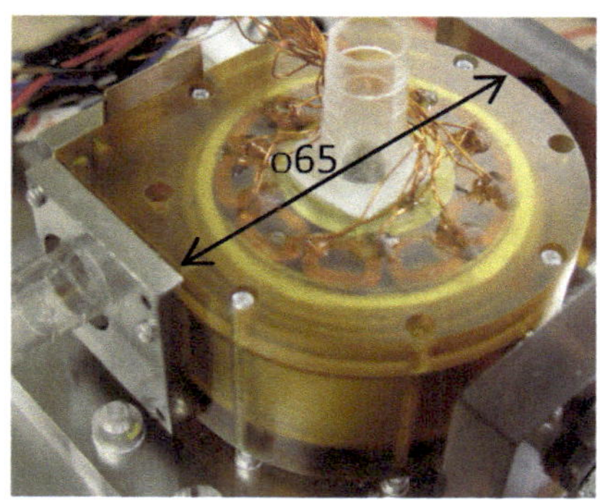

(c) Assembled pump

Figure 18.7 Prototype of an implantable pump using one degree of freedom controlled magnetic bearing.

Halbach magnet arrays arranged between the inner and outer permanent magnet rings in the rotor generate a magnetic flux in the axial direction. The built-in motor consists of air-core motor coils in the stator and Halbach arrays. Figure 18.7b,c shows that the prototype has an impeller/rotor of 50 mm in diameter and achieves non-contact levitation and rotation from 0 to 2600 rpm. It also achieves the required pump performance of more than 5 L/min and 100 mmHg.

This configuration has the advantage that the number of displacement sensors and positioning electromagnets can be minimized because only one-direction control is required. However, the rotor vibrates easily due to the disturbance generated by the fluid because the bearing stiffness is small in the passively supported directions. The pump design should be improved to reduce the disturbance forces and increases the stiffness in the passively supported directions using fluid analysis and electromagnetic field analysis.

18.3.2 Disposable VADs

Disposable VADs are placed outside the body and are used in heart surgery as bridges to heart transplantation and implantable VADs. Although they are not required to be as durable and compact as implantable VADs, low hemolysis and no thrombus formation are required. Furthermore, the pump head needs to be disposable. Therefore, it is necessary to be able to attach and detach easily, and to reduce the cost. In addition, extracorporeal VADs are often used in connection with artificial lungs. The maximum output pressure is more than 250 mmHg, which is higher than that of implantable VADs.

Figure 18.8 shows a prototype of an extracorporeal VAD [8]. The impeller/rotor is levitated by a two degrees of freedom controlled magnetic bearing, the same as that shown in Fig. 18.5a. The measured radial displacement is fed back to the controller. The torque from the motor to the impeller/rotor is transmitted via a magnetic coupling disk. Figure 18.9 shows the magnetic coupling disk, which consists of gear-shaped rings, and the ring magnet placed inside the rotor.

This prototype, using an impeller with a diameter of 50.6 mm, achieved non-contact levitation and rotation from 0 to 3600 rpm without step-out of the magnetic coupling disk, and a pump performance of 5 L/min and 400 mmHg at 3600 rpm.

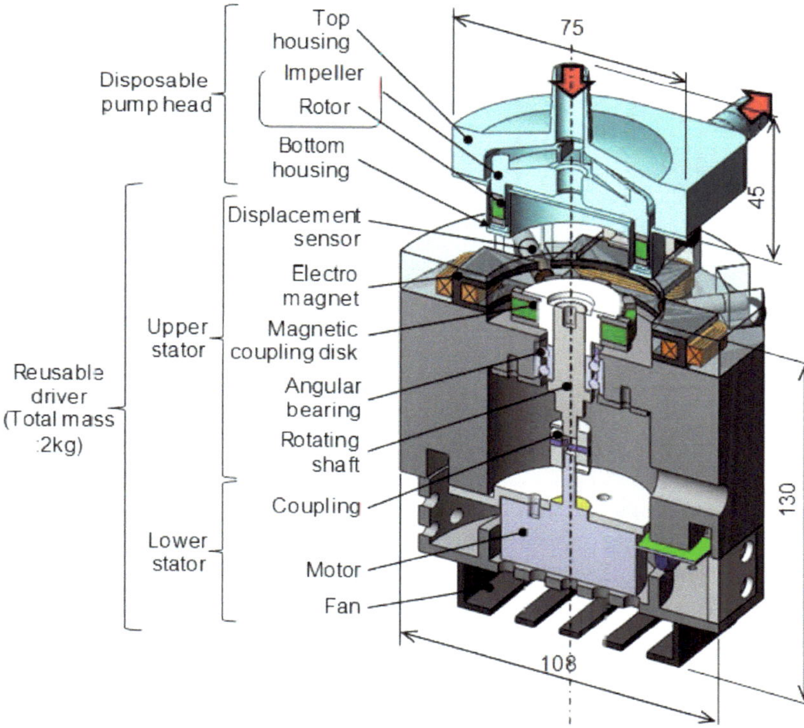

(a)Configuration of a disposable VAD using magnetic bearing

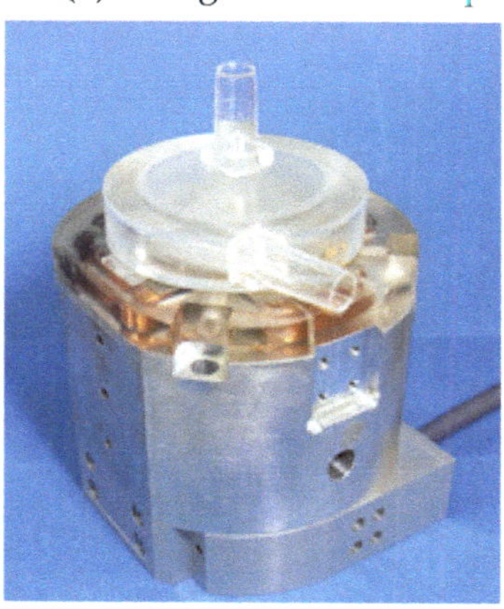

(b) Assembled prototype

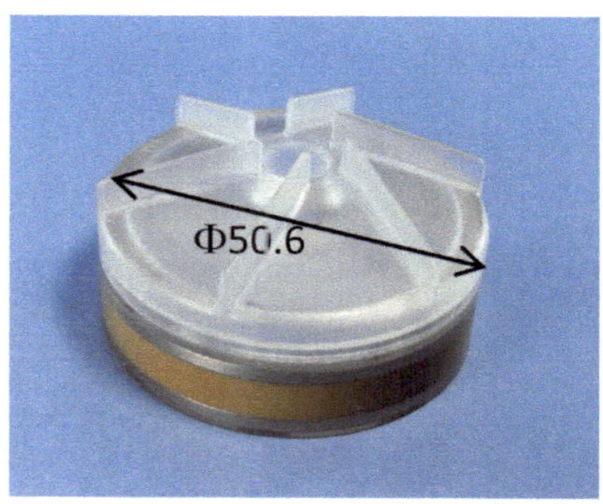

(c) Disposable rotor

Figure 18.8 Prototype of a disposable VAD using magnetic bearing.

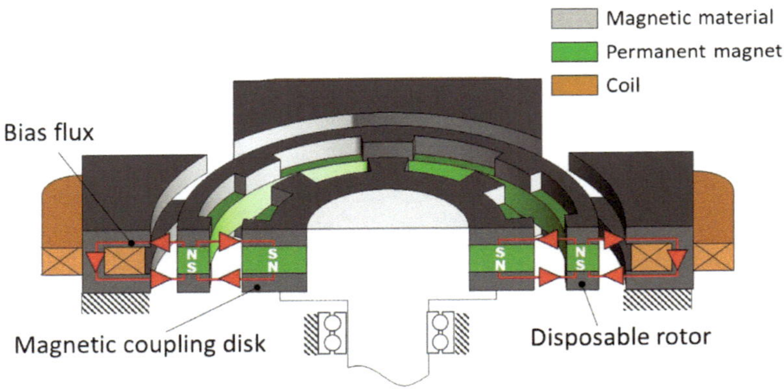

Figure 18.9 Principle of a disposable maglev VAD.

A rotor without a permanent magnet is also proposed, in order to reduce the cost of the disposable pump head, as shown in Fig. 18.10 [9]. As shown in Fig. 18.11, without a permanent magnet in the rotor, the structure of the magnetic coupling has been changed to provide a magnetic bias flux to the magnetic bearing. This impeller/rotor can also be levitated and rotated from 0 to 3750 rpm, and the same pump performance was achieved. Furthermore, a disposable pump using a bearingless motor with a magnet-free rotor has been also studied [10].

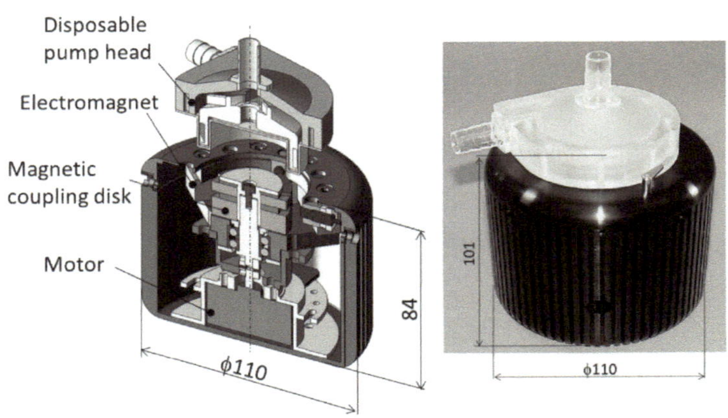

(a)Configuration of a maglev disposable VAD using a magnet-free rotor

(b) Assembled prototype

Figure 18.10 Prototype of a maglev disposable VAD using a magnet free rotor.

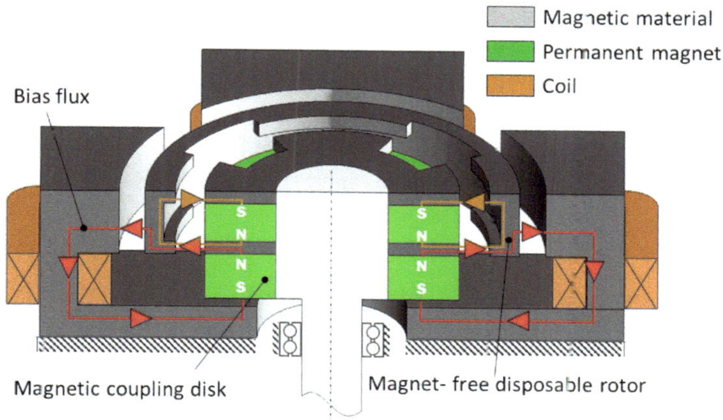

Figure 18.11 Principle of a maglev disposable VAD using a magnet free rotor.

18.3.3 Durability and Biocompatibility

For the practical use of a VAD, it is essential to evaluate its durability and biocompatibility. Under pulsatile flow simulating a ventricular assist condition, a long-term pumping test is necessary. It is also necessary to perform shock and vibration tests assuming patient activity and transportation by vehicles [11]. Needless to say, there should be no possibility of short circuits and rust of devices due to blood leakage.

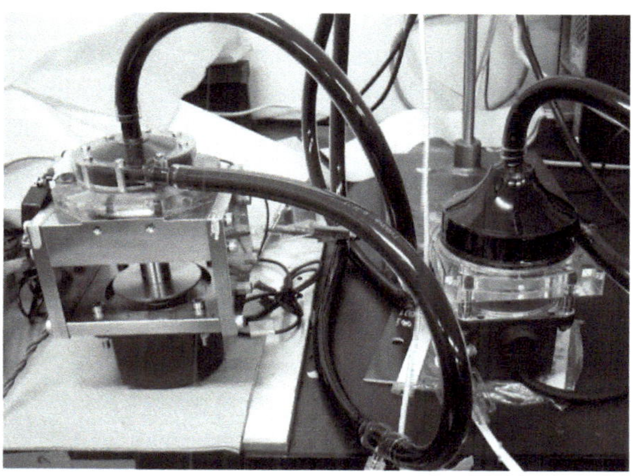

Figure 18.12 In vitro hemolysis test using porcine.

Hemolysis and thrombus formation have been evaluated by simulation. However, hemolysis tests using animal blood and thrombus tests using animals, as shown in Fig. 18.12 and 18.13, respectively, are still indispensable before clinical trials [12, 13].

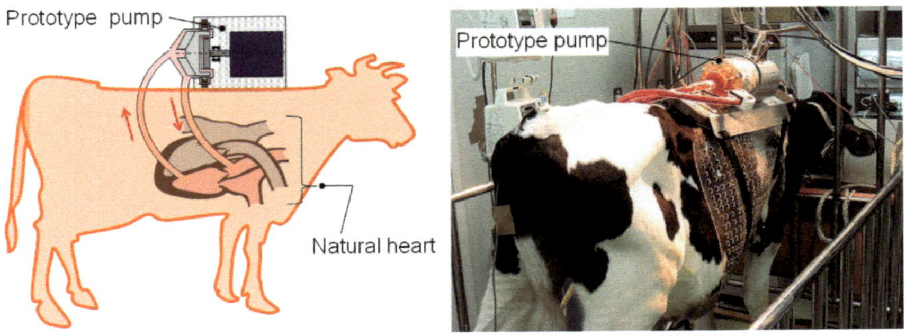

Figure 18.13 Animal test for evaluating durability and biocompatibility.

18.4 Multifunctional Maglev VADs

Magnetic bearings can not only support the impeller/rotor but also be used to measure its displacement and measure the forces acting on it. By utilizing these measurements, new functions can be added to maglev VADS.

In blood circulation, the impeller/rotor rotates at a constant rotational speed. Adjusting the rotational speed according to the state of the living heart is desirable. However, this has not yet been realized due to problems such as flow measurement.

The pulsatile flow of the living heart gives a periodic disturbance force to the impeller/rotor. It may be possible to estimate the pulsatile flow by measuring the force on the impeller. Observer-based measurements of the forces on the impeller have been made [14]. In addition, measuring the variation in blood viscosity by positively vibrating the impeller with a magnetic bearing [15] has been studied to predict the occurrence of thrombus.

Acknowledgments

The author thanks Prof. S. Takatani of Tokyo Medical and Dental University, Prof. J. Asama of Shizuoka University, Prof. W. Hijikata of Tokyo Institute of Technology, and Dr. J. Yumoto of Nippon Steel. This chapter was supported in part by the Ministry of Education, Science, Sports and Culture, Grant-in Aid for Scientific Research and the Japan Science and Technology Agency.

References

1. Yamane, T. (2016) *Mechanism of Artificial Heart* (Springer, Japan).
2. Hoshi, H., Shinshi, T., Takatani, S. (2006). The third generation blood pumps: Mechanical non-contact with magnetic levitation, *Artif. Organs*, **30**(5), pp. 324–338.
3. Chiba, A. (2005) *Magnetic Bearings and Bearingless Drives* (Newnes, MA).
4. Schweitzer, G., and Maslen, E. H. (2010) *Magnetic Bearings Theory, Design, and Application to Rotating Machinery* (Springer, Dordrecht).
5. Ulbrich, H., and Ginzinger, L. (2010) *Motion and Vibration Selected papers from Movic 2008* (Springer) pp. 357–366.
6. Asama, J., Shinshi, T., Hoshi, H., Takatani, S., and Shimokohbe, A. (2004). New design for a compact centrifugal blood pump with a magnetically levitated rotor, *ASAIO J.*, **50**(6), pp. 550–556.
7. Yumoto, A., and Shinshi, T. (2012). A compact centrifugal blood pump utilizing an axially-controlled magnetic bearing motor, *JSME J. C*, **78**(792), pp. 345–353 (in Japanese).
8. Hijikata, W., Shinshi, T., Asama, J., Li, L., Hoshi, H., Takatani, S., and Shimokohbe, A. (2008). A maglev centrifugal blood pump with a simple-structured disposable pump head, *Artif. Organs*, **32**(7), pp. 351–540.
9. Hijikata, W., Mamiya, T., Shinshi, T., and Takatani, S. (2011). A cost-effective extracorporeal magnetically-levitated centrifugal blood pump employing a disposable magnet-free impeller, *Proc. Inst. Mech. Eng. Part H J. Eng. Med.*, **225**, pp. 1149–1157.
10. RAO, J., Hijikata, W., and Shinshi, T. (2015). Bearingless motor utilizing a permanent magnet free structure for disposable centrifugal blood pumps, *J. Adv. Mech. Des. Syst. Manufacturing*, **9**(3), pp. 1–15.
11. Hijikata, W., Shinshi, T., Someya, T., Arai, H., Takatani, S., and Shimokohbe, A. (2010). A disposable magnetically levitated centrifugal blood pump for extracorporeal circulation support –improvement of pump performance for animal experiment, *JSPE J.*, **76**(9), pp. 1064–1069 (in Japanese).

12. Nagaoka, E., Someya, T. Kitao, T., Kimura, T., Ushiyama, T., Hijikata, W., Shinshi, T., Arai, H., and Takatani, T. (2010). Development of a disposable magnetically levitated centrifugal blood pump (MedTech Dispo) intended for bridge-to-bridge applications two-week in vivo evaluation, *Artif. Organs*, **34**(9), pp. 778–783.

13. Fujiwara, T., Nagaoka, E., Watanabe, T., Miyagi, N., Kitao, T., Takota, D., Mamiya, T., Shinshi, T., Arai, H., and Takatani, S. (2013). New generation extracorporeal membrane oxygenation with MedTech mag-lev, a single-use, magnetically levitated, centrifugal blood pump: Preclinical evaluation in calves, *Artif. Organs*, **37**(5), pp. 447–456.

14. Pai, C. N., Shinshi, T., and Shimokohbe, A. (2010). Sensorless measurement of pulsatile flow rate using a disturbance force observer in a magnetically levitated centrifugal blood pump during ventricular assistance, *Flow Meas. Instrumentation*, **21**(1), pp. 33–39.

15. Hijikata, W., Rao, J., Abe, S., Takatani, S., and Shinshi, T. (2015). Sensorless viscosity measurement in a magnetically-levitated rotary blood pump, *Artif. Organs*, **39**(7), pp. 559–568.

Index